IP-14   16x4(08)

Kundalini Yoga Meditation:

Techniques Specific for Psychiatric Disorders,
Couples Therapy, and Personal Growth

Kundalini Yoga Meditation:

Techniques Specific for Psychiatric Disorders, Couples Therapy, and Personal Growth

David Shannahoff-Khalsa

W. W. Norton & Company

New York • London

The techniques and protocols taught in this book are not meant to be a substitute for medical care and advice. You are advised to consult with your health care professional with regard to matters relating to your health, including matters that may require diagnosis or medical attention. In particular, if you have been diagnosed with anxiety disorders, panic disorder, phobias, obsessive-compulsive disorder, depression, bipolar disorders, an addictive disorder, impulse control disorder, eating disorder, insomnia or any other sleep disorder, chronic fatigue syndrome, attention deficit hyperactivity disorder, attention deficit disorder, posttraumatic stress disorder or any related disorder, or if you are taking or have been advised to take any medication, you should consult regularly with your physician regarding any changes in medication use.

Photos by Suzanne Pitts

For reader comments or to order a video mentioned in the book, please visit the author's web site at *www.theinternetyogi.com* (to order videos), or email him at dsk@ucsd.edu (for reader comments).

For information about permission to reproduce selections from this book, write to Permissions, W. W. Norton & Company, Inc., 500 Fifth Avenue, New York, NY 10110

Composition and book design by Martha Meyer
Manufacturing by Quebecor World Fairfield
Production Manager: Leeann Graham

Library of Congress Cataloging-in-Publication Data

Shannahoff-Khalsa, David.
    Kundalini yoga meditation : techniques specific for psychiatric disorders, couples therapy, and personal growth / David Shannahoff-Khalsa.
        p. cm.
        Includes bibliographical references and index.
        ISBN-13: 978-0-393-70475-4
        ISBN-10: 0-393-70475-0
        1. Psychotherapy. 2. Kundalini—Therapeutic use. I. Title.
RC480.5S442 2006
616.89'14—dc22   2006045331
ISBN 13: 978-00-393-70475-4
ISBN 10: 0-393-70475-0

W. W. Norton & Company, Inc., 500 Fifth Avenue, New York, N.Y. 10110
www.wwnorton.com
W. W. Norton & Company Ltd., Castle House, 75/76 Wells St., London W1T 3QT
    2 3 4 5 6 7 8 9 0

This book is dedicated to

Raj Yog Guru Ram Das, my Guru in the Divine;

Raj Yog Yogi Bhajan, Master of Kundalini Yoga,
my Spiritual Teacher;

David and Sarah Shannahoff, my parents, for their
life-long loving support;

Patrick, JJ, and Bubba, my three Golden Sons,
for their endless loving devotion.

CONTENTS

PART IV
Appendices

Acknowledgments

First and foremost, I want to thank Yogi Bhajan for the teachings that have made my scientific work and this book possible. Virtually all of the yogic knowledge and techniques in this book are the result of his commitment to share publicly the sacred knowledge of Kundalini yoga. Secondly, I want to thank Floyd E. Bloom, MD, for his efforts as my first scientific collaborator on yogic research when we were both at The Salk Institute, and for helping to launch this work and make it a respectable and important scientific endeavor. His active participation inspired many others to collaborate. I am truly grateful for the many years of his support and guidance that have followed. He gave me the idea of establishing a nonprofit foundation to help fund this work, and committed to be the first vice president on the board of directors and first scientific advisor in the early years. I am also grateful to Drs. David Schubert, Tony Hunter, and Walter Eckhart, who gave me many years of institutional support at The Salk to help establish my scientific career. I am indebted to Sheldon S. Hendler, MD, PhD, for his role as my first scientific mentor and for facilitating my initial engagement at The Salk, his role as a vice president of The Khalsa Foundation for Medical Science, and his sage advice over the last 38 years. I am grateful to Michael G. Ziegler, MD, for nearly 20 years of collaboration on pioneering physiological studies in his laboratory and at the General Clinical Research Center at the University of California, San Diego (UCSD). Michael's keen mind led to the discovery of the ultradian rhythms of alternating lateralization of catecholamine activity throughout the periphery. I am immensely grateful to F. Eugene Yates, MD, University of California, Los Angeles (UCLA), for his mentoring in time-series analysis and managing multivariate physiological data sets, and for his many years of collaboration, scholarship, and guidance that have helped lead to new insights for defining psychophysiological states. I am grateful to the late J. Christian Gillin, MD, Department of Psychiatry, UCSD, for his years of sleep-research collaborations and generous collegial tutoring in the arena of NIH grant applications. I am grateful to Liana Beckett, MA, MFCC, Department of Psychiatry, UCSD, for the first invitation to collaborate using Kundalini yoga meditation techniques for treating obsessive compulsive disorder (OCD). I am grateful to Saul Levine, MD, Departments of Psychiatry, UCSD and Children's Hospital, San Diego, for his interest and collaboration to help further the OCD clinical trial work and making possible the controlled study funded by the National Institute of Health (NIH). I want to acknowledge with gratitude Christopher C. Gallen, MD, PhD, for his collaboration on the second OCD trial, for study design, and professional guidance throughout. I am also grateful to Chris for initiating the research opportunities employing magnetoencephalography (MEG) for studying OCD patients, healthy controls, and the study of the OCD breath technique when he directed the MEG lab at The Scripps Research Institute. His collaborative support and sage advice over the years have been priceless. I am grateful to Leslie Ellen Ray, MA, MFCC, for running the control group in the OCD clinical trial, and to Barry J. Schwartz, PhD, when at The Scripps Research Institute, and John

Sidorowich, PhD, UCSD, for collaboration on the OCD trial. In addition, I am grateful to Henry D. I. Abarbanel, PhD, Director of the Institute for Nonlinear Science (INLS), UCSD, for providing institutional support and a most wonderful, open, rigorous, creative, and productive atmosphere in which to conduct this scientific work. I want to thank my other colleagues in INLS, Drs. Jon A. Wright, Roy Schult, Evgeny Novikov, Barry J. Schwartz, and Matthew B. Kennel for collaboration on pioneering MEG studies. I also want to thank Drs. Luigi Fortuna, Maide Bucolo, Manuela La Rosa, Mattia Frasca, and Francesca Sapuppo at the University of Catania in Sicily, Dipartimento di Ingegneria Elettrica Elettronica e dei Sistemi, Catania, Sicily, for their enduring and creative collaborative efforts on MEG signal processing for the study of yogic meditation techniques, normals, and OCD patients. I am grateful to Stuart W. Jamieson, MB, Head of the Division of Cardiothoracic Surgery, UCSD, and B. Bo Sramek, PhD, Czech Technical University Prague, Department of Mechanical Engineering, for collaboration on yogic techniques for altering cardiovascular function and for novel work on defining hemodynamic states. I am indeed grateful to Brian Fallon, MD, Columbia University, Department of Psychiatry, and New York State Psychiatric Institute, for inviting me to present at a 2003 symposium on OCD at the Annual American Psychiatric Association (APA) Conference. This event led to my teaching other APA workshops and courses on Kundalini yoga meditation techniques specific to treating psychiatric disorders. I want to acknowledge Sidney Zisook, MD, Department of Psychiatry, UCSD, for his departmental support and help to further our OCD and posttraumatic stress disorder (PTSD) clinical trial efforts, and his patience and sage advice on designing and applying for NIH grants. There are many other scientific collaborators and support staff who have helped to make this work possible over the last 30 years, and I am grateful to all of them for their key roles. I am grateful to Guru Singh for transmitting the three techniques for bipolar disorders and the protocol for chronic fatigue syndrome.

I especially want to acknowledge with my deepest gratitude Mr. John DeBeer and Dr. Mona Baumgartel for providing financial support to The Khalsa Foundation for Medical Science every year since its inception in 1984. Their generosity has made the continuation of this work possible. In addition, I want to thank the Fetzer Institute, the Waletzky Charitable Lead Trust, Earl Bakken, and the National Institutes of Health for funding some of the scientific studies described in this book.

And last but not least, I am very grateful and indebted to my editor, Deborah Malmud, Director of Norton Professional Books at W. W. Norton & Company, for the invitation to write this book and her patience and creative support during the process.

Preface

The intent of this book is twofold. First is to bring the numerous unique Kundalini yoga meditation techniques specific for the treatment of psychiatric disorders, and those specific for couples therapy, to the attention of the medical, scientific, and therapeutic communities. The second purpose is to provide the reader with enough evidence to consider this knowledge as an important ancient science, which today is perhaps best described as an "ancient technology of the mind." This of course implies that the ancients who developed the original system of yoga were highly evolved, in fact, much more so than Westerners might think. However, for those who have their origins in the East, and in particular India, the concepts of being adept at altering states of consciousness, achieving states of transcendence and enlightenment, and wielding the mystical abilities of the saints are common throughout their history. Clearly the axiom "extraordinary claims require extraordinary proof" is as important and relevant here as it might be anywhere. However, proof can come in one of two ways. One way is through scientific insight, and the other is through personal experience. The best proof comes through both. My initial convictions about the uniqueness of Kundalini yoga came in the summer of 1974 at the age of 26. My very first experience was remarkably compelling, and it became clear to me through further study that Kundalini yoga was a highly structured science that took an untold number of generations to develop. Over the past 31 years, I have practiced more than a 1,000 different Kundalini yoga meditation techniques, and many that are supposedly specific for treating psychiatric disorders. I have also learned a great deal about yogic concepts that have led to extraordinary scientific insights into how the mind and body work. While the yogic knowledge in this book goes back many thousands of years, these teachings have their more recent origins from The House of Guru Ram Das and the teachings of Kundalini yoga as taught by Yogi Bhajan.

Introduction

This book is designed for use by psychiatrists, psychothera-
pists, psychologists, social workers, physicians, other clinicians, and for yoga therapists who have an interest in
working with psychiatric patients. This book is also written to help
supplement marital therapy, and for those who want to enhance
their personal growth, performance, and mental health. Scientists
who have an interest in yoga, mind-body relations, consciousness,
and theoretical aspects of health and disease may also find the
topics included in this book of interest. The presentation of material, including the definitions of the respective disorders and their
prevalence rates, will be especially useful to those who lack formal
study in these disorders, but may also be useful as reasonably
current summaries for trained clinicians and others in the public
health sector.

Chapter 1 introduces a number of landmark scientific discoveries that were based on concepts from the ancient science of
Kundalini yoga. These discoveries demonstrate that yoga can be a
useful source of insight into both the areas of basic science and
preclinical science, independent of what we can learn from
employing yogic techniques in clinical trials. To date, this work has
led to an entirely new perspective on the dynamics of mind-body
interactions during both waking and sleep, as well as a novel under-

standing of physiological states and how the body's major systems are integrated and co-regulated by the hypothalamus. In addition, studies presented here demonstrate that yoga can provide insight into endogenous mechanisms that have not been previously discovered in the West, and how these insights can be applied toward self-regulation and healing. One such natural mechanism now exploited through the use of selective unilateral autonomic activation has recently been discovered as a correlate of a yogic technique called *unilateral forced nostril breathing* (UFNB), where sympathetic tone is selectively activated on one side of the body. The correlate now being tested is called *vagal nerve stimulation*, which employs an implanted pacemaker for selectively stimulating the vagus nerve on one side of the body, and which has generated considerable evidence for the efficacious treatment of epilepsy as well as limited data to date for treating depression and obsessive compulsive disorder (OCD). The yogic technique has been shown to selectively stimulate the contralateral cerebral hemisphere and has been used to treat OCD. In addition, this use of selective autonomic activation has also been shown to have differential effects on heart rate, eye-blink rates, glucose levels, and intraocular pressures. The scientific discoveries reported here have all been previously published in peer-reviewed scientific journals.

Chapter 1 also introduces additional yogic concepts that may lead to other important breakthroughs in the understanding of mind-body interactions, the nature and dynamics of the mind, personality structure, levels of consciousness, and other basic concepts that may help us to better comprehend health and disease beyond the molecular, cellular, and genetic levels. This chapter introduces the yogic concept of the *chakras* that helps to define the eight basic levels of human consciousness, which have yet to be defined in a practical way by Western science. The concept of the rhythm of the 11 *moon centers*, or erogenous zones, that is unique to women, can, for example, give us fascinating insight into a new dimension and a deeper understanding of the female psyche as observed by yogis in ancient times. The simple male correlate of the female rhythm is also described. A highly complex model of the human mind that includes 81 practical facets and which is unique to the teachings of Kundalini yoga is also presented. In addition, this chapter explains how mantras may work and how languages may affect us beyond the Western notions of linguistics. Lastly, the concept of the five *elements*, or *tattvas*, commonly called earth, water, fire, air and ether, are presented in their conceptual framework in yogic medicine, which has correlates in other ancient systems of health and wellness. These concepts may all help advance our understanding of the dynamics and structure of the brain, the mind and personalities, and consciousness, and how they are all linked in health and disease.

Chapters 2 through 8 present 50 different meditation techniques that are each specific to one of the following: anger, anxiety, fatigue, fear, obsessive compulsive disorder (OCD), panic attacks, phobias, depression, bipolar disorders, grief, addictions, impulse control disorders, insomnia, nightmares, inducing super-efficient sleep, dyslexia, patience and temperament, releasing childhood anger, long-lasting deep inner anger, self-esteem, and a half-dozen techniques for the abused and battered psyche that can be used with children, adolescents, and adults. In addition, Chapters 2 through 8 include eight unique multipart protocols specific for the respective disorders in the following chapters: Chapter 2, OCD, acute stress disorder; Chapter 3, major depressive disorder, bipolar disorder; Chapter 4, addictions, impulse control, and eating disorders; Chapter 6, chronic fatigue syndrome; Chapter 7, attention deficit hyperactivity disorder and co-morbid disorders (conduct disorder and oppositional defiant disorder); Chapter 8, posttraumatic stress disorder. This last protocol can be used by individuals who have been sexually abused or physically abused through war or other traumas. This protocol can also be used by trauma victims at either early or late stages of the disorder, or as a means to help prevent or minimize the onset of this disorder immediately after trauma.

Chapter 9 provides insight into how to employ these protocols and techniques effectively for treating psychiatric patients. A variety of options are presented to help augment traditional treatment programs.

Chapter 10 includes 14 different meditation techniques that are specific for couples therapy, and which can also be used simply to enhance otherwise healthy relationships. All of the techniques in Chapters 2 through 8 can be helpful and practiced by individuals for the purpose of personal growth and wellness. Since these techniques can be of benefit to nearly everyone, there is no single chapter that addresses personal growth per se. I leave it to the individual to decide which area or ability they may choose to improve or explore in their lives.

Chapter 2 also includes the description of two clinical trials, a pilot uncontrolled trial and a randomized controlled trial funded by the National Institutes of Health. Both trials employed the Kundalini yoga meditation protocol specific for OCD described in detail in Chapter 2. The results of this trial may help set a precedent for the further testing of the efficacious effects of Kundalini yoga meditation techniques (or protocols) for a wide range of disorders. Chapters 2 through 8 also each include a number of case histories that offer insight into the efficacious use of each protocol. Chapter 2 includes the case histories for many of the patients who were involved in the two OCD clinical trials. Chapter 8 includes a very lengthy and detailed case history of a young woman who suffered from OCD, posttraumatic stress disorder, borderline personality disorder, eating disorders, depression, and self-mutilation. This case history is an edit of the patient's own self-described ordeal throughout her psychiatric history, both using conventional modalities and Kundalini yoga meditation techniques. In part, the value here is that a large percentage of patients present with a range of disorders, not just a single disorder, and, therefore, Kundalini yoga meditation techniques may provide a solution for the treatment of the more complicated cases with poly-disorder conditions and histories. In fact, a number of case histories in this book describe patients presenting with multiple disorders.

Introduction

The epilogue provides further argument for why Kundalini yoga meditation techniques should to be considered for use as a first-line modality for treatment, but more so because of their extraordinary value as a means of prevention. It presents further support for why funding should be directed more toward prevention, an almost completely neglected area of public health when compared to the national spending rates for research on disease treatment.

What this book is *not*: this book is not a review of the scientific literature on yoga, meditation, or other complementary and alternative modalities for treating psychiatric disorders. Nor does it expound on the trade publications on these topics. Therefore, I apologize to any researchers who find that their very important articles are not cited in this book. Due to length limitations and the scope and intent of this book, such reviews would be simply overwhelming within the space and time required to do justice to these topics. In addition, many other areas of important conventional information that would lend further insight into the treatment of the disorders in this book are also not covered or described in appropriate detail. This book is limited in its scope in terms of using Kundalini yoga for the treatment of other psychiatric disorders and conditions. No chapters are written on how to treat the psychotic disorders, pervasive developmental disorders, traumatic brain injuries, stroke patients, and other important areas where these techniques may prove to be useful. This book is primarily directed at making the case for a further and rigorous investigation of the concepts and techniques of Kundalini yoga as taught by Yogi Bhajan. I attempt here to make the case for exploring the potential wealth of information and practical techniques this ancient technology of the mind offers for improving our future in a world of ever-increasing complications resulting from the human failings of ignorance, greed, lack of tolerance, and limited awareness and self-control. Videos are being prepared to assist in the teaching of the techniques and protocols in this book and will be available through the following web site: www.theinternetyogi.com.

PART ONE

THE ANCIENT SCIENCE OF
KUNDALINI YOGA

ONE

Yogic Insights into Mind-Body Medicine and Healing

The origins of Kundalini yoga date back to the time of the rishis in ancient India more than 5,000 years ago, a time before the advent of the world's formal religions. The rishis were people of spiritual power who over an untold number of generations had developed through experimentation a highly advanced understanding of how the mind and body work. This understanding led to the body of knowledge called *yoga*. During that ancient era, yoga did not have the many branches or subspecialties that are common today. Yoga was a comprehensive, technical, and highly integrated system, and the physical movements, static postures, breathing patterns, mantras, and meditation techniques formed the basis of a vast integrated science. In addition, the perceived difference today between *yoga* and *meditation* was nonexistent. Prior to about 1,000 B.C. the knowledge and technical know-how of this vast science was taught openly. However, in the last 3,000 years, this sacred and secret knowledge has been taught intact only from master to selected disciples. During this latter era there were limits on what was taught openly or what was available through some yogic lineages. Yoga is described here as "Kundalini yoga as taught by Yogi Bhajan," a master of the ancient system and the yogi responsible for teaching this system again as it was taught openly in ancient times. Yogi Bhajan came to the West in late 1968 and began teaching Kundalini yoga to anyone who had an interest. From 1968 to 2004 he taught approximately 5,000 different meditation techniques as well as hundreds of different sets of yoga exercises, each set with a specific sequence, and all claiming to have a unique therapeutic value.

The intent in this chapter is to briefly inform the reader of some of the major concepts inherent to this ancient knowledge that can give us deeper insight into the mind and body and how yogis perceive these relationships for purposes of healing and as a means for understanding the nature of consciousness itself. All foreign systems of medicine, healing, or physiology include terms that are not readily translatable into the modern concepts of Western science and medicine, and these terms may therefore appear to be primitive and perhaps naïve from a Western scientific viewpoint. Even though remarkable and fascinating advances have been made in the last 100 years that have led to this fascinating new era of the genome, with a much more vast knowledge of the molecular nature of the cell, along with the novel instrumentation for imaging the dynamics of the brain, the West has made limited progress in the fields of macrosystems biology and understanding physiological states, or in elucidating much of the natural and endogenous mechanisms for self-activating the body's healing machinery, or in understanding consciousness. The latter is clearly the last great frontier, and of course any new concepts and insights may be useful for this exploration if they can prove to have practical value.

This chapter will introduce the yogic concepts and correlates of *ida* and *pingala* that have led to a greater understanding of physiological states and mind-body dynamics, as well as basic endogenous mechanisms for self-regulation. Additional concepts to be covered include: the eight states of consciousness defined by the chakra system; female rhythms of the 11 erogenous centers that influence the psyche, and the male correlate; the 81 facets of the mind; the five elements (earth, water, fire, air, and ether) that play

2

a fundamental role in healing and add a level of refinement to the chakra system; and finally a basic physiological mechanism that in part helps explain how mantras work.

The chapters on clinical treatment will describe a broad array of techniques for activating the body's healing and self-regulatory systems. Chapter 1 is only meant to be an elementary introduction to selected yogic topics and is not intended to be either a thorough or in-depth treatise on these topics, which are each much deeper and more complex in practice. When these topics are taken together, they present an astonishingly advanced vision of the make-up of the human psyche and mind-body relations.

Defining Physiological States: Insights Based on the Yogic Physiological Concepts of *Ida* and *Pingala*

In the ancient yogic system, *nadis* are defined as "astral tubes" that carry *prana* or "life force" energy. They are the equivalent of the energy *meridians* in the acupuncture system. There are supposedly 72,000 nadis in the body, and they are related but not equivalent to nerves. *Ida, pingala,* and *sushumna* are the three major and most important nadis. Sushumna is the central nadi and it is represented in the figure of caduceus—the universal symbol for healing—by the center rod that is symbolic of the spinal canal. The ida and pingala nadis are represented in the caduceus by the two entwined snakes that cross at six central points, with their origins at the spinal base along with the sushumna nadi. These six points of intersection are symbolic of the six lower chakras, or primary energy centers in the body (see discussion on chakras, page 31). However, the ida and pingala nadis also have importance in the yogic system for defining physiological states. The ida nadi correlates to the state of the nervous system, energetics, and the physiological state that is identified when airflow dominates through the left nostril. The pingala nadi correlates to the state when airflow dominates through the right nostril. In the yogic system, these two subtle variations are actually polar, complementary physiological states that correlate to the two polar phases of what is called the *nasal cycle*. Note, in the caduceus figure, the two snake heads meet at the region comparable with the two nostrils. What yogis knew about the nasal cycle and its correlates has led to an array of exciting and novel studies that today present a new and comprehensive view of both mind-body dynamics and physiological states.

The nasal cycle was first noted in the West at the turn of the 19th century by Kayser, a German physician (Kayser, 1889, 1895). Kayser's observation led to sporadic studies throughout the 20th century (Beickert, 1951; Cole & Haight, 1986; Eccles, 2000; Heetderks, 1927; Kennedy, Ziegler, Shannahoff-Khalsa, 1986; Keuning, 1968; Shannahoff-Khalsa, 1991a; Shannahoff-Khalsa, Kennedy, Yates, & Ziegler, 1996; Werntz, Bickford, Bloom, & Shannahoff-Khalsa, 1983). These references are selected highlights on the topic and are not all-inclusive of the nasal-cycle literature. The nasal cycle is defined as an alternating congestion in one nostril with simultaneous decongestion in the other nostril, which is manifested by vasodilation in one nasal turbinate paralleled by vasoconstriction in the other, respectively. Airflow dominates through the decongested nostril for a period and then congestion and decongestion switch. This alternation in dominance is continuous throughout both waking and sleep. The cycle has been measured to last from as short as 25 minutes (Werntz et al., 1983) up to 8 hours (Keuning, 1968). Keuning reviewed numerous studies on the nasal cycle during waking and concluded that the average cycle length is about 3 to 4 hours but ranges from 2 to 8 hours and appears to be partly related to age and health (Keuning, 1968). Hasegawa and Kern (1978) studied 50 human subjects and found a mean duration of 2.9 hours, ranging from 1 to 6 hours. The nasal cycle literature reports the same uncertainty, wobble, nonstationarity, and intermittency as do the other ultradian phenomena (Shannahoff-Khalsa et al., 1996). Yogis claim that the healthy human has 10 complete cycles in 24 hours. The nasal mucosa are densely innervated with autonomic fibers and the dominance of sympathetic activity on one side produces vasoconstriction in the turbinates allowing for greater airflow, while the contralateral nostril exhibits a simultaneous dominance of parasympathetic activity that causes swelling and restricted airflow. Kayser described the nasal cycle as a marker of "the alternation of vaso-motor tone throughout the periphery on the two sides of the body" (Kayser, 1889, 1895). However, from the time of its discovery in the West, with several exceptions (Beickert in 1951 on half-sided rhythms of the nasal cycle with some organ systems, and studies on posture and the nasal cycle [Cole & Haight, 1986; Rao & Potdar, 1970] and on lateralized patterns of perspiration with nasal patency [Kawase, 1952]), the nasal cycle was primarily studied as a phenomenon independent of other physiological systems until the work of Werntz, Bickford, Bloom, and Shanna-hoff-Khalsa in 1983. However, the basic autonomics of sympa-thetic and parasympathetic regulation of the nasal cycle were well understood (Bamford & Eccles, 1982; Eccles, 2000; Keuning, 1968). Stoksted first speculated that the nasal cycle was "regulated by a central sympathetic centre possibly situated in the hypothal-amus" (1953). Later, a detailed clock-like model for hypothalamic regulation was proposed for how the hypothalamus via the auto-nomic nervous system (ANS) regulates the nasal cycle along with the coupled ultradian ("hourly" domain) rhythms of the body's major systems, including the neuroendocrine system, cardiovas-cular system, central nervous system (CNS), immune system, gastrointestinal system, and energy regulation through the pancreas (Shannahoff-Khalsa, 1991b; Shannahoff-Khalsa et al., 1996). The nasal cycle has also been demonstrated in rats and rabbits (Bojsen-Moller & Fahrenkrug, 1971), in anesthetized pigs (Ashley & Lea, 1978), and cats (Bamford & Eccles, 1982), and no doubt occurs in all mammals.

Prior to the studies described below demonstrating the unique physiological correlates of ida and pingala, the latest major insight into physiological states was that proposed by Kleitman in the 1960s, when he first postulated the *basic rest-activity cycle*, or BRAC, hypothesis (Kleitman, 1961, 1967, 1982). Kleitman's BRAC hypothesis had its origins in the discovery of how EEG and eye-movement patterns change in concert during sleep, giving rise to the concept of the *rapid eye movement* (REM) and *non-rapid eye movement* (NREM) sleep stages, and how eye movements, dreaming, and body motility are temporally organized during sleep (Dement & Kleitman, 1957). Other physiological events were also found to be coupled to REM and NREM sleep activity (Kleitman, 1967, 1982). Kleitman's BRAC concept was supposed to explain why some psychological and physiological activities are integrated and account for the obvious patterns of intermixed locomotor activity and quiescent states observed during sleep and how related changes continue during the waking state (Kleitman, 1967). Kleitman concluded "the BRAC is probably a fundamental variation in the functioning of the central nervous system, increasing in duration with phylogenetic progression" where "in each species of mammal studied, the BRAC also lengthens during ontogenetic development" (Kleitman, 1967). He proposed the BRAC to be a reflection and variation of integrated events during the 24-hour period that served both the needs for rest and activity.

Yogi Bhajan taught a range of yogic concepts that give us insight today into physiological states that are based on the concepts of ida and pingala and which now present a new dynamical view of mind-body physiology governed by CNS–ANS relations. Listed here are six major concepts that he taught that are relevant to the topic, and all have been studied in the laboratory and proven valid. Following this list, each concept will be presented separately along with the published scientific studies that support it.

1. The nasal cycle is a marker for the ultradian rhythm of alternating cerebral hemispheric activity during both waking and sleep. When airflow dominates through the right nostril, this

correlates to greater cerebral activity in the left hemisphere (the pingala state), and when airflow dominates through the left nostril, this correlates to greater cerebral activity in the right hemisphere (the ida state).

2. The nasal cycle is a marker for the dynamic lateralization of ANS function. That is, when sympathetic activity prevails on the left side of the body, parasympathetic activity prevails on the right side of the body. These two modes alternate in dominance.

3. Right-nostril dominance correlates to REM sleep and greater activity in the left hemisphere, and left-nostril dominance correlates to NREM sleep and greater right-hemispheric activity.

4. The nasal cycle is a marker for physiological states. Greater airflow in the left nostril correlates with the *resting phase*, and greater airflow in the right nostril correlates with the *activity phase*. Yogis defined ida as the "moon" or "female-like" energetic state (the equivalent of the resting phase of the BRAC), and pingala as the state when "sun energy" or "male energy" dominates (the equivalent of the activity phase of the BRAC).

5. The hypothalamus integrates and regulates the two polar physiological states of rest and activity.

6. Unilateral forced nostril breathing, that is, forcing the breath through only one nostril, stimulates the contralateral hemisphere and ipsilateral sympathetic nervous system via the hypothalamus.

1. The nasal cycle is a marker for the ultradian rhythm of alternating cerebral hemispheric activity during both waking and sleep.

When Yogi Bhajan first stated the significance of the nasal cycle in the early 1970s, claiming that it was a marker for physiological states and coupled to the alternating dominance of the two cerebral hemispheres, the concept of alternating cerebral dominance during the waking phase had yet to be discovered in the West.

However, there was some preliminary evidence for alternating cerebral dominance during sleep in humans (Goldstein, Stoltzfus, & Gardocki, 1972). In 1979, Klein and Armitage first observed the ultradian rhythms of alternating cognitive-performance efficiency by studying changes in verbal and spatial skills in naïve subjects. They tested eight subjects with a verbal and spatial task every 15 minutes for 8 hours. They noted ultradian variations with the most significant peaks at 37, 96, and 240 minutes, and the respective oscillations with each task were 180 degrees out of phase with each other (Klein & Armitage, 1979). The studies that demonstrate the ultradian rhythm of alternating cerebral hemispheric activity during both waking and sleep in a variety of species have been reviewed (Shannahoff-Khalsa, 1993), along with a selected review on unihemispheric sleep in Cetaceans, eared-seals, manatees, and birds (Rattenborg, Amlaner, & Lima, 2000).

Experimental verification of the first yogic postulate on the relationship of the nasal cycle and the ultradian rhythm of alternating cerebral hemispheric activity during waking was first reported in 1980 and in greater detail in 1983 (Werntz et al., 1980, 1983). Alternating dominance of cerebral hemispheric activity was demonstrated in humans by use of the electroencephalogram (EEG). Relative changes of electrocortical activity were found to have a direct and tightly coupled relationship with changes in the nasal cycle. Werntz et al. (1980, 1983) observed during waking rest in young naïve healthy male and female subjects that the efficiency of breathing alternates predominantly through the right or left nostril with a periodicity ranging from 25 to greater than 200 minutes. Relatively greater EEG power in one hemisphere was found to correlate with predominant airflow in the contralateral nostril. They concluded that this observation defines a new inter-relationship between cerebral dominance and peripheral autonomic nervous function. Figure 1.1 shows three subjects during waking and how the periodicity can vary widely under passive resting conditions.

FIGURE 1.1

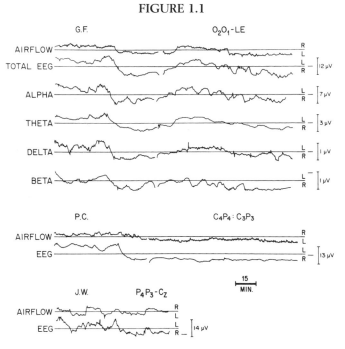

FIGURE 1.1. Airflow tracings: Points above the baseline indicate greater right-nostril airflow and points below indicate greater left-nostril airflow. Total EEG is 1–35 Hz. Alpha (8–13 Hz), Theta (4–8 Hz), Delta (1–4 Hz), and Beta (13–35 Hz) tracings were filtered through an analog filter before integration. This baseline is drawn to visually enhance the similarity of the basic correlation of the two phenomena. The dash to the right of the EEG tracings indicates the true zero line where the right and left EEG amplitudes are equal. The bar and its numerical equivalent next to the integrated EEG tracings represent the actual calibrated amplitudes in microvolts. Subject GF's EEG montage (O2O1-LE) is right and left occipital compared to linked ears; subject PC is bipolar central-parietal; and subject JW is parietal compared to central midline. (From "Alternating Cerebral Hemispheric Activity and the Lateralization of Autonomic Nervous Function," by D. A. Werntz et al., 1983, *Human Neurobiology* 2(1), 39–43. Reprinted with permission.)

In addition, the ultradian rhythm of alternating cerebral hemispheric activity is further demonstrated during sleep in 10 young (ages 20 to 30) normal healthy males (Shannahoff-Khalsa, Gillin, Yates, Schlosser, & Zawadzki, 2001). Figure 1.2 plots the left-minus-right EEG power for all subjects.

FIGURE 1.2

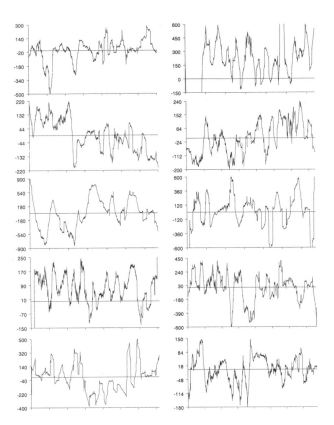

FIGURE 1.2. The time series for subjects 1–10 are presented for L-R-total EEG power for the entire recording period after lights out to awakening. The plots are not detrended and are of the RMS of each C3 and C4 treated for artifacts, moving average at 500, normalized means, and subtractions. The y-axis scaling is adjusted for each to maximize the visual appearance of the fluctuations. The y-axis value is the difference of power between left and right hemispheres and 100 units is the equivalent of 0.61 microvolts. The average variation from the largest negative peak to the largest positive peak for the 10 subjects ranges across approximately 800 units total or about 5 microvolts. Subject 1 starts at the left top and goes down through subject 5, and subject 6 starts at the right top. The x-axis lengths (tic marks in hours) for subjects 1-10 are similar and are: 7.08, 6.99, 6.75, 7.09, 7.20, 6.50, 6.86, 6.79, 7.71, 7.96 hours, respectively. (From "Ultradian Rhythms of Alternating Cerebral Hemispheric EEG Dominance Are Coupled to Rapid Eye Movement and Stage 4 Non-Rapid Eye Movement Sleep in Humans" by D. S. Shannahoff-Khalsa et al., 2001, *Sleep Medicine 2*, 333–346, 2001. Reprinted with permission.)

The tightly coupled relationship of the nasal cycle and cerebral rhythm was also demonstrated during sleep in a multivariate physiological study that measured the nasal cycle (4 Hz sampling rate), left and right EEG (sampling rate 256 Hz), and several beat-to-beat cardiovascular measures in normal healthy males (Shannahoff-Khalsa & Yates, 2000). Figure 1.3 shows the data for a sleeping subject with the left-minus-right nasal airflow in the top panel and the left-minus-right EEG power in the lower panel. Note, in Figure 1.1, the left-minus-right nasal airflow and right-minus-left EEG power are plotted and thus show a direct relationship in coupling, while Figure 1.3 shows the inverse relationship. However, the only difference here is in how the lefts and rights are plotted. Both figures demonstrate that when airflow is greater in one nostril, there is relatively greater EEG power in the contralateral hemisphere.

Figure 1.3

NC

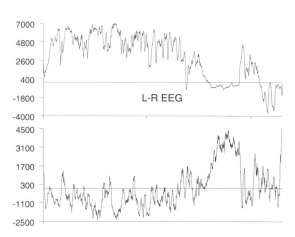

Figure 1.3. The primary time-series data for a subject are plotted from top down for the nasal cycle (left-minus-right nostril dominance), and left-minus-right hemisphere EEG power. The scaling is adjusted for each to maximize the visual appearance of the fluctuations. The x-axis is for 4.78 hr and the y-axis values for the left-minus-right NC measures are in arbitrary electronic units related to differential thermistor activity. Data above the midline indicates left-nostril airflow dominance, LREEG is scaled as the difference of the root mean square (RMS) calculations after a normalization of left and right means for RMS values over the night.

Figure 1.4

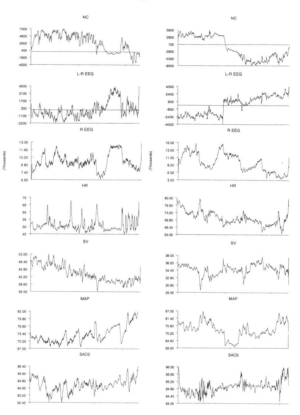

Figure 1.4. The primary time-series data for subject 3, night 2 (left side of figure), and subject 2, night 3, are plotted from top down for the nasal cycle (left-minus-right nostril dominance), left-minus-right hemisphere EEG power, right hemisphere EEG power, heart rate, stroke volume, mean arterial pressure, and hemoglobin-oxygen saturation. The scaling is adjusted for each to maximize the visual appearance of the fluctuations. These time series were not detrended here. The x-axis is for 4.78 hrs for subject 3 and for 6.04 hrs for subject 2. The y-axis values for the left-minus-right NC measures are in arbitrary electronic units related to differential thermistor activity, data above the midline indicates left-nostril airflow dominance, LREEG is scaled as the difference of the RMS calculations after a normalization of left and right means for RMS values over the night; REEG is scaled as the RMS calculation from the raw primary data; the HR values are in beats/min; SV is in mls/beat; MAP is in mm Hg; and SAO2 is in % hemoglobin-oxygen saturation. (From "Ultradian Sleep Rhythms of Lateral EEG, Autonomic, and Cardiovascular Activity Are Coupled in Humans," by D. S. Shannahoff-Khalsa and F. E. Yates, 2000, *International Journal of Neuroscience 101* (1–4), 21–43. Reprinted with permission.)

This study also shows how the ultradian rhythms of the cardiovascular system are coupled to the nasal cycle and cerebral rhythm (Shannahoff-Khalsa & Yates 2000). A total of 11 parameters (left-right EEG power [LREEG], left EEG power [LEEG], right EEG power [REEG], the nasal cycle [NC], heart rate [HR]], stroke volume [SV], cardiac output [CO], systolic blood pressure [SBP], diastolic blood pressure [DBP], mean arterial pressure [MAP], and hemoglobin-oxygen saturation [SAO2]) were measured simultaneously and then subjected to time-series analysis. Figure 1.4 shows how the NC, LREEG, REEG, HR, SV, MAP, and SAO2 are coupled in two separate subjects.

Figure 1.5 shows the coupling with two additional subjects with the same multi-variate measures.

One unique element of this study is that it compared the dynamics of multiple systems during sleep with earlier multi-variate results during waking under strict resting conditions (Shannahoff-Khalsa et al., 1996, 1997). Three consecutive nights of data were collected from three healthy adult males for: left and right central EEGs; the 4 Hz measured NC; beat-to-beat measures of CO, SV, HR, SBP, DBP, MAP, and hemoglobin-oxygen saturation. Time series analysis detected periods at 280–300, 215–275, 165–210, 145–160, 105–140, 70–100, and 40–65 minute bins with the greatest spectral power in longer periods (see Figure 1.6). We found statistical significance across subjects with all parameters at 280–300, 105–140 (except left EEG power, left-minus-right EEG power, and HR), 70–100, and 40–65 minutes. Statistically significant periods (see Figure 1.7) were reported during waking for the NC, pituitary hormones (luteinizing hormone, adrenocorticotropin hormone), catecholamines (norepinephrine, epinephrine, dopamine), insulin, and cardiovascular function in five bins at 220–340, 170–215, 115–145, 70–100, and 40–65 minutes, with 115–145, 70–100, and 40–65 minutes common across all variables (Shannahoff-Khalsa et al., 1996, 1997). Note, Klein and Armitage (1979) found three dominant peaks for alternating cerebral hemispheric rhythms at 37, 96, and 240 minutes, and their results are

Figure 1.5

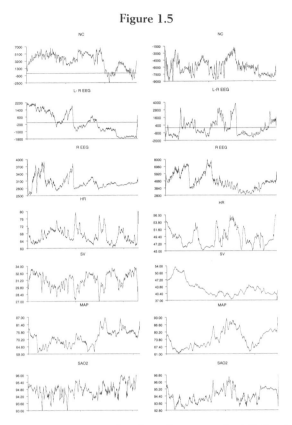

Figure 1.5. The primary time-series data for subject 1, night 1 (left side of figure), and subject 3, night 3, are plotted from top down for the nasal cycle (left-minus-right nostril dominance), left-minus-right hemisphere EEG power, right hemisphere EEG power, heart rate, stroke volume, mean arterial pressure, and hemoglobin-oxygen saturation. The scaling is adjusted for each to maximize the visual appearance of the fluctuations. These time series were not detrended here. The x-axis is for 5.83 hrs for subject 1 and for 5.29 hrs for subject 3. The y-axis values for the left-minus-right NC measures are in arbitrary electronic units related to differential thermistor activity. Data above the midline indicates left-nostril airflow dominance; LREEG is scaled as the difference of the RMS calculations after a normalization of left and right means for RMS values over the night; REEG is scaled as the RMS calculation from the raw primary data; the HR values are in beats/min; SV is in mls/beat; MAP is in mm Hg; and SAO2 is in % hemoglobin-oxygen saturation. Note, subject 3's NC shows only relative shifts in right-nostril dominance during the entire night. (From "Ultradian Sleep Rhythms of Lateral EEG, Autonomic, and Cardiovascular Activity Are Coupled in Humans," by D. S. Shannahoff-Khalsa and F. E. Yates, 2000, *International Journal of Neuroscience 101*, 21–43. Reprinted with permission.)

commensurate with the multivariate waking and sleep studies (Shannahoff-Khalsa et al., 1996, 1997; Shannahoff-Khalsa & Yates, 2000; Shannahoff-Khalsa et al., 2001). In addition, for the sleep analysis of EEG parameters in young healthy normal males, significant peaks were found for all C3, C4, and L-R frequency (delta, theta, alpha, beta, and total EEG) bands at the 280–300, 75–125, 55–70, and 25–50 minute bins, with power dominating in the 75–125 minute bin, and LREEG rhythms were observed for all frequency bands (Shannahoff-Khalsa, Gillin, et al., 2001).

The spectral density plots for the time series of the various parameters from the multivariate sleep study are another way to demonstrate the rhythmic linkage of the different systems (Shannahoff-Khalsa, & Yates, 2000). When the "hourly" ultradian frequencies are studied using spectral analysis (see Figure 1.6), it is clear that the NC, LREEG, LEEG, REEG, CO, SV, HR, SBP, DBP, MAP, and hemoglobin-oxygen saturation values all show similar profiles during sleep.

In addition, Figure 1.7 shows us how these systems are coupled during waking rest in 10 different subjects. Note the similarity of the spectral plots for both waking and sleep.

These results suggest that lateral EEG power during sleep has a common pacemaker (the hypothalamus), or a mutually entrained pacemaker, with the cardiovascular system and ANS, and that waking ultradians of the neuroendocrine and fuel-regulatory hormones (insulin) are also coupled to the cerebral rhythm. Taken together, these results present a new perspective for the BRAC and the physiology and dynamics of the ANS–CNS during both waking and sleep.

2. The nasal cycle is a marker for the dynamic lateralization of ANS function.

In addition to the nasal cycle being a marker for the alternating lateralization of ANS function in the two nasal cavities, additional support for this phenomenon throughout the periphery comes

Figure 1.6

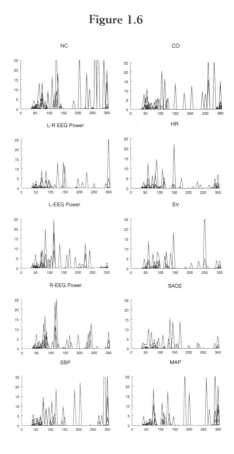

Figure 1.6. Spectral density plots of three subjects for all three nights using Fast Orthogonal Search time-history analysis of the nasal cycle (NC), left-minus-right hemisphere EEG power (LREEG power), left hemisphere EEG power (LEEG power), right hemisphere EEG power (REEG), systolic blood pressure (SBP), cardiac output (CO), heart rate (HR), stroke volume (SV), hemoglobin-oxygen saturation (SAO2), and mean arterial pressure (MAP). X-axis is 0–300 min with data of 0–40 min not included; y-axis is in 0–25% total mean square error (TMSE) accounted for by that period. Plots of SAO2 are missing subject 2's data for night 2. (From "Ultradian Sleep Rhythms of Lateral EEG, Autonomic, and Cardiovascular Activity Are Coupled in Humans," by D. S. Shannahoff-Khalsa and F. E. Yates, 2000, *International Journal of Neuroscience 101* (1–4), 21–43. Reprinted with permission.)

Figure 1.7

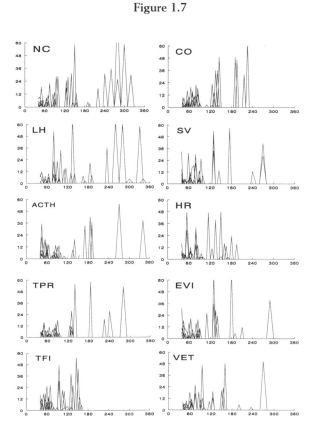

Figure 1.7. Spectral density plots of 10 subjects from FOS time-history analysis of the nasal cycle (NC), luteinizing hormone (LH), adrenocorticotropic hormone (ACTH), total peripheral resistance (TPR), thoracic fluid index (TFI), cardiac output (CO), stroke volume (SV), heart rate (HR), ejection velocity index (EVI), and ventricular ejection time (VET). X-axis is O–360 min with data of O–40 min not included; y-axis is in O–60% TMSE. Plots of CO, TPR, SV, HR, VET, EVI, and TFI are from 9 subjects; one subject's data was lost. (From "Ultradian Rhythms of Autonomic, Cardiovascular, and Neuroendocrine Systems Are Related in Humans," by D. S. Shannahoff-Khalsa et al., 1996, *American Journal of Physiology 270*, R873–87. Reprinted with permission.)

from a landmark study showing how the catecholamines (norepi-nephrine, epinephrine, dopamine) in the peripheral circulation differ and alternate in dominance in humans when measured over time under strict resting conditions (Kennedy et al., 1986). This study demonstrated through venous sampling in completely passive, resting, immobile humans sitting upright that cate-cholamines can be elevated in one arm and lower in the other arm when sampled at 7.5-minute intervals, and the levels alternate in dominance. Figure 1.8 shows how norepinephrine (NE), a plasma marker for sympathetic activity, can be elevated in one arm and lower in the other, and how the left-minus-right values can plot similarly to the typical ultradian profiles observed in other studies.

In addition, this study demonstrated how the NC in fact paral-lels the left-minus-right pattern of NE in peripheral circulation. Figure 1.9 demonstrates how the NC and left-minus-right values of NE closely parallel each other even when the NC shows a highly irregular nonsinusoidal pattern. This clearly indicates that the sympathetic nervous system throughout the periphery, as gauged by venous circulation in the arms and the modulation of the NC, supports the yogic claim of the NC being a marker for how the ANS alternates dominance on the two sides of the body. This result is contrary to the dogmatic view today that sampling blood cate-cholamines in one arm obviously would give the same result regardless of sides. Similar profiles for epinephrine and dopamine have been demonstrated (Kennedy et al., 1986). A comprehensive review has been published on the lateralized rhythms of the CNS and ANS and how other organ systems also exhibit lateralized differences (Shannahoff-Khalsa, 1991a).

3. Right-nostril dominance correlates with REM sleep and left-nostril dominance correlates with NREM sleep.

The third yogic postulate that right-nostril dominance correlates with REM sleep and greater activity in the left hemisphere (the active phase of the BRAC during sleep) and left-nostril dominance

Figure 1.8

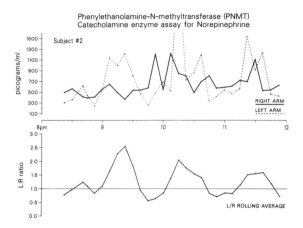

Figure 1.8. Top graph: Variations in plasma NE levels (pg/ml) were measured at 7.5-minute intervals in both right (unbroken line) and left (hatched line) arms. Raw data for subject 1 is represented from 8 A.M. to 12 noon. NE was measured by radioenzymatic assay with phenylethanolamine-N-methyltransferase and ([3H]SAM). Bottom graph: The left-right ratio of the values of the two arms in the top section are presented as a rolling average using the formula (1:2:1). Values in the curve above 1.00 represent greater levels of NE in the left arm and values below 1.00 are greater levels in the right arm. Time scale is the same as the top section. Note that the values plotted in the ratio have been transformed by the smoothing function and therefore, as in the first point, an obvious inconsistency seems apparent. (From "Alternating Lateralization of Plasma Catecholamines and Nasal Patency in Humans," by Kennedy, Shannahoff-Khalsa, & Ziegler, 1986, *Life Sciences* 38(13), 1203–1214. Reprinted with permission.)

correlates with NREM sleep stages and greater right-hemispheric activity (the resting phase of the BRAC during sleep) is inferred from the following data. We have observed how during sleep right-nostril dominance is coupled to relatively greater left-hemisphere EEG power and vice versa in Figures 1.4 and 1.5 (Shannahoff-Khalsa & Yates, 2000). In Figure 1.10 we observe how the left hemisphere shows relatively greater power during REM sleep and how the right hemisphere shows relatively greater power during stage 4 NREM sleep. Overall, across all 10 subjects, greater right-

Figure 1.9

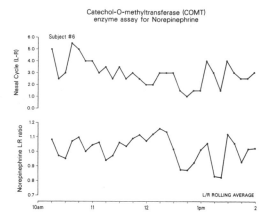

Catechol-O-methyltransferase (COMT)
enzyme assay for Norepinephrine

Figure 1.9. Top graph: The nasal-cycle determination of subject 6 is plotted as the raw data of the left-minus-right (L-R) value versus time. The (L-R) value was assessed at each time point for blood sampling, every 7.5 minutes. The subject fluctuates in left-nostril dominance during the entire recording period. The time scale is from 10:15 A.M. to 2:00 P.M. The nasal cycle has been shifted 15 minutes to the right. Bottom graph: The left-right ratio of the two arms is generated by dividing the average of the triplicate value of one arm by the other. The rolling average is presented here using the formula (1:2:1). Points greater than 1.0 represent greater levels of NE in the left arm and values below 1.0 represent greater levels of NE in the right arm. NE was determined by radioenzymatic assay with catechol-O-methyltransferase and ([3H]SAM). (From "Alternating Lateralization of Plasma Catecholamines and Nasal Patency in Humans," by Kennedy, Shannahoff-Khalsa, & Ziegler, 1986, *Life Sciences 38*(13), 1203–1214. Reprinted with permission.)

hemisphere EEG dominance was found during NREM stage 4 sleep, and greater left during REM for total EEG, delta and alpha bands (Chi-squares, P < 0.001). Theta was similar, but not significant (P = 0.163), and beta was equivocal (Shannahoff-Khalsa, Gillin, et al., 2001). They concluded that since earlier ultradian studies show that lateral EEG and LREEG power have a common pacemaker, or a mutually entrained pacemaker with the autonomic, cardiovascular, neuroendocrine, and fuel-regulatory hormone systems, the results for LREEG coupling to sleep stages

Figure 1.10

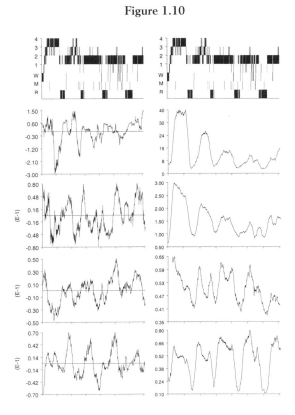

Figure 1.10. Left column: The sleep hypnogram for subject 1 is at the top. In the hypnogram vertical axis, "R" indicates REM sleep, "M" indicates movement, "W" indicates waking, and 1, 2, 3, and 4 indicate the various stages of NREM sleep. The time-series data for subject 1 for the L-R for the four different frequency bands—delta, theta, alpha, and beta—are presented below the hypnogram, respectively. These data are not detrended and are from the FFT power per 4-second intervals for the entire night (7.08 hrs). The respective C3 and C4 were treated for artifacts, moving averages at 500, left and right means normalized, and subtracted. The scaling is adjusted for each to maximize the visual appearance of the fluctuations, and the x-axis has markers for 1-hour intervals. The y-axis values are in microvolts/Hertz. Right column: The sleep hypnogram followed by the left-hemisphere C3 counterpart to the left column L-Rs presented for delta, theta, alpha, and beta bands, respectively. The y-axis values are in microvolts/Hertz. (From "Ultradian Rhythms of Alternating Cerebral Hemispheric EEG Dominance Are Coupled to Rapid Eye Movement and Stage 4 Non-rapid Eye Movement Sleep Stage in Humans," by D. S. Shannahoff-Khalsa et al., 2000, *Sleep Medicine*, 2, 333–346. Reprinted with permission.)

and multivariate relations help present a new perspective for Kleitman's BRAC and for diagnosing potential variants of pathopsychophysiological states (Shannahoff-Khalsa, Gillin, et al., 2001).

4. The nasal cycle is a marker for physiological states.

The inclusion of the yogic concepts of ida and pingala and the experimental studies that now support these concepts, along with the BRAC hypothesis, provides both a new perspective and a new organizing principle for structural features and temporal activities in humans and other higher vertebrates. This leads to a more comprehensive understanding of physiological states per se. While metabolic activities in the body can be viewed as a sea of rhythmic changes, the ultradian rhythms of lateralized neural (derived from the concepts of ida and pingala) activity may be viewed as a fundamental stage in the evolution of organizational development (Shannahoff-Khalsa, 1991a). The emergence of lateralized neural rhythms with evolution reflects the integration of the structural and temporal aspects of an organism's metabolic activities to enhance survival in an ever-changing environment (Shannahoff-Khalsa, 1991a). While lateralized neural rhythms are not incorporated in Kleitman's BRAC hypothesis, the BRAC concept reflects one of the most elementary requirements of any organism— expending energy and resting. Aschoff and Gerkema stated, "In considering the functional significance of ultradian rhythms, one should first keep in mind that a rhythmic organization (of whatever frequency) is one of the means to keep temporal order within the organism. Where many processes have to be maintained which to some degree are mutually exclusive, but nevertheless cooperate, a temporal compartmentalization by rhythmic alternation is an obvious solution" (1985). They concluded, "It is impossible to postulate one common mechanism for all ultradian rhythms." However, when the phenomenon of the lateralized neural rhythms of both the CNS and ANS are included, a broader perspective can be conceived for the functional significance of these numerous ultradian rhythms and a structure-function model becomes more apparent (Shannahoff-Khalsa, 1991a, 1991b; Shannahoff-Khalsa et al., 1996, 1997; Shannahoff-Khalsa & Yates, 2000; Shannahoff-Khalsa et al., 2001).

5. The hypothalamus integrates and regulates the two polar physiological states of rest and activity.

A single oscillator model for hypothalamic regulation and integration of these various rhythms has been proposed (Shannahoff-Khalsa, 1991b; Shannahoff-Khalsa et al.,1996). This model is an extended BRAC hypothesis that includes lateralized neural rhythms playing an integral role in the organization and function of this more general phenomenon. I proposed that this phenomenon has evolved as "a neural matrix for coupling mind and metabolism" (1991b). I argued that these lateralized rhythms manifest as a pendulum of ANS–CNS activity to help maintain homeostasis, "not as a single homeostatic state, but as a continuous alternation between two polar conditions for both mind and metabolism. The alternating dominance of two polar states of mind (two modes of intelligence) would be advantageous compared to a static state of cerebral activity, as alternating cerebral activity can thus accommodate different specific tasks more efficiently. This alternation can be coupled to metabolic states such as the ergotrophic and trophotropic states described by Hess, or the active and resting states of the BRAC, respectively." Hess (1954) coined the terms of *ergotrophic* and *trophotropic* to describe ANS functions. Ergotrophic reactions are "coupled with energy expenditure," and an endophylactic-trophotropic system "provides for protection and restitution." Gellhorn (1967) discussed these concepts at length in his discourses on ANS–somatic integration. The key concept here is the antagonistic relationship of the sympathetic and parasympathetic systems in maintaining balance between these two polar states.

In sum, the multivariate studies during waking and sleep show similar periodicities using spectral analysis and thus the coupling of the ANS, CNS, cardiovascular, neuroendocrine, and fuel regulatory systems under these experimental conditions provide support for Kleitman's BRAC model and argue for a physical coupling via the hypothalamus, thus also supporting the fifth yogic postulate. In addition, these results argue for support of the yogic postulate for how the activity of ida (left-nostril dominance) and pingala (right-nostril dominance) help mark physiological states. The lateral dimensions and dynamics of the ANS–CNS rhythm broadens the concept of the BRAC. In part, it can be concluded that the NC is a useful noninvasive marker for better understanding the dynamics of physiological states (Shannahoff-Khalsa et al., 1996). It has now been shown that the ultradian rhythms of pituitary hormones and catecholamine secretion, cardiovascular function, and fuel regulation are also tightly coupled to the NC. This work as a whole demonstrates a lack of autonomy for different systems and suggests that the hypothalamus plays the primary regulatory and integrative role for mind-body states. Four detailed tables are published that list the relationships of the two phases of the nasal cycle with a wide range of autonomic activities, cerebral relations, neuroendocrine relations, and behavioral relations that further help define the physiological states represented by ida and pingala dominant modes (Shannahoff-Khalsa, 1991a). Furthermore, it has been demonstrated that there are nearly identical ultradian rhythms in humans in the immune system since cytokines show periodicities ranging from 80 to 240 minutes when sampled at 20-minute intervals for 8 hours (Bouayd-Amine, Cupissol, Nougier-Soule, Bres, Gestin-Boyer, et al., 1993). Their result, which is temporally coincident with the above cited studies, suggests that the immune system is also coupled to the other major bodily systems. I stated, "Left nostril/right brain dominance is unlikely to underlie the fight-or-flight response as it appears to represent the resting state of generalized increased parasympathetic tone which is antithetical to the stress response. It is also likely that peaks of immune function, regeneration, and healing occur during the increased parasympathetic state of right brain/left nostril dominance" (Shannahoff-Khala, 1991a). Neveu (1998) reviewed how lateralized lesion studies in the neocortex of the rat can demonstrate how the two hemispheres play profoundly different roles in regulating activities of the immune system. He stated "The asymmetry in the cerebral control of immune responses should represent a phylogenetic advantage which has to be elucidated." He summarizes the effects of lateralized neocortical lesions on spleen weight, thymus weight, number of T cells, percent of helper T cells, percent of cytotoxic/suppressive T cells, antibody production, T and B lymphocyte proliferation, and natural killer cell activity. A later and more comprehensive review on cerebral lateralization and immunity has been published (Meador, Loring, Ray, Helman, Vazquez, & Neveu, 2004). These lateralized differences in immunomodulation suggest that cerebral rhythms also play an important role in the health and homeostasis of immunity (Shannahoff-Khalsa, 1991a). Our understanding of psychoneuroimmunology may be increased by considering how the ANS acts as a neural matrix for coupling mind and immunity. I stated that "Different stressors may play key roles in how the pendulum of CNS–ANS activity affects immune functions. Over-stimulation or abnormal activity of one hemisphere may over- or underactivate different immune functions. It is even possible that a selective stimulation of one side of the brain may have beneficial effects on specific immune disorders" (1991a). In fact, a left-nostril-specific yogic breathing technique has been published that is claimed to be effective for enhancing antiviral and antibiotic activity (Shannahoff-Khalsa, 2001). It has been predicted that if these subsystems diverge from a "dynamic equilibrium" with each other, a new and fascinating basis for studying disease states may arise (Shannahoff-Khalsa et al., 1997). Indeed, according to yogic teachings on physiology, the balance of ida and pingala plays a vital role in health and disease.

6. Unilateral forced nostril breathing stimulates the contralateral cerebral hemisphere and ipsilateral sympathetic nervous system.

The sixth yogic postulate states that forcing air through one nostril selectively stimulates the contralateral cerebral hemisphere and the ipsilateral branch of the sympathetic nervous system. This technique entails more than a simple passive redirection of airflow using a plug, and requires that the inspiration and expiration are made with various degrees of intensity. The first example of using unilateral forced nostril breathing (UFNB) to selectively stimulate the contralateral hemisphere was demonstrated in young naïve healthy subjects using EEG (Werntz et al., 1981, 1983; Werntz, Bickford, Shannahoff-Khalsa, 1987). This study involved a continuous measurement of EEG activity in the two cerebral hemispheres using a variety of homologous electrode sites to compare left and right power. Subjects were asked to force breathe through the more congested nostril for 11 to 20 minutes followed by one, two, or more periods, alternating sides throughout the experiment (Werntz et al., 1987). Figure 1.11 shows the results from one subject with six complete periods of UFNB and it is clear how the EEG power drifts toward the contralateral hemisphere regardless of the endogenous phase of the nasal cycle. This phenomenon was observed in five out of five untrained subjects. "These results suggest the possibility of a non-invasive approach in the treatment of states of psychopathology where lateralized cerebral dysfunction have been shown to occur" (Werntz et al., 1987).

One study suggested that the electrographic activity generated by nasal (versus oral) breathing is produced by a neural mechanism in the superior nasal meatus (Kristof, Servit, & Manas, 1981). This activating effect could also be produced by air insufflation into the upper nasal cavity without inflating the lung. Local anesthesia of the mucosal membrane suppressed the cortical effects of airflow stimulation. Another study showed how deep breathing through one nostril could activate abnormalities in epileptic patients with unilateral focal or lateralized paroxysmal abnormalities in the fronto- or occipitotemporal region. "The abnormalities of this type were significantly more activated from the ipsilateral nasal cavity" (Servit et al., 1981). However, these paroxysmal abnormalities were also generated with contralateral breathing to the foci in 60% of the patients. These paroxysmal abnormalities are not equivalent

Figure 1.11

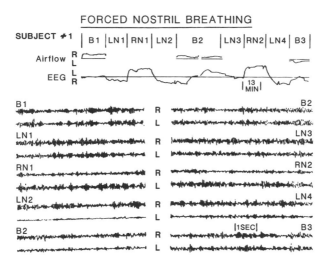

Figure 1.11. Effect of unilateral forced breathing on EEG asymmetry. Subject 1, trial 2. Top: "Airflow" tracing: points above the baseline indicate greater right-nostril airflow and points below indicate greater left-nostril airflow. Periods of forced nostril breathing are indicated. "EEG" tracing points above the baseline indicate relatively greater left-hemisphere EEG amplitude, points below relatively greater right-hemisphere amplitude. B = baseline. LN = left-nostril breathing. RN = right-nostril breathing. Montage, (02-P4:01-P3). Bottom: Representative segments of the primary EEG that were integrated and subtracted to produce the tracings in the top section. For each pair, the top tracing is from the right hemisphere and the bottom is from the left hemisphere. (From "Selective Hemispheric Stimulation by Unilateral Forced Nostril Breathing," by Werntz et al., 1987, *Human Neurobiology*, 6(3), 165–71. Reprinted with permission.)

to the sustained contralateral increases in EEG power that were produced in the UFNB studies cited above (Werntz et al., 1981, 1983, 1987), since this paroxysmal activity manifests only as intermittent spikes in a small fraction of the record with epileptic patients. However, it is an example of how lateralized EEG activity can be affected by unilateral nasal airflow.

The contralateral increase in relatively greater EEG power as a marker of greater or lesser mental activity was controversial. The yogic postulate states that UFNB activates the contralateral hemisphere and would result in an increase of cognitive performance efficiency in that hemisphere. One study (Klein, Pilon, Prosser, & Shannahoff-Khalsa, 1986) showed under resting conditions that right nasal dominance is coupled to relatively greater verbal performance, or left-brain activity, and left-nasal dominance is coupled with relatively greater spatial or right-hemispheric skills. This study, however, was not successful at demonstrating the effects of UFNB on changes in cognition, possibly due to the experimental design. Their comparison cognitive task testing was post-UFNB rather than during the active breathing. However, two later studies (Shannahoff-Khalsa, Boyle, & Buebel, 1991; Jella & Shannahoff-Khalsa, 1993) using 30 minutes of UFNB showed that right UFNB increased left-hemispheric cognitive performance and that left UFNB increased right-hemispheric performance, as predicted. Both of these studies employed UFNB prior to and during task assessment. The study by Klein et al. (1986) also used tasks that may not have been as well lateralized and some of their data included breathing-exercise periods of only 15 minutes.

A pilot study used whole-head 148 channel magnetoencephalography (MEG) to explore the effects of left and right UFNB at one breath per minute using the pattern with the four respective phases of 15 seconds slow inspiration, 15 seconds breath retention, 15 seconds slow expiration, and 15 seconds breath hold out phase for 31 consecutive minutes. This study showed differential hemispheric effects (Baglio, Bucolo, Fortuna, Frasca, La Rosa & Shannahoff-Khalsa, 2002). The left-nostril version of this specific four-phase pattern was found by yogis to be effective for treating OCD (see Chapter 2), and the technique is referred to here as the OCD breath (OCDB).

Preliminary MEG brain imaging results of the OCDB technique and the right nostril correlate at one breath per minute for 31 minutes are presented in color figures C.1 through C5. C.1 shows the effects of the left and right nostril patterns for the gamma band power (34 Hz to 50 Hz) averaged per channel over the respective recording periods using an adjusted energy scale for comparing the three respective plots per experiment. The same subject was employed in both experiments. In the three panels on the right, 31 minutes of the OCDB exercise (left-UFNB) (middle plot) is compared to 10 minutes of pre-exercise rest (top plot) and 10 minutes post-exercise rest (bottom plot). The same rest-exercise-rest sequence is presented on the left side of the figure, using the right nostril instead of the left, again using the one-breath-per-minute pattern of 15 seconds inhalation, 15 seconds breath retention, 15 seconds exhalation, and 15 seconds breath held out, for 31 consecutive minutes. Compared to rest phase 1, the left-nostril breathing pattern clearly activates greater right-frontal hemispheric activity. The reverse is observed for the right-nostril pattern. In addition, both breath patterns produce a greater bilateral and diffused hemispheric activation in the rest 2 phase. However, in rest 2 there is substantially greater bilateral activation using the right-nostril breathing pattern. This is consistent with the yogic view that right-nostril breathing is more "stimulating" compared to the left. This work is a preliminary result from a collaboration of the author with a group at the University of Catania, Sicily (La Rosa, Bucolo, Frasca, Fortuna, & Shannahoff-Khalsa).

In Figures C.2 through C.5, during the 10-minute rest 2 phase of the study, the channels with the top 20% of the power were identified and arrows are drawn from the respective channels to the channel site in the respective hemisphere. It is clear in C.2 that during total MEG power (0.1 Hz to 54 Hz) the majority of channels with the greatest energy are contralateral to the activated nostril. C.3 shows this to be the case for the delta frequency band (0.1 Hz to 4.0 Hz), C.4 shows it for the beta frequency band (12 Hz to 16 Hz), and C.5 shows it for the gamma frequency band (34 Hz to 54 Hz). The results were the same for the theta frequency band (4 Hz to 8 Hz) and also the alpha frequency band (8 Hz to 12 Hz). All frequencies showed a pattern of greater contralateral

MEG power activation with UNFB at one breath per minute in the rest 2 phase of the study. The same results were observed in multiple recording sessions with the same subject over a period of three months (Sapuppo, Umana, Frasca, La Rosa, Shannahoff-Khalsa, Fortuna, & Bucolo, 2006). These results further support the contralateral activation patterns observed with the EEG and cognitive performance efficiency using UFNB. However, the MEG results provide a greater insight to the location of activation.

The interpretation of the expected functional relationships based on the lack of crossover by autonomic fibers (Saper, Loewy, Swanson, & Lowan, 1976) coincides with the yogic interpretations. It appears that nasal airflow may stimulate sympathetic dominance on the homolateral (ipsilateral) body-brain half. Therefore, it is possible that direct stimulation of one-half of the cortex may occur by sympathetic stimulation and thus result in vasoconstriction. And it is likely that increased parasympathetic activation may occur simultaneously in the contralateral hemisphere to compensate for the contralateral sympathetic activation, thus helping to maintain adequate cerebral perfusion in the brain in total (Shannahoff-Khalsa, 2001). For an extensive review of all other studies on UFNB, see Appendix 2, page 320.

Defining States of Consciousness:
The Concepts of the Chakra System

Perhaps the most controversial topic in science today is that of the nature of consciousness. There are two core questions that are central to the arguments on the nature of consciousness. Does consciousness transcend time and space? Is consciousness only an epiphenomenon of the brain? A recent review on the psychobiology of "altered states of consciousness" concludes that these states "have tended to defy systematic elucidation" (Vaitl, Birbaumer, Gruzelier, Jamieson, Kotchoubey, et al., 2005). Clearly, even the definition of *consciousness* is controversial.

Ages ago, yogis devised a practical and systematic view of consciousness that involves eight discrete levels. Each level is related to what yogis call *chakras*, repositories or centers of psychic energy, and an individual's consciousness is then determined and affected by the amount of energy and activity in these eight centers. Each chakra or center is both symbolic for and instrumental in determining the mode of behavior, personality structure, and level of awareness. Chakras are not related to the gross, or physical body alone, but are mainly situated in the subtle, or *etheric*, bodies. The intensity of activity in any one chakra imparts an effect that reflects a world perspective, understanding of cause and effect, and source of motivation and desire that is unique to each center.

The consciousness of an individual who lives mainly in the **first chakra** is concerned primarily with survival. His or her actions and values are based solely on the need to survive. Fears and paranoia coincide with this center, as do instincts, concerns about elimination, destructive sexual activities, and habitual and addictive activities. Blocks and imbalances here can lead to a rigid and stubborn mentality and a range of diseases. The **second chakra** reflects mentality directed mainly toward reproduction and sexual activities. Overactivity here leads to sexual neuroses, whether it is in the form of abnormal sexual indulgence or that of a puritanical mentality. A balanced second chakra helps establish a creative and expressive mentality. The **third chakra** is the center of power, territory, and ego; the "me" mentality prevails to the exclusion of the well-being of others. This center is the source of physical well-being and when it is weak it leads to a wide range of illnesses and a weak character, drive, and willpower. The first three levels of consciousness are the nature of the beast and prevail throughout the animal kingdom; they are not unique to the human. And indeed much of society's ills are the result of an imbalance in the first three chakras.

The biggest step in human development is from the third level of consciousness to the fourth. The **fourth chakra**, the heart center, embraces the human element of compassion, the attitude to nurture and give without consideration of the cost to one's self. This center is considered to be the first level of *higher consciousness*, where the human can experience a true expansion in awareness. Love is born through activity in this center. When the heart chakra is not awakened, greed, selfishness, and ego dominate. The **fifth chakra** is the center for creative communication through expression. When this center is active, the individual can speak and live a blunt truth; when it is blocked, that person will feel stifled and unable to be direct and truthful with others. A quality of higher consciousness that manifests with this center is that of clairaudient awareness. The **sixth chakra** allows for both sides of the coin to be seen and the dual nature of life to be understood beyond the polarity of right and wrong. This center is responsible for intuition and clairvoyant abilities. Supernatural abilities are also said to be governed by this center. The **seventh chakra** is the center for pure thoughts and saintly intelligence, where actions are based on concern for the highest good for all. This center is called the "thousand-petalled lotus" and is the seat of universal consciousness, the doorway through which one experiences the connectedness of all. The **eighth chakra** is the aura, and how it functions is representative of the relationship of all other chakras. This chakra acts both as a shield and source of attraction for events in our lives. This center can act as a guard against illness and calamity. Awareness in this center takes one's consciousness beyond the realm of time and space into the realm where past, present, and futures merge. It is said that if an individual lives in the consciousness of this center too long, the world will pass him by.

Each chakra, or energy center, also has a physiological correlate in the body. The first chakra is related to the area of the rectum (sacro-coccygeal plexus); the second chakra is related to the sex organs (sacral plexus); the third chakra is related to the navel point region (solar plexus); the fourth chakra is the *heart center* (cardiac plexus); the fifth chakra is related to the thyroid and parathyroid, or *throat center* (laryngeal plexus); the sixth chakra is related to the activity of the pituitary gland and is called the *third eye*; the seventh chakra is related to the pineal gland and cerebral cortex and is called the *crown center*; and the eighth chakra is the *aura*, or the psychoelectromagnetic field that surrounds the body.

The fully awakened yogi has the ability to consciously activate any and all chakras, and to choose the appropriate combination of chakra activities that can lead to the most effective outcome under any given situation. However, every individual has one chakra that predominates to establish his or her personality, and over time this center may change as a personality matures. All chakras are equally important. There are many meditation techniques in Kundalini yoga that are specific for activating one chakra and correcting an imbalance. Many diseases also result from an imbalance in one or more centers. There are also meditation techniques that work on multiple chakras and some that work to awaken and heal all chakras simultaneously.

Female Rhythms of the 11 Erogenous Centers That Influence the Psyche

One topic of study of the ancient yogis communicated by Yogi Bhajan involves a rhythm of activity in the 11 erogenous centers or zones (Bhajan, 1982). This phenomenon pertains exclusively to women. Yogis called these 11 centers *moon centers*, and each center is coupled with a specific psychological and emotional correlate that predominates when that center is the most active center. The 11 centers are the frontal hairline, eyebrows, pink of the cheeks, earlobes, lips, back of the neck, breasts, navel region or corresponding area on the back, clitoris, vagina, and inner thighs. There is also a sequence where each center dominates for two and a half days for a total cycle length of 28 days and then the same entire sequence repeats. The sequence can differ in each woman and the cycle remains the same throughout life unless there is a major emotional shock that can then alter the sequence. According to Yogi Bhajan, the psychological and emotional correlates of the respective centers are the following: (1) Hairline: "The woman is most stable and nothing can move her an inch, she is most real." The frontal hairline also relates to what yogis call the *arcline* or *halo region* of the aura. (2) Eyebrows: the woman is "most imaginative, illusionary and builds sand castles." (3) Cheeks: "When it is around the pink of the cheeks the woman is absolutely almost out of control, this is a dangerous time," a time that is similar in mood to a woman's premenstrual syndrome. (4) Earlobes: "She discusses values" and is more self-reflective. (5) Lips: "Communication is either excellent or troubled," and much here depends on her diet. (6) Back of the neck: "You want to communicate on a very romantic frequency, this is such a foolish time that one little flower or little gesture can make you go nuts." (7) Breasts: "When it is around your breasts you are compassionate and giving to the extent of foolishness." (8) Navel region or corresponding area on the spine: "You are most insecure." (9) Clitoris and (10) vagina: "You are eager to socialize, talk, meet; basically you are very external; your extracurricular activity is very charming." (11) Inner thighs: "You are very confirmative, you want to confirm everything" (1982).

Clearly, this proposed phenomenon is highly complex, and the moods that supposedly dominate with the respective moon centers would pose a challenge to study in the laboratory because the individual rhythmic sequence in women no doubt varies widely. The level of subtlety required here in awareness would also pose a challenge to verify this phenomenon.

In men, a weekly cycle, called the 30/70 cycle, is perhaps the closest correlate to the 11-center cycle exclusive to women. According to Yogi Bhajan, "In one week you are 30% up, in another week you are 70% up. It is called the projection of the sun. Sometimes it flames over and sometimes it flames under. It is always there and it is on a weekly basis. It changes week to week. In one week there are certain things you want to do. In one week you want to eat something. In one week you want to go out. In one week you want to do everything, and the next week, in the same environments, you don't want to do anything. On a certain week you promise everything on the phone. The next week you say 'nay' to all those things which last week you promised. That is called the sun caliber, 30/70. Most of the things you admit before a woman, you do when you are on a 30% rhythm. She can get anything out of you. When you are on a 70% rhythm, she will try a lot but you are the king and there is nobody else. On the 30% rhythm, forget it, you are nobody" (1982). Perhaps the "30/70 sun caliber rhythm" is the easiest to study and verify. Whether we consider it folklore or truth, in the West, there is clearly the conception that the woman is far more complex in nature than the man. The 11-center cycle in women and the 30/70 sun caliber rhythm in men present us with fascinating concepts for future study.

The 81 Facets of the Mind

Yogi Bhajan has proposed an elaborate model describing the complexity of the mind (Bhajan & Khalsa, 1998a). This model first assumes an undifferentiated, formless *universal consciousness*, what yogis also call the *universal mind*, or *cosmic consciousness*, or *chitta* in Sanskrit. This universal, undifferentiated mind manifests itself through the properties of the three *gunas* called *sattva*, *rajas*, and *tamas*, which each represent separate qualities of the so-called primary awareness or universal cosmic consciousness. The qualities of the sattva guna are purity, neutrality, and clarity. The qualities of the rajas guna are activity, rapid transformation, and fiery change. The qualities of the tamas guna are heavy, slow, habitual, and impurity. The gunas are the foundation of a differentiation that lends qualities to the a material realm. When the universal mind is first differentiated by the three gunas, the result gives rise to the three "impersonal minds" called *manas*, *ahangkar*, and *buddhi*. Manas recognizes, records, and creates sequences. Ahangkar establishes boundaries and categories and contains data and labels. Buddhi discerns values and reality. These three impersonal minds each influence the individual human mind, which has three "functional minds" called the *negative mind, positive mind*, and *neutral mind*. The negative mind is always the first to react and it gauges the danger and potential harm in any given situation and thus plays a protective role. The positive mind searches for pleasure and sees the good in any given situation; it is constructive. The neutral mind is intuitive and it balances the input of both the negative mind and positive mind to produce the "big picture." When the neutral mind engages, it is objective and neutral and helps put actions into perspective to achieve a higher and just goal. The negative, positive, and neutral minds each have three *aspects* as a result of the influence of the three impersonal minds (manas, ahangkar, and buddhi). The influence of manas, ahangkar, and buddhi on the negative mind leads to the three aspects described as the *defender*, the *manager*, and the *preserver*, respectively. The same three influences on the positive mind lead to the *artist*, the *producer*, and the *missionary*, and the three influences on the neutral mind lead to the *strategist*, the *leader*, and the *teacher*.

At this level of complexity, there are nine characters or aspects of the mind. Each of these nine aspects are then influenced by one of the impersonal minds combined with either the negative, positive, or neutral mind, thus leading to 27 divisions of mind. The impact of the negative mind and manas on the defender informs how one deals with a threat, which gives birth to the *soldier*. The impact of the positive mind and manas on the defender informs how one deals with an accident, which gives birth to the *ombudsman*. The impact of the neutral mind and manas on the defender is how one deals with a coincidence, which gives birth to the *prospector*. The impact of the three functional minds and ahangkar on the manager leads to the relay of a past memory, which gives birth to the *historian*, the phase of mental projection, which gives birth to the *chameleon*, and the shadow of a mental projection, which gives birth to the *judge*. Finally, the effects of buddhi and the three functional minds on the preserver lead to the deep memory of a past projection (the *runner*), the mental intersection (the *integrator*), and the mental outer projection (the *apostle*). The influence of manas and the three functional minds on the artist respectively leads to the art of memorizing creativity (the *actor*), the art of creating art (the *doer*), and the art of creating creativity (the *originator*). The influence of ahangkar and the three functional minds on the producer leads to creating art through past memory (the *gourmet*), creating art through environmental effects (the *architect*), and creating art by projecting into the future (the *entrepreneur*). The influence of buddhi and the three functional minds on the missionary are, respectively, pursuing the cycle of success (the *devotee*), pursuing the cycle of artistic attributes (the *enthusiast*), and pursuing the art of cohesiveness (the *creator*). The influence of manas and the three functional minds on the strategist are, respectively, judging environments through the senses (the *scout*), judging environments (the *coach*), judging positive environments through intuition (the *guide*). The influence of ahangkar and the three functional minds on the leader are the assessment of the position (the *protector*), the assessment of the successful (the *commander*), and the assessment of personality and facets through intuition (the *pathfinder*). The influence of buddhi and the three functional minds on the teacher are the intuitive assessment of personality defects to be covered (the *educator*), the interpretations of all facets of life (the *expert*), and the assessment of personality of overlords and their projections to be controlled (the *master*).

These lead to 27 *projections* of the mind, and each of these 27 projections is again influenced by the three functional minds (negative, positive, neutral) to yield, for example, the *negative soldier*, the *positive soldier*, and the *neutral soldier*, and so on. So we then have three possible facets for each projection or personality type, leading finally to 81 total facets of the mind. This scheme is somewhat daunting and takes some study. However, the model is clearly unique, highly structured, practical, and may prove to have definite merit as an accurate rendition of the human mind. The 27 projections range from the soldier personality to the master personality, with the latter representing the highest evolved state of mind, according to this model.

The Tattvas or Five Elements
(Earth, Water, Fire, Air, and Ether)

In yogic healing, one ultimately learns to gain control over the *tattvas*, or *five elements*—earth, water, fire, air, and ether. While these terms appear to the Western scientific mind as naïve concepts for understanding nature, the five elements are in fact a classification scheme based on perceptions of experience within one's own consciousness, and can be used in a range of healing modalities in which the practitioner becomes aware of the workings of the five elements within his own consciousness. In this regard, a healer has an experience within his own awareness or conscious space just as if he were having an experience of the five senses. So, the experience of an element is as much a sensory experience for a trained healer as vision, hearing, taste, touch, and smell are for others. A healer may experience that an element is out of balance in a patient. This obviously presumes that fields of consciousness are contiguous. For example, a person who has experienced a traumatic event may not be fully "in his body" and present with symptoms of dissociation. In addition, this person may frequently bump into things because he is not body aware or may have difficulty following what's going on in a conversation or other activities. In part, the diagnosis is a lack of the earth element, which instills the property of being grounded. While this behavior will be apparent to the Western therapist, the approach of the yogic healer for treatment will differ. He will employ techniques that help to increase the earth element to bring the patient into balance. With another patient who feels stuck in life and is overly rigid and unwilling to change, the healer may sense the patient has too much earth, detecting this through feelings within his consciousness of being heavy and dense. Either the lack, or excess of the earth element, or any of the other four elements, reduces a person's ability to deal with life. Therefore, one agenda in yoga is to balance the five elements.

The elements also have relationships to each chakra. The first chakra relates to the earth element. The water element is experienced as flow, or lack of flow, and may manifest in a person's creativity, related to the second chakra. For example, a writer suffering from writer's block may manifest an imbalance in the water element, experienced as a lack of flow in the energy of the second chakra, and with proper treatment creativity may be restored. Fire, the element that rules the third chakra, may show up in the consciousness of the healer as excess heat or light. Air or wind, ruler of the heart chakra, may be experienced as a breeze on the skin, and the lack of it as stillness. Excess ether, ruler of the fifth chakra, produces dreaminess in the conscious space of the healer. Ether is also related to communication, which may be experienced as blocks in the throat chakra by the healer. This may appear when the healer is working on a patient who was raised as a child "to be seen and not heard," thus stifling his or her expression through speech.

While this approach to healing has great merit, it is complex and requires extensive training. The development of this unique sensitivity can lead to a useful approach to working with patients. This approach requires less formal verbal input and response from the patient, and so the diagnosis is much less dependent on information relayed by the patient. In addition, the wide range of yogic techniques known for affecting the balance of the elements can be more easily and specifically prescribed.

In addition to the chakras, the elements are also related to the fingers, brain regions, and the planets, as well as other aspects of nature. In respect to the fingers, the thumb is related to the earth element, which helps define one's ego nature, and its primitive mentality is related to the brainstem. The index finger is related to water, which relates to brain regions involving knowledge and awareness. The middle finger relates to fire and the personality qualities of patience and temperament. The ring finger relates to air and one's vitality and strength. And the little finger relates to the ether element and to the frontal cortex controlling communication and executive functions. A variety of meditation techniques employ the use of the fingers to help bring a balance to the elements and thus the personality. In addition, earth, water, fire, air, and ether are related to qualities of the respective planets Earth, Jupiter, Saturn, Sun, and Mercury.

These relationships help to define another view of our interconnectedness through fingers, brain regions, chakras, and aspects of our personalities. In addition, these schemas help to define a broader relationship between ourselves and the macrocosm. While these supposed relationships may challenge the Western gestalt, they may help to explain how and why some of the Kundalini yoga meditation techniques work.

A Basic Physical Mechanism That Helps to Explain How Mantras Work

Mantras are fundamental tools in yogic technology for altering the psyche, and they are used in some of the meditation techniques described in this book. However, the mystical properties of mantras that are claimed to help heal the psyche, lead to elevated states of consciousness, transcendence, or non-ordinary realms of reality, clearly present us with the question about *how* they work. One concept of the mechanism of their effects was communicated by Yogi Bhajan in the 1970s (Shannahoff-Khalsa & Bhajan, 1988, 1991; Shannahoff-Khalsa, 1996). This concept is portrayed in Figure 1.12 with a diagram of the upper palate and its 84 meridian points. It was believed that this map of 84 points (2 points located by each of the 16 teeth on the upper palate, 2 rows of 25 points along the center, and 2 points in the very center) explained, in part, the basic physical mechanism for how sounds have various effects

Figure 1.12

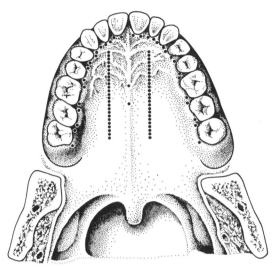

Figure 1.12. The 84 Meridian Point System: The Mechanistic Basis for Mantras
Note that next to each tooth on the upper palate are 2 points, 32 points along the perimeter, 25 points in each of 2 parallel rows, a single central point that relates to the anterior fontanel, and another point that relates to the posterior fontanel. There are 84 points total. (© Shannahoff-Khalsa, 1991; Shannahoff-Khalsa & Bhajan, 1991.)

on the psyche. The idea is that the tongue, through both the tip and broader areas, interacts with the upper palate in a discrete and specific way, imparting a series of stimulations in which different sounds act like codes for an array of points the tongue touches, much like how fingers interact with a keyboard. The sequential and repetitious stimulation of these points then transmits effects to higher brain centers through the hypothalamus and thalamus (Shannahoff-Khalsa & Bhajan, 1988).

Besides the various sacred mantras and how they effect the five elements, each language also relates primarily to one (and sometimes more) of the elements (Shannahoff-Khalsa & Bhajan, 1988). For example, supposedly French is a water language, German a fire language, and Dutch mostly air. Some ancient languages, particularly Sanskrit, Gurmukhi, and Japanese (before mixing with Chinese) were specifically constructed and coded with this understanding by those who mastered Nad yoga, the yoga of sound. And in these coded languages, both the meaning and effect on the psyche were the same. For example, mother: *ma*, "resurrection," and *dar*, "gate" or "door," together make "gate of resurrection" or "door of rebirth." *Man* is "mind," and *woman* is "wo," an expression of wonder, plus *man*, together relating to the female in her totality and meaning "great mind." This indicates an awareness of the elevated woman in her full capacity. Human: *hu* is "light" and *man* is "mind." Therefore, *human* means the "being with the mind of light." The word *guru* is made up of two sounds, *gu* and *ru*. *Gu* means "darkness" and *ru* means "light." Therefore, *guru* means the technique that takes one from the darkness into the light. Many words have meaning and an impact on the psyche that we do not understand. The ancient yogis discovered the code for which sounds are elevating and healing.

People of different nationalities pronounce certain vowels and consonants in a similar but slightly different way. The way the Dutch pronounce "sa ta na ma," for example, is different from the way Americans pronounce the same sounds. The Dutch *t* is like the Punjabi *t* and is pronounced with the tongue farther forward in the mouth than it is with the American *t*. When speaking languages, these differences have different effects. But when one learns to use sounds in meditation, the tongue adjusts to the correct position after repetition, eventually touching the correct meridian points with a universal effect on everyone. Even dialects have different effects. There are many that believe that the personalities of people from various nations and regions differ, and in part, if this is true, it may be that their respective languages help lead to these differences.

Therefore, the tongue supposedly plays a key role in the development of the psyche. In addition, Yogi Bhajan taught that the placement of the tongue can help lead to the experience of each of the five elements in a unique way. If the tongue is resting solely

148 Channel MEG–Power in the Gamma Band (34–50 Hz)

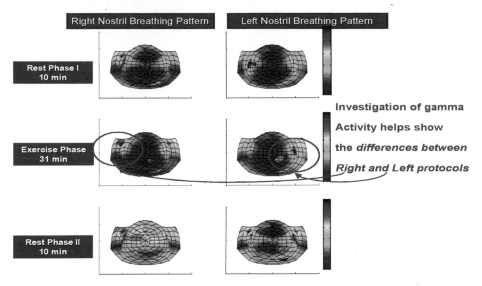

Figure C.1. Gamma band (34 Hz–50 Hz) activity is presented for whole-head MEG power. Comparatively increased power is induced during the exercise period in the frontal and prefrontal areas of the contralateral hemisphere. Greater overall diffused hemispheric power is observed with both left- and right-nostril breathing patterns in the rest 2 phase of the study compared to rest 1 and the exercise phase.

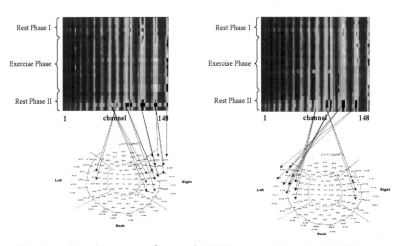

Figure C.2. Broadband response for total MEG power (0.1 Hz–54 Hz) is presented in channel-space. Channels within 20% of maximum power in the post-exercise rest period are mapped with arrows to their spatial locations in the lower part of the figure. Note here that the left-nostril breathing pattern is presented on the left side of the figure and the right-nostril breathing pattern is presented here on the right side of the figure. C.2 demonstrates the contralateral activation patterns for either the left- or right-nostril breathing patterns for total energy power.

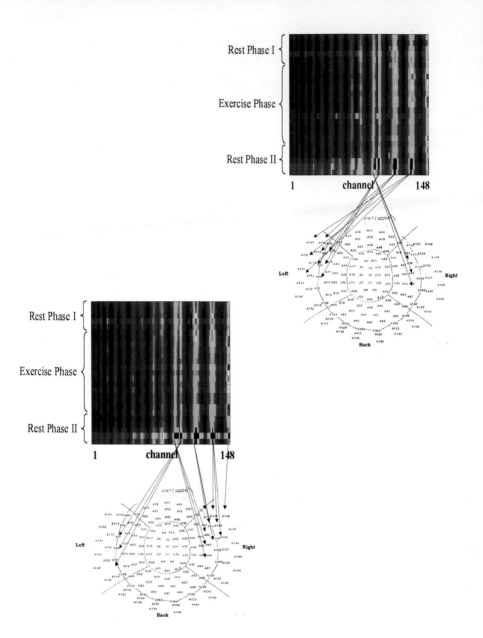

Figure C.3. Delta band (0.1 Hz–4 Hz) MEG power is presented in channel-space. Channels within 20% of maximum power in the post-exercise rest period are mapped with arrows to their spatial locations in the lower part of the figure. The left-nostril breathing pattern is presented on the left side of the figure and the right-nostril breathing pattern is presented here on the right side of the figure. Note the contralateral activation patterns for either the left- or right-nostril breathing patterns for the delta frequency band.

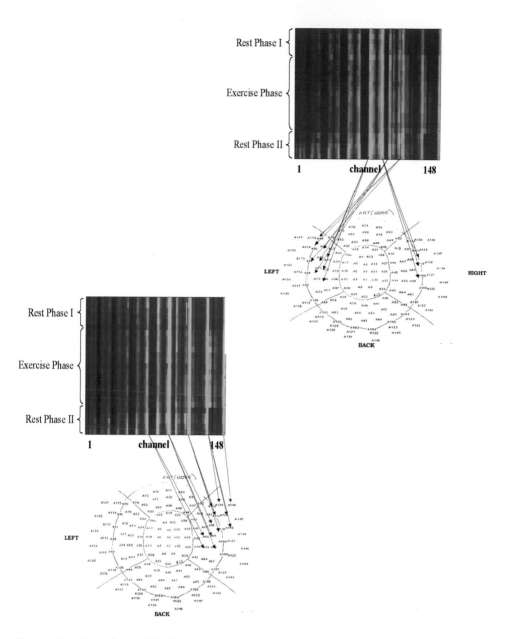

Figure C.4. Beta band (12 Hz–16 Hz) MEG power is presented in channel-space. Channels within 20% of maximum power in the post-exercise rest period are mapped with arrows to their spatial locations in the lower part of the figure. The left-nostril breathing pattern is presented on the left side of the figure and the right-nostril breathing pattern is presented here on the right side of the figure. Note the contralateral activation patterns for either the left- or right-nostril breathing patterns for the beta frequency band.

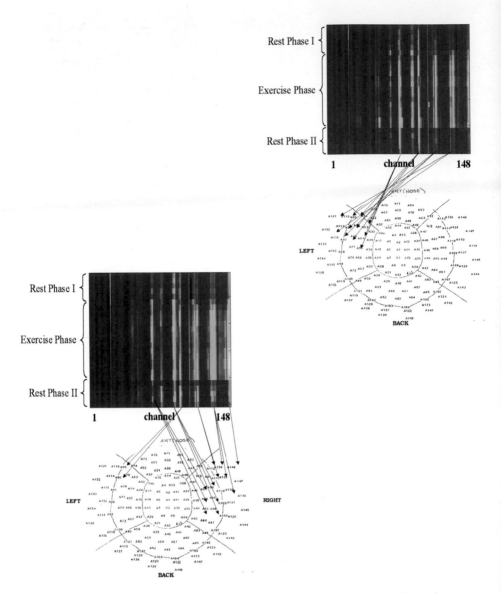

Figure C.5. Gamma band (35 Hz–54 Hz) MEG power is presented in channel-space. Channels within 20% of maximum power in the post-exercise rest period are mapped with arrows to their spatial locations in the lower part of the figure. The left-nostril breathing pattern is presented on the left side of the figure and the right-nostril breathing pattern is presented here on the right side of the figure. Note the contralateral activation patterns for either the left- or right-nostril breathing patterns for the gamma frequency band.

on the lower palate without touching the front teeth, it will help lead to the experience of the earth element. If the tongue tip is placed on the roof of the mouth, back behind the hard palate in the area leading to the throat, this position can help induce the experience of the water element. When the tongue tip is placed on the roof of the mouth, this position helps induce the experience of the fire element. When the tongue tip is placed on the upper palate and touching the back of the front teeth, this relates to the air element. Finally, the experience of the ether element can be induced when the tongue tip is placed under the upper lip touching the front of the front teeth. These tongue postures can be used to develop sensitivity to the five elements or tattvas.

In sum, in addition to all the Western knowledge about the psychology of the human, we are now faced with the possibility of incorporating the phenomena of the 2- to 3-hour cerebral rhythm that influences mood, emotions, modes of intelligence, and the efficiency of mental performance; the chakra system, which is relatively stable over time for defining states of consciousness and personality structure; the 2.5-day female rhythm that varies with the 11 moon centers and its weekly male correlate that effects the psyche; the 81 facets of the mind, providing a highly detailed conceptual framework of an individual's mental and personality structure that is also relatively stable over time; and the concepts of the elements for understanding personalities and disease states, another relatively stable factor. These phenomena offer a whole new framework for understanding ourselves and our patients. Where can it lead? Can a therapist compute in therapy "my patient is currently left-nostril dominant, but exhibits tendencies of an overactive second chakra that reflect his/her unusual and highly destructive promiscuous sexual behavior"? If in the case of a woman client, can the therapist determine that her moon cycle may now be dominant in the clitoral/vagina zone; she by nature has all the qualities of a "pathfinder"; and her fire element is also excessive? What would a therapist do in this case? A good starting point is the "Gan Puttee Kriya" technique, which will help the patient to balance out all of her chakras and elements. In addition, this patient could be taught the "Jupiter-Saturn" meditation technique for depression (Chapter 3), as it will help her reduce and eliminate her self-destructive behavior and gain patience and a refined temperament. Clearly, we are faced here with new challenges and opportunities in therapy. The following chapters help to guide the therapist by describing highly effective protocols for many different disorders and conditions, and single techniques for specific conditions.

PART TWO

TREATING PSYCHIATRIC DISORDERS

TWO

Treating the Anxiety Disorders

As a group, the anxiety disorders are the most common of all psychiatric and other medical disorders (APA, 1994). This group includes phobias, the most common anxiety disorder, with variants exceeding more than 500 in number; panic disorder; obsessive compulsive disorder (OCD); posttraumatic stress disorder (PTSD); generalized anxiety disorder (GAD); and acute stress disorder (ASD) (APA, 1994). This chapter gives a brief explanation and facts about each disorder and its prevalence rate, then describes one or more specific meditation techniques or a specific protocol for each disorder, as well as case histories of treatment. In the section for OCD, readers might also like to refer to Appendix Three, which contains a description of two published peer-reviewed clinical trials that employed an 11-part Kundalini yoga meditation protocol that also includes specific techniques for treating fear and anger, turning negative thoughts into positive thoughts, and meeting mental challenges, which of course have utility with other disorders. All of these disorders can range in severity from only "being persistently and excessively anxious," as with GAD, to the sheer acute terror that is the hallmark of a panic attack and often occurs with PTSD and OCD.

In this chapter, only the most appropriate formulas for treatment are provided. All of the formulas outlined here can be practiced by anyone to help prevent these and related disorders after a traumatic event, and each can lead to significant improvements in wellness, mental health, mental performance, and mental competence for those who are not afflicted by a specific disorder. From the yogic point of view, there is no upper limit on what can be achieved in respect to mental clarity and mental stability. While PTSD is an anxiety disorder, this condition will be addressed in Chapter 8 ("Treating the Abused and Battered Psyche"), since PTSD is more prevalent with those who have been battered, abused, or traumatized.

Treating Obsessive Compulsive Disorder and Obsessive Compulsive Spectrum Disorders

While OCD and the obsessive compulsive (OC) spectrum disorders are not the most common of the anxiety disorders, this chapter will first address these disorders because there are now two published clinical trials testing Kundalini yoga meditation techniques (Shannahoff-Khalsa & Beckett, 1996; Shannahoff-Khalsa, Ray, Levine, Gallen, Schwartz & Sidorowich, 1999) that demonstrate high success rates with "perhaps the most disabling of the anxiety disorders" (Rapoport, 1990). These results help set a precedent for testing the efficacy of meditation techniques with other psychiatric disorders (see Appendix Three).

OCD has a lifetime prevalence rate of 2.5% to 5% in the United States, and is estimated to be the fourth most common psychiatric disorder following phobias, substance-abuse disorders, and the major depressive disorders (Rasmussen & Eisen, 1990). OCD is prevalent throughout all cultures and is understood to be a chronic and lifelong illness. It is now known to be the tenth most disabling disorder worldwide, according to the World Health Organization (Murray & Lopez, 1996b). OCD is marked by the waxing and waning of recurrent and persistent obsessions that occur in the form of thoughts, ideas, impulses, or images that are all unpleasant, negative, disruptive, and senseless. These recurrent obsessions are then almost always followed by a compulsive urge to perform stereotypical behaviors or rituals according to rules that the person makes up. The person believes that by performing his rituals, the feared obsession can be avoided. The rules for performing the rituals are always rigid and time-consuming. However, the rituals only temporarily abate some of the lingering anxiety that emerges during the obsession(s). Rituals do not prevent the fears from reemerging, as these fears are always lurking like the grim-reaper of death not far from the forefront of the mind. The official psychiatric definition of OCD states: "The obsessions and compulsions cause marked distress, are time-consuming (take more than an hour a day), or significantly interfere with the person's normal routine, occupational functioning, or usual social activities or relationships with others" (APA, 1994). The qualifying terms here are "more than an hour a day" or "significantly interfere."

Both children and adults can develop OCD. The manifestations are the same for all ages and the symptoms have been observed in children as early as age two. While it seems to start earlier in boys, the numbers of the sexes are eventually equal. The mean age of the onset for males is 17.5 years and 20.8 years for females. About 65% of people develop OCD prior to age 25 and less than 15% develop it after the age of 35 (Rasmussen & Eisen, 1990).

Following are descriptions of OCD symptomology taken from my clinical trials that help convey the nature of this disorder. Additional case histories are also reported, published from the trials (using fictitious names), with their progress reported (Shannahoff-Khalsa, 1997). Perhaps the best collection of individual cases was reported by Judith L. Rapoport, MD, chief of the child psychiatry branch at the National Institute of Mental Health, in an insightful and entertaining book called *The Boy Who Couldn't Stop Washing* (Rapoport, 1989). This book is probably the best introduction for the nonprofessional and has been read by virtually all serious scholars in the field.

Carl's Mental Checking and Mental Repeating Rituals

Carl's compulsions are all mental, whereas most patients perform rituals that can be noticed by others. Carl has a range of obsessions and fears that form a complex web of mental interactions. In his own words, Carl describes the manner of his bizarre checking rituals as:

> Repetitious obsessional thinking of constantly checking my most recent thoughts to make sure they are in order. If I can't remember the sequence of thoughts properly, I experience anxiety and frustration which leads to depression. Looking over my notes I see a phrase that I was repeating yesterday. I can't remember why I was repeating the phrase, i.e., what the trigger was. So I search and search until I remember exactly what I was thinking the moment the phrase entered my mind. Of course this can be quite exhaustive. If I can't remember the sequence of thoughts that triggered the phrase I get moody, depressed, or anxious. If I can remember what the trigger was, or sequence, I experience an incredible feeling of relief and peace. I feel safe and positive and I know everything is going to be all right until the next compulsion or doubt. Then the cycle starts all over again. The trigger or reminder can be a word in conversation (dead, splatter, axes), objects (ropes, knifes, pens), sounds (a scream, gurgling, tearing or ripping sounds), names (a loved one, especially children), photographs (especially children), anatomical areas (eyes, throat, neck, ears, etc.), or other objects (seat belts, bridges, tall buildings, poles, sticks, antennas). A series of repetitive phrases and words must then accompany these objects or thoughts to neutralize them. Of course these phrases become a large part of the problem. Some examples of the phrases are: no more setup, healing process, fill up (with the holy spirit), change scenario, kitt kat, hanging out, relief and freedom, uncle God, uncle action, all right, don't set up, tools of the program, contact, most recent, good news, add to the fear or confusion.

Carl's obsessions are about his safety and that of others. For him this translates to keeping his thoughts in order. He holds himself accountable for what he is doing in an overbearing way. He must therefore remember the sequences of his thoughts and the reminders and triggers that gave rise to each thought. The whole process becomes a vicious cycle. Anyone without OCD is immediately taken by the bizarre dynamics of Carl's mind and why his mental bookkeeping is so painfully debilitating.

Myrtle's Case of Hoarding: An Example of the Complications of Living with an OCD Patient

OCD patients never advise others to do what they do, but frequently attempt to get others to accommodate their own special needs. This becomes a major complication for other household members, and a family where more than one person has OCD can become an extremely complex, impaired, and chaotic environment. Imagine three people living together where two have OCD and both have hoarding as a primary obsession. This was the case for Myrtle. *Hoarding* is the term used to describe the classic pack-rat, the person who continuously collects usually useless objects, frequently leaving them in disarray, and can't throw them away. Prior to Kundalini yoga therapy, Myrtle spent hours gathering, sorting, storing, and trying to organize her "collections," which ended up not only in the house but in both her yard and a broken-down car parked on the street, all as eyesores to her neighbors. Myrtle "saved these valuable items for both her own use and to give away later to needy people." However, during the course of her therapy she told me they got soaked from the rain because they were not suitably protected. After the rain she had the urgent need to again reorganize and "salvage" what she could. Myrtle and her housemate hoarder had their own piles, stacks, and sheds that suffered from the downpour. Now everything was growing mildew and some things had to be separated out to dry. Imagine the hoarding headaches that definitely led to extreme household friction. In this case, Myrtle was in treatment and her housemate was not! Such cases are not that unusual, and are best described as a living nightmare.

In fact, hoarding is one of the more difficult-to-treat forms of OCD because it always includes the final homework of cleaning up and discarding the "valuables." The most extreme hoarding cases are those of people who have their homes so cluttered that there are only pathways between the rooms, and the valuables are piled so high that the walls become obscured from view. There have even been cases where people save their own feces and urine in jars for years on end. Both of these extremes are rare but stand as some of the worst examples of how people can suffer from this unique disorder. The other forms of OCD do not have this complication. For example, when you have stopped excessively washing, that's it, you have stopped.

Catherine's Interpersonal Checking Symptoms

One of the most common forms of OCD is called *checking,* and it can manifest so that one mate is endlessly asking the other if they are loved. This was one of Catherine's checking symptoms. Checking soon appears to be a neurosis when the question has been asked again and again and again all in one evening even after getting a full positive and thoughtful confirmation the first time. However, Catherine's husband understood her disorder and showed great tolerance. Sometimes it was triggered by seeing her mate look at another woman, or just by her own insecurities and doubts that came from her imagination. This neurotic checking obsession was only one of Catherine's OCD symptoms.

Jeannette's Lonely Life with Her Ordering and Arranging Rituals

People with OCD statistically have fewer partners and for obvious reasons. They are difficult to live with and likewise find the behaviors of others often overly complicating. The ordering and arranging rituals are a perfect example. People with the severe form of this disorder must have things in just "their right places."

They can never be moved or something terrible will happen. Jeannette, one of my patients, suffered with this symptom. Her house had a lot of knickknacks all around. Her husband eventually moved out because he could no longer tolerate not being allowed to pick things up or to move them. He felt like a prisoner in his own house. Before arriving at the official terminology of OCD, many physicians described this disorder as obsessional neurosis.

Dorothy's Unique Touching Rituals

Dorothy, had *touching* rituals. If she was touched by someone or something on the left side of her body, she had to have the right side touched as well in the same place. This was not the case if Dorothy only had her right side touched. However, if she saw that her children were touched on one side she made sure that they also got touched on the other side. This occasionally meant pushing the child into the initial object. Of course, whenever possible, Dorothy attempted to perform the rituals without being noticed. Her family members were well aware of her disorder. Dorothy also had a childhood history of aggressive, contamination, and religious obsessions. As an adult she had obsessions for symmetry and exactness, a need to know, and fear of not saying the right things, with rereading and rewriting compulsions. Otherwise Dorothy was a very loving, well-educated, and devoted wife and mother. I found her to be a very pleasant person.

Most people with OCD keep their behaviors hidden whenever possible. However, when they are prevented from performing their rituals, the tensions build. The gold standard for diagnostic tests in the field for determining the severity of OCD is called the Yale-Brown Obsessive-Compulsive Scale, or the Y-BOCS (Goodman, Price, Rasmussen, Mazure, Fleischmann, Hill, et al., 1989, 1989b). One of the questions asks "How would you feel if prevented from performing your compulsion(s)?" The answers regarding the degrees of anxiety range, in brief, from none, slightly anxious, moderate but manageable, severe and very disturbing, to extreme incapacitating anxiety. The other questions for severity with this rating scale are related to the amount of time occupied by obsessive thoughts, interference due to obsessive thoughts, distress associated with obsessive thoughts, how much effort is made to resist obsessive thoughts, and the degree of control over obsessions. Similar questions are asked regarding compulsions. The total score for obsessions and compulsions determines whether someone has a mild, moderate, severe, or extreme form of the disorder. (The range of scores for each of the 10 questions is from 0 to 4, or 40 points total for both of the obsession and compulsion subscale scores, which each have five questions or 20 points total.)

Don, a Classic Washer

One of the most common OCD profiles is that of a *washer*. Don feared contamination by germs, viruses, dirt, sticky substances, and environmental products, especially pesticides and normal household cleaning agents. It was not that Don was allergic, but he feared that he would be poisoned because he was so "sensitive" to these agents. He also feared that he would succumb to a dreaded illness due to contact. Don was then driven by a compelling urge to wash his hands incessantly, or whatever part of his body that he thought became contaminated. Frequently, washers do this to the extent of drawing blood on their skin where they have already become raw from past washing. Fortunately, Don's washing routines were not this severe. However, Don also suffered from fears of saying the wrong thing, sexual obsessions, hoarding, religious, somatic, and six other less-common obsessions. He also suffered from depression, learning disabilities, and chronic fatigue syndrome.

When suspect of contamination, some people may have a routine of what to do with their clothes. For example, in Don's case, upon returning home, he first entered the garage, deposited all his contaminated items in the washer, and then proceeded to the shower for decontamination. The showering was then followed by wiping the floor from the bathroom back to the garage and then depositing the wiping agents in a safe area for later disposal. Then, of course, he would wash his hands again. Washers' lives can become a futile and senseless attempt to live in a near-sterile environment where they only have less fear of becoming contaminated and getting ill.

Frequently, those with fears of contamination fear that they might also contaminate others. A common obsession is the fear of being contaminated by the HIV virus. When we enter the winter seasons, when the flu bug is spreading, doctors suggest washing our hands more often after touching door knobs, shaking hands, and other places that can be a real source of contagion. Don's tendency was to isolate himself more during this time of year. These types of fears and behaviors can become endless and debilitating to the point where people are spending more than eight hours a day cleaning the house seven days a week. Imagine, for example, wiping and polishing the coffee table 16 times in one day when it was never used. It happens. I met a woman who told me about this obsession and she appeared to have an intellectual understanding of it but could not overcome her need to clean.

Sundari, a Washer, and Her Unavoidable Trigger

Some washers spend two to three hours in the shower at any one time methodically cleaning themselves. Sundari was such a case. She was a woman seeking treatment with our protocol but lived on the East Coast and could not enter the trial. Sundari is a 61-year-old wife and mother born in India with otherwise normal behavior except that of her late-onset OCD involving washing rituals. When she was 50, her father died suddenly and unexpectedly. From that day forward she had a terrible fear of contamination after performing normal routines in the bathroom. She had only one obsession and one ritual. After every bowel movement, she had to spend 2 to 3 hours in the shower to clean herself. This disability made traveling very difficult for Sundari, and no doubt ran up her water bill. Besides this "habit," Sundari was completely normal. What is atypical here is the late onset of the disorder. She was taking medication for the disorder, but when I asked if she derived benefit from the drug (Anaphranil), she said, "Yes, it keeps me constipated and limits my movements to once a day." Constipation from Anaphranil is common; however, it is rarely considered a benefit. But in her case it probably saved her from spending several more hours a day in the shower. There was no means of persuading Sundari to shorten her routine or that her washing was excessive, even though intellectually she understood how it looked to others. Sundari still had to follow through with her cleaning rituals to overcome her fears of contamination.

Some clinicians may believe that the father's death and Sundari's OCD onset are coincidental and unrelated. However, much of my own work shows that a specific traumatic event can act as a trigger for the onset of OCD. The relationship of trauma and the onset of OCD symptoms, a fear-based disorder, deserves much further study. One study is consistent with some evidence from previous studies that suggest that childhood trauma plays a role in the development of these disorders with a "greater severity of childhood trauma in general, and emotional neglect specifically, in the patient groups compared to the controls" (Lochner, du Toit, Zungu-Dirwayi, Marais, van Kradenburg, et al., 2002).

A Few Novel Examples of Checking and Repeating Rituals

People with OCD do not trust their own physical senses. They can check 15 times to see if they have locked the car door while other members of the family are waiting to go into a restaurant. It is also not unusual for that person to get up in the middle of the meal, excuse himself, and check again. The lingering doubt comes back. One woman was never sure if she had turned off the light in the walk-in closet. She would stand in the closet for 5 to 30 minutes every morning after getting dressed turning the light on and off and then finally leaving the closet still in doubt. OCD is frequently referred to as a disease of doubt.

Going in and out of a doorway or getting up and down from a chair until it is done just right can be another form of OCD, and these behaviors are examples of *repeating* rituals. A well-documented and famous case is that of Samuel Johnson, a famous poet, playwright, and scholar in the eighteenth century, who had his own unique and extraordinary hand gestures and antics whenever he entered a passageway: he would proceed to twirl about in a circular motion in just the right way before entering with just the right number of steps and placing just the right foot first before going across the threshold. Some clinicians later thought these antics to be tics of the mind. If he missed doing it correctly, he would repeat the entire sequence. Accuracy here is the key and any deviation from perfection calls for a new round of rituals.

The case of Carl, described above, included only mental rituals that involved trying to keep his thoughts in order. Another mental ritualizer in one of my studies was Frank, a psychologist who feared that if he forgot the clinical definition of how to classify a child with attention-deficit/hyperactivity disorder he would lose his job. Frank would spend 3 to 4 hours during his most severe episodes mentally reciting the same list of rules for this particular classification. Consequently, Frank became quite distant from his family during the more difficult years of his disorder prior to treatment. In addition to his own torment, it put a strain on his marriage and made him feel guilty about the time that he did not spend with his wife and children. In these two cases of mental repeating rituals, and with OCD in general, stress exacerbates the disorder and, in turn, the disorder creates more stress and dysfunction. Life then becomes a vicious cycle and mixture of obsessions, compulsions, stress, and dysfunction. Performing simple tasks in life often becomes painfully complex and very lengthy. Imagine what can happen if you are a checker and you are employed as a banker, accountant, or computer programmer. The work definitely begins to slow down as someone is checking for mistakes. This was the case for Jeannette, the woman described above with ordering and arranging rituals. However, she was not noticed by her fellow bank employees because checking was expected, and fortunately she was not a teller. This part of her disorder was only moderate and could be disguised as part of her occupation. Jeannette never made mistakes, and you can be sure that the things on her desk were always in the same place.

Some "repeaters" mentally have to recite complex sets of numbers or lists of names in a particular order every time they encounter a trigger. The trigger could be seeing the color pink or certain number, even or odd. If the repeater makes an error in his recitation, he must start all over until it is done just right. Sometimes the "rules" require two, three, or any number of complete and accurate repetitions. Repeating rituals can also be performed outwardly, and the range of possibilities for how they can manifest is infinite. Sometimes patients start as washers and later become checkers, or hoarders, or any combination of the above. Most patients have multiple obsessions and compulsions. The specific obsessions and rituals are frequently transitory, even if this means over decades. However, the old ones are always replaced with new ones. Each patient has his or her own unique evolution, although there are many similarities across patients.

Other Disorders Commonly Occurring with OCD

Some patients have OCD along with other related impulse-control disorders like trichotillomania, body dysmorphic disorder (BDD), or Tourette's syndrome. These disorders are thought to be related to OCD because their frequency of occurrence in OCD patients is much higher than in the normal population. Trichotillomania is the irresistible impulse to pull out one's own hair. Hairs are plucked from any part of the body but most commonly from the head, eyelashes, eyebrows, and pubic areas. Trichotillomania has a mean age of onset at 11 and usually "causes severe social discomfort, interferes with daily activities, and may lead to social isolation" (Jenike, 1990). Jenike also states that its prevalence in the U.S. may reach as high as 8 million (Jenike, 1990). One of the five patients in the second Kundalini yoga trial who had trichotillomania was hospitalized due to a car accident some years before the trial.

During her bed-ridden stay and traction for broken bones, she was so stressed out that she pulled out every hair from her head, eyelashes, and eyebrows.

The following quote is a personal report by a female patient (age 20) who underwent Kundalini yoga therapy seeking relief primarily for her BDD, but also for OCD and a social phobia (Shannahoff-Khalsa, 2003). Her OCD symptoms began at age 10 and her BDD and social anxiety started at age 17. Her OCD symptoms included an obsession with the fear of harming others (she was convinced that if she called a relative or friend on their cell phones, she would cause a car accident, or something horrific). The fear, she felt, was "paralyzing." Her most prevalent OCD fear came in the form of not saying the correct thing in any situation, something that left her "constantly fearful and in check of her own thoughts and words." However, her BDD involved rituals—that of looking in a mirror, sometimes for several hours a day. She had the fear that her right eye and right side of her face were distorted. Before entering Kundalini yoga therapy, she had undergone insight-oriented psychotherapy with several therapists for approximately one year. After seeing me the first time and not following through with Kundalini yoga treatment, she again saw a therapist while at university. Prior to seeing me the second time, she also started using fluoxetine hydrochloride for about 6 weeks, and the side effects became too severe to tolerate so she was switched to paroxetine hydrochloride for 3 weeks. However, she found the side effects again too severe to continue. In my experience, her short-term response to Kundalini yoga therapy is typical. How she was treated using Kundalini yoga techniques is described after the extract below.

> I first began my work with David Shannahoff-Khalsa and the Kundalini yoga practice during spring break of the year 2001. The break was taken from the university I was currently attending, where I am now still enrolled as an undergraduate student. I consulted David for various reasons; the main (and most difficult)

ones being anxiety (in general social situations), stress (in the competitive nature of the academics at college), and body dysmorphic disorder. I had also been previously diagnosed 3 years before with OCD and depression, both of which I was still struggling with.

The very first session that I had with David altered my experience of anxiety, so much that the rushing of thoughts that seemed so constantly harrowing before had dissipated to a state of calm and relaxation. In addition to this, the body dysmorphic disorder I was experiencing totally disappeared for the remainder of the day. And, finally, the OCD disappeared completely and the results again lasted for the remainder of the day.

Despite the immediate advantages, though, within a week, vacation had ended and I returned to my dorm room at college, complete with roommate, and my practice suffered. I rarely found the opportunity to continue with what David had taught me, and the anxiety became a major problem in my life again. The BDD flourished, consuming nearly 2 hours per day in front of the mirror. This was extremely difficult to manage, particularly in light of the fact that my homework often took a back seat to my obsessions.

After this period, and another painful year following that (this time with four other roommates, and no practice of the yoga), I finally decided in the summer of 2002 to return to David, this time with the knowledge and certainty that I would dedicate myself to improving my state of mind.

Before seeing David at this time, my life had completely fallen apart. Up at my university, I had decided to consult a psychologist through a program at the university, and she had suggested that I try medication. Following that advice, I later consulted a psychiatrist who prescribed Prozac for me at 20 mg a day. Even under the influence of the drug for many weeks, I was so completely anxious and depressed simultaneously that I began to harm myself by self-mutilating my arm. First I started with the ends of cigarettes, and then, with a razor, cutting so deep on two places on my arm that they required stitches. I also had a severely diminished interest in eating to the point that I would actually avoid two meals per day and I started losing weight, and my mother began to question whether I was also becoming anorexic. It was at this point that my doctor was suggesting hospitalization to my parents that I went back to see David.

On this second meeting, everything became manageable again. At this time I also gave up use of the medication. The yoga put me in a state of balance, and gave me peace of mind immediately. I was able to quit cigarettes, and discontinue the self-mutilation as I worked at focusing on my breath and the exercises. I also started to have a normal appetite again. This all happened within a week of meeting with David and continuing the practice. The most beneficial aspect of the experience, however, was the immediate release from anxiety, depression, and OCD that I received upon meeting with him again. The continuation of the practice led to a greater state of peace and general strength that has continued up to this day.

Therapy with this patient included the entire Kundalini yoga protocol used in both clinical trials (see the 11-part Kundalini protocol for treating OCD on pages 71–80), along with the later inclusion of techniques called "Meditation to Help Understand, Focus, and Create a Clear Consciousness," (page 99), "When You Do Not Know What to Do" (page 102), and "Meditation to Balance the Jupiter and Saturn Energies: A Technique Useful for Treating Depression, Focusing the Mind, and Eliminating Self-Destructive Behavior" (page 119).

The OCD patient's life can also be complicated by one or more of the following disorders: schizophrenia, phobias, panic disorders, eating disorders, alcohol abuse, sleep disorders, organic mental disorders, and the major depressive disorders, such as seasonal affective disorder, unipolar depression, and bipolar disorder. Also, what is called monosymptomatic hypochondriasis presents more frequently with OCD patients. This syndrome can manifest as dysmorphophobia (delusional beliefs that one's body parts are distorted) or olfactory reference syndrome (delusional belief that one emits foul body odors), or even as a delusional parasitic infection (Jenike, 1990). What seems somewhat rare is a patient who only suffers from OCD. In one major clinic, the majority (57%) of patients had at least one other current psychiatric diagnosis (Rasmussen & Eisen, 1990). These additional disorders obviously complicate treatment. When one disorder gets worse, like depression, the OCD symptoms almost invariably get worse, and vice versa. Major depression is usually the most common co-morbid diagnosis with OCD, followed by simple phobias, social phobia, eating disorders, alcohol abuse, panic disorder, and Tourette's syndrome (Rasmussen & Eisen, 1990). Tourette's syndrome "is a neuropsychiatric disorder characterized by the waxing and waning of motor and phonic tics" (Pauls, 1990). It can present as facial distortions, hand waving, convulsive movements of any part of the body, repeating what others have just said (echolalia), and blurting out obscenities (coprolalia; see the story of Louis below). In our two studies totaling 33 patients, five (15%) of the total presented with trichotillomania and 31% of the total presented with major depressive disorders.

Louis's All-too-Common Case of Tourette's Syndrome

Louis interviewed for our study but refused to enter due to his own intense fears and concerns about being in a group. He had both OCD and Tourette's. Louis's convulsive hand movements were sometimes expressed as an uncontrolled tapping of the leg or back of the head of someone driving him in the car. This tic-like tapping in fact victimized his father whenever they were in the car together. Long trips can become quite unpleasant with these people even when the disorder is well understood by family members. However, the most awkward, unpleasant, and socially stigmatizing form of Tourette's syndrome is called coprolalia. This is where the patient suffers from frequent short bursts and uncontrolled outbreaks of speaking obscenities. An OCD patient may fear blurting out obscenities, but people with Tourette's actually do. Under stressful conditions, these patients often use the "f" and "s" words in a very uncontrolled manner. It happened to me while interviewing Louis. In fact, his first outbursts occurred only 30 seconds into our first conversation. It can happen to an unsuspecting stranger passing on the street, or during a phone conversation with someone they do not know, and even with a loved one. Louis described how he once was thrown off a public bus by the bus driver for using the "n" word with an African-American male passenger who was beginning to lose his patience. People just don't assume that such outbursts are the result of an illness. Recent studies show that 32% to 90% of people with Tourette's also suffer from OCD (Pauls, 1990).

Treating OCD with Conventional Therapies

Except in very rare cases, OCD has not been effectively treated with talk therapy (also called insight-oriented or traditional psychotherapy) (Jenike, Baer, & Minichiello, 1986). However, there are two well-accepted therapeutic approaches for treatment, behavior therapy (BT), in the form of exposure and response prevention (ERP), and pharmacological. In 1966, Victor Meyer first reported an uncontrolled but seminal study on exposure and response prevention, suggesting that short, effective treatment was possible. This led to controlled trials by Isaac Marks (1981) on ERP and paved the way for modern cognitive behavior therapy (CBT), which added cognitive restructuring to exposure exercises. The next major advance was the effectiveness of clomipramine suggested in Spain (Lopez-Ibor, 1968) and confirmed in subsequent controlled studies. More recently, both gamma knife surgery and deep brain stimulation using implanted electrodes show some benefits in a small number of patients (Rasmussen, Greenberg, Noren, Marshano, & Eisen, 2003) as well as unilateral vagal nerve stimulation (Husted & Shapira, 2004).

Patients who can tolerate medication usually respond with only a 30% to 60% reduction in symptoms (White & Cole, 1990). This improvement requires a continued use of medication and the majority of patients experience unpleasant drug-induced side effects and some patients also show regression after the initial success. Approximately 30% of patients treated do not benefit to any significant degree even after adequate treatment with medication, thus defining the "drug treatment resistant patient" (Goodman, McDougle, Barr, Aronson, & Price, 1993). Some experts claim that 40% to 60% of patients exhibit only minimal improvement or no change with selective serotonin re-uptake inhibitors (SSRIs) (Goodman, McDougle, & Price, 1992), the current favored class of drugs for treating OCD. For most responders, a "20% to 35% decrease in mean Y-BOCS scores may represent a clinically meaningful change in symptom severity" (Goodman et al., 1993). A multicenter study (Goodman, Kozak, Liebowitz, & White, 1996) comparing one of the most recently approved SSRI drugs for treating OCD (fluvoxamine) showed only a 17.5% improvement (Y-BOCS) for drug-treated patients in a randomized double-blind placebo-controlled trial (fluvoxamine, $n = 78$; placebo, $n = 78$). The mean improvement in the fluvoxamine group was 3.95 (Y-BOCS total) and 1.71 for the placebo group on the Y-BOCS 0 to 40 point scale. Discontinuation of pharmacological treatment also poses problems as reported in two double-blind substitution or withdrawal studies (Pato, Zohar-Kadouch, Zohar, & Murphy, 1988; Leonard, Swedo, Lenane, Rettew, Cheslow, et al., 1991). Pato et al. (1988) observed a relapse rate of 90% within two to four months following abrupt discontinuation of clomipramine in 18 remitted patients, and desipramine was substituted for clomipramine in a crossover design (Leonard et al., 1991). A high percentage of these patients relapsed within two months of beginning desipramine. Similar results were found in an open-label study of 35 OCD patients who discontinued fluoxetine after having a good initial response (Fontaine & Chouinard, 1989). Preliminary evidence suggests that relapse after discontinuation of the drug is associated with increased resistance to treatment (Maina, Albert, & Bogetto, 2001). A recent meta-analysis compared the results from four multicenter placebo-controlled trials of clomipramine, fluoxetine, fluvoxamine, and sertraline, and found Y-BOCS improvements of 39%, 27%, 20%, and 26% for the "best dose comparisons," respectively (Greist, Jefferson, Kobak, Katzelnick, & Serlin, 1995). A recent meta-analysis compared BT to the SSRIs and concluded that "BT was comparable to the serotonin reuptake inhibitors" (Kobak, Greist, Jefferson, Katzelnick, 1998). But only about 10% of the clinical centers skilled in the treatment of OCD have programs for BT. All the SSRIs have significant side effects, the most common being sedation, sexual dysfunction, and weight gain (Rasmussen, Eisen, & Pato, 1993). Other side effects can include nausea, memory loss, a worsening of OCD symptoms, headaches, diarrhea, night sweats, sleeplessness, seizures, and numerous others that make the choice between diminishing the OCD symptoms and living with the side effects a major dilemma for the patient. Additionally, the long-term effects of these drugs are unknown.

Considerable interest has also been given to the combination of pharmacotherapy and ERP. However, one report suggests that the efficacy of combined ERP and pharmacotherapy for OCD is controversial (Simos, 2002), and a review of relevant studies concluded that this combination has shown little advantage over ERP alone (Steketee, 1993). Preliminary findings from a trial also supported this point of view (Kozak, Liebowitz, & Foa, 2000). However, one study showed that a combination of fluvoxamine plus ERP, compared with placebo plus ERP, gave better results at 3 months on rituals and at 6 months on depression, with equivalent results at 12 and 18 months (Cottraux, Mollard, Bouvard, & Marks, 1993). Patients who received ERP were less likely to take antidepressants at a 1-year follow-up (Cottraux et al., 1993). A small sample study comparing medication with CBT showed evidence in favor of both (O'Connor, Todorov Robillard, Borgeat, & Brault, 1999). One controlled trial with 122 patients compared very intensive ERP, clomipramine, their combination, and pill placebo (Foa, Liebowitz, Kizak, Davies, & Campeas, et al. 2005). The trial was conducted at a center known for its expertise in pharmacotherapy, a center known for expertise in ERP, and a third with expertise in both treatments. Interventions included 4 weeks of

ERP with exposure sessions lasting 2 hours each weekday over a 3-week period (15 sessions), along with additional daily exposure and ritual-prevention homework (up to 2 hours a day). In the fourth week, therapists visited the patients' homes twice (4 hours total) to promote generalizability of treatment gains by conducting exposures in contexts relevant to the patient's functioning. For the remaining 8 weeks, 45-minute sessions were conducted weekly to promote maintenance. The patient and therapist discussed the patient's remaining OCD symptoms and how to combat them; no new in-session exposure exercises were assigned, only 8 weekly maintenance sessions. Another group compared the same regimen and clomipramine administered for 12 weeks with a maximum dose of 250 mg per day, and two additional groups consisted of drug alone or placebo. At 12 weeks the effects of all active treatments were superior to placebo, but ERP did not differ from that of ERP plus clomipramine, and both were superior to clomipramine alone. Twelve-week Y-BOCS results showed 55% improvement for ERP, 31% for clomipramine, 59% for ERP plus clomipramine, and 11% for placebo. Clomipramine, ERP, and their combination were all efficacious treatments for OCD. The authors suggested that intensive ERP might be superior to clomipramine and, by implication, to other SSRIs. It should be noted that these results were achieved by a very intensive program. Several researchers have stated "This may be impossible to implement in most therapeutic settings, and requires very compliant patients" (Cottraux, Bouvard, & Milliery, 2005). The study authors stated "This may represent the gold standard for patients who fail to benefit from a less intensive form of treatment" (Foa et al., 2005).

While the Foa et al. (2005) trial is exemplary, three meta-analyses have examined the effects of drugs and/or CBT. The first study combined 86 trials (from 1970 to 1993) and found no difference between antidepressants alone, CBT, and their combination (Van Balkom, Van Oppen, Vermeulen, Van Dych, Nauta, et al., 1994). Another meta-analysis (combining 77 trials between 1973 and 1997, yielding 106 comparisons) found that CBT was equivalent or better than treatment with SSRIs (Kobak et al., 1998), and another found SSRIs, CT, and ERP to be equally effective (Abramowitz, 1997).

In summary, of the current state of affairs for treatment, Cottraux, Bouvard, and Milliery conclude: "Initial management of OCD relies on potent SSRIs and CBT, used separately, sequentially, or concurrently: as severity increases, it is recommended to add medications. However, the response rate is still too low, and some patients remain refractory to any kind of treatment. Therefore, further basic research, both psychological and biological, is needed to understand and better manage this chronic condition. Over the last 20 years much has been accomplished for understanding and treating OCD, but a fresh start is now needed" (2005).

Discovering the efficacy of Kundalini yoga meditation techniques in the treatment of OCD constitutes a completely new approach or, "fresh start," for treatment in the West. In addition, this discovery has important implications for the thousands of different Kundalini yoga meditation techniques. This chapter and this book suggest the possibility of a new era in psychiatry. Two clinical trials on the benefits of Kundalini yoga for treating OCD are presented in Appendix 3.

Preliminary Comments on the Kundalini Yoga Protocol for Treating OCD

Each technique in this protocol can lead to a profound experience. Patients in our studies have made comments during their first experience with the protocol such as "I almost forgot that I had OCD, my mind is so quiet." The woman that made this comment did so after 15 minutes in her first session. She was thoroughly amazed, especially since she was in a doctoral program for clinical psychology. In fact, once you become experienced with the protocol, you can usually achieve some significant relief within several minutes. Knowing this from one's own experience is itself a source of great relief. After this awareness, the patient decides how much torture or relief they can tolerate or enjoy, respectively. Some people make an early commitment to practice every day, some take weeks to commit, some take months, some only practice when they come to the group, and of course some drop out so they do not have to test their own will to commit even after achieving relief while participating in the group. The first axiom in our group was "If you fall down (in your discipline) get up." The star pupil in the second study was Terry. She was asked by another patient after several months, "How is it that you manage to practice every day?" Terry said, "I have had OCD since I was five. I have suffered with it almost all of my life. I have tried medications that only gave me terrible side effects. BT did not help. I tried different religions. I even tried other forms of meditation. Nothing else has worked. This [Kundalini yoga therapy] does and I just want to get well." Terry enjoyed the great benefits that she got from a daily discipline. She appreciated the extraordinary contrast. Her baseline Y-BOCS total score was 24, which meant that Terry had a moderate to severe case of OCD. Her end Y-BOCS totals were 1—on a scale of 40. This protocol also produces delightful feelings throughout the body. There is an increase in energy and a new sense of comfort devoid of the constant tension that leaves OCD patients feeling temperamental and tense. The patient also experiences renewal and rejuvenation. Everyone that comes to the group feels completely refreshed, even before we reach the halfway point. Their sense of well-being only increases after that time and grows as the weeks of therapy progress.

Age is not a critical factor even though it plays a role. The younger subjects who innately have more physical ability to comply with the protocol usually are less mature in their commitment. Dominique, on the other hand, was 66 years of age when she entered the study. Her spine was much less flexible, and she had mild scoliosis (abnormal spinal curvature). She also had osteoporosis. Her lung capacity was diminished. She initially had problems with one of the eye postures and she definitely had the signs of an aging nervous system. But Dominique's will was enormous and she was extremely grateful for the opportunity to participate. She had been waiting years for a solution for her OCD. She was waiting for a cure in her lifetime. An hour a day was not too much for what Dominique had gained from it. The techniques also increased their sense of well-being, vitality, and the experience of their own spirituality. She felt like she was getting a taste of enlightenment.

This protocol includes eight primary techniques to be used on a daily basis and three additional techniques to be used at your personal discretion. Most patients also found two of the three supplementary techniques (techniques 9 and 10) to be useful adjuncts to their daily routine. They require very little extra effort, and the benefits are well worth a few additional minutes.

The protocol has a specific order that we always followed in the trials. In fact, I suggest you follow it exactly as it is prescribed. Some people, due to disabilities, cannot perform some of these techniques. However, all Kundalini yoga meditation techniques start with the first technique. This technique for "tuning in" should never be left out. There is a reason for the order prescribed. Whenever someone altered the order, or left techniques out, they soon realized that they got diminished returns. They would observe within a few weekly sessions how others seemed to be progressing more rapidly, or that they did not achieve the same benefit that they had in earlier weeks. There are no shortcuts, except that of a daily discipline. Once you have the time-tested experience of the techniques, patients learn how much good the protocol can do for them. A video has also been produced to aid those who prefer to learn in that mode. However, the figures that accompany the techniques below will suffice.

The first technique, called "tuning in," helps induce a meditative state of mind and provides the patient with the experience of being in a "womb of healing energy." The second and third techniques increase metabolism, uplift the spirit, and induce the healthy glandular changes that give the experience of vitality. These are helpful precursors to the others. The fourth technique is a powerful technique that induces a calm and quiet mind. It works even if the patient is feeling absolutely insane. In fact, in ancient times it was used to treat insanity. The fifth also helps to alleviate emotional stress. It also rejuvenates the nervous, glandular, and cardiovascular systems. This one is very important because it helps develop the ability to do the one breath technique specific to OCD (see technique 8). Technique 5 will help build the respiratory capacity. Technique 6 takes about 75 seconds once learned and helps strip away any residual mental tension. Technique 7 takes 3 minutes and is extremely useful for managing fears, especially if the patient is actually in a state of intense fear. It is almost effortless. (I first learned the value of this technique when using it to treat a 38-year-old woman dying of metastatic breast cancer who was suffering from extreme anxiety. The cancer had traveled to her lungs, brain, spine, neck, and liver. Her breathing became so impaired that she was living in a constant state of anxiety. She had a tremendous fear of her pending death. After 3 minutes use, the maximum prescribed time, she began to smile and she commented that every negative thought seemed to change to a positive thought. Her husband who was watching commented, "This is the first time that I have seen you smile in 2 months.") Technique 8 is the yogic technique specific for treating OCD, now called the OCD breath (OCDB). It would suffice by itself if practiced perfectly, but only a few patients would ever survive a program that only included this technique. All the other techniques are included to help facilitate the practice of the OCDB. Technique 9, the victory breath, is for facing mental challenges. It seems too simple to be effective, but 3 to 5 minutes of proper use yield a small miracle. All patients learned to use this technique and they relied on it when they were unable to sit down and practice the others. It can be practiced anywhere and at anytime. Technique 10 can be used to transform negative thought patterns into positive thoughts. This technique produces so much healing energy that bliss can be the ultimate result. On occasion we would practice it for 11 minutes in the group. The first time Myrtle tried it for 11 minutes, she said she felt like she had a golden light surrounding her head. These kinds of experiences are transforming. The last technique is usually used only when patients are experiencing significant anger. It is a wonderful option to be able to tranquilize an angry mind. There are at least a half-dozen Kundalini yoga meditation techniques for anger and this one, in my opinion, is by far the simplest and most effective. Results can last up to 3 days. Everyone ought to carry it around in their mental tool chest.

The 11-Part Kundalini Yoga Protocol for Treating OCD[*]

1. Technique to Induce a Meditative State: "Tuning In"

Sit with a straight spine and with the feet flat on the floor if sitting in a chair (see Figure 2.1). Put the hands together at the chest in "prayer pose"—the palms are pressed together with 10 to 15 pounds of pressure between the hands (a mild to medium pressure, nothing too intense). The area where the sides of the thumbs touch rests on the sternum with the thumbs pointing up (along the sternum), and the fingers are together and point up and out at a 60-degree angle to the ground. The eyes are closed and focused on the third eye (imagine a sun rising on the horizon, or the equivalent of the point between the eyebrows at the origin of the nose). A mantra is chanted out loud in a 1½-breath cycle. Inhale first through the nose and chant "Ong Namo" with an equal emphasis on the Ong and the Namo. Then immediately follow with a half-breath inhalation through the mouth and chant "Guru Dev Namo" with approximately equal emphasis on each word. (The O in *Ong* and *Namo*

---

[*] This protocol was first published in full in Shannahoff-Khalsa (1997) and later in Shannahoff-Khalsa (2003).

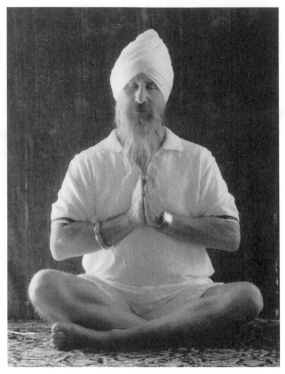

Figure 2.1
Technique to Induce a Meditative State: "Tuning In"

are each a long "o" sound; *Dev* sounds like *Dave*, with a long "a" sound.) The practitioner should focus on the experience of the vibrations these sounds create on the upper palate and throughout the cranium while letting the mind be carried by the sounds into a new and pleasant mental space. This should be repeated a minimum of three times. We employed it in our group about 10–12 times. This technique helps to create a "meditative state of mind" and is *always* used as a precursor to the other techniques.

2. Spine-Flexing Technique for Vitality

This technique can be practiced while sitting either in a chair or on the floor in a cross-legged position. If you are in a chair, hold the knees with both hands for support and leverage. If you are sitting cross-legged, grasp the ankles in front with both hands. Begin by pulling the chest up and slightly forward, inhaling deeply through the nose at the same time. Then exhale as you relax the spine down into a slouching position. Keep the head up straight, as if you were looking forward, without allowing it to move much while flexing the spine. This will help prevent a whip effect in the cervical vertebrae. All breathing should only be through the nose for both the inhalation and exhalation. The eyes are closed as if you were looking at a central point on the horizon, the third eye. Your mental focus is kept on the sound of the breath while listening to the fluid movement of the inhalation and exhalation. Begin the technique slowly while loosening up the spine. Eventually, a very rapid movement can be achieved with practice, reaching a rate of one to two times per second for the entire movement. A few minutes are adequate in the beginning. Later, there is no time limit. Food should be avoided just prior to this exercise. Be careful and flex the spine slowly in the beginning. Relax for 1 minute when finished.

3. Shoulder-Shrug Technique for Vitality

While keeping the spine straight, rest the hands on the knees if sitting in a cross-legged position or with hands on the thighs if sitting in a chair. Inhale and raise the shoulders toward the ears, then exhale, relaxing them down. All breathing is done only through the nose. Eyes should be kept closed and focused on the third eye. Mentally focus on the sound of the inhalation and exhalation. Continue this action rapidly, building to three times per second for a *maximum* of 2 minutes. This technique should not be practiced by individuals who are hyperactive.

4. Technique for Reducing Anxiety, Stress, and Mental Tension

Sit and maintain a straight spine. Relax the arms and the hands in the lap. Focus the eyes on the tip of the nose even though you cannot see it. When you are unsure about where this is, start by placing the tip of your index finger on the very end of your nose. You will not be able to see the tip of your finger, but this is the area of your visual focus. You can only see the sides of the nose and they will appear blurred while focusing on the tip. Open the mouth as wide as possible, slightly stressing the temporal-mandibular joint, the jaw joint. Touch the tongue tip to the upper palate where it is hard and smooth in the upper center. Breathe continuously through the nose only, while making the respirations slow and deep. Mentally focus on the sound of the breath; listen to the sound of the inhalation and exhalation. Remember to keep the eyes focused, the jaw stretched, and the tongue on the upper palate throughout. In the beginning, remembering to do every-thing correctly is sometimes challenging. Maintain this pattern for at least 3 to 5 minutes with a maximum of 8 minutes on the first trial. With practice it can be maintained for 31 minutes maximum. This technique can be used to curb a restless mind and bring an inner stillness and extraordinary experience of mental silence.

5. Technique for Reducing Anxiety, Stress, and Mental Tension

Sit and maintain a straight spine (see Figure 2.2). The hands are in front of the chest at heart level. The left hand is 2 inches away from the chest and the right is about 2 inches behind the left (4 inches away from the chest), the left fingers point to the right. The right palm faces the back of the left hand with the right fingers pointing to the left. The thumbs of both hands point up without tension. The eyes are open and focused on the tip of the nose (see technique 4). All breathing is done through the nose only. Inhale, then keep the breath in as long as possible, then exhale and keep the breath out as long as possible without creating undo discom-fort at any stage. The inhalation and exhalation phases are each short. Only the holding in and holding out stages are stressed. When finished, inhale while still maintaining the eye and hand posture and then tense every muscle in the body for about 10

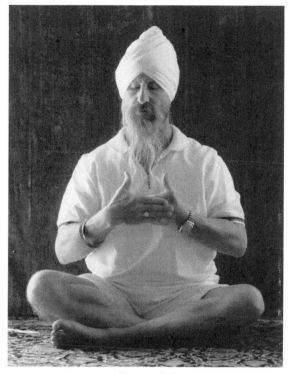

Figure 2.2
Technique for Reducing Anxiety, Stress, and Mental Tension

seconds. Exhale and repeat two times. Build the capacity for this technique to a maximum time of 15 minutes. Avoid this exercise if you have high blood pressure or are pregnant. This technique was taught for relaxing the mind when there is emotional stress or mental tension.

6. *Technique for Reducing Anxiety, Stress, and Mental Tension*

Sit as in technique 5. Eyes are open and focused on the tip of the nose during the *entire* exercise. Attempt to pull the nose down toward the upper lip by actually pulling the upper lip down over the upper front teeth using the muscles of the upper lip. The mouth is left open during this exercise while keeping constant tension on the upper lip. This upper-lip tension is maintained during, in between, and throughout all six rounds. There are three steps to this exercise. Step one: Start with the hands and arms up and out to the sides at 45 to 60 degrees, then inhale deeply and tightly clench the fists (this also produces tension in the arms and shoulders) and slowly pull them down toward the abdomen, the navel-point region. Step two: (Remember to keep the breath in, eyes focused, and lip pulled down.) Maintaining the tension in the fists, arms, and shoulders, bring the shoulders up toward the ears, tensing the shoulders and neck as they go up. Step three: Exhale and relax (but keep the lip pulled down and the eyes focused on the tip of the nose). Repeat the entire sequence six times. Avoid this exercise if you have high blood pressure or are pregnant. This short exercise is claimed to be so effective that if it is done correctly it can relieve the most tense person.

7. Technique for Managing Fears

Sit with a straight spine (see Figure 2.3). Close the eyes. Place the left hand with the four finger tips and thumb grouped and pressed very lightly into the navel point, like a plug. Place the right hand with the four fingers pointing left over the third eye point (on the forehead just above the root of the nose), as if feeling your temperature. Play the audio musical tape of Chakkra Chattra Varti (*Ancient Healing Ways*, 2006) for 3 minutes while assessing all your fears and consciously relating to the mental experience of each fear. This technique helps to manage acute states of fear and eliminate fearful images and negative emotions that have developed due to fearful experiences. The effect is that the negative emotions related to specific fears are replaced with positive emotions, thereby slowly creating a new and different mental association with the stimulus. Only the musical tape recommended here will actually produce this unique effect.

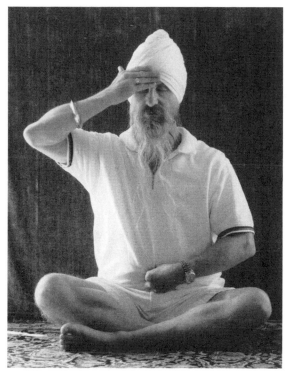

Figure 2.3
Technique for Managing Fears

8. Technique for Treating Obsessive Compulsive Disorders (OCDB)[*]

Sit with a straight spine in a comfortable position, either with the legs crossed while sitting on the floor or in a straight-back chair with both feet flat on the ground. Close the eyes. Use the right thumb tip to block the end of the right nostril, other fingers point up straight. Allow the arm to relax (the elbow should not be sticking up or out to the side, creating unnecessary tension). A small cork or secure plug made of wet or dry tissue paper can also be used to plug the right nostril. Inhale very slowly and deeply through the left nostril, hold the breath in for a long time, exhale

[*] This meditation technique was first published in Shannahoff-Khalsa (1991b).

77

out slowly and completely through the same nostril only (left nostril), and hold the breath out for a long time. The mental focus should be on the sound of the breath. Continue this pattern with a maximum time of 31 minutes for each sitting. Initially, begin with a comfortable rate and time, but where the effort presents a fair challenge for each phase of the breath. The length of time a person can hold out his or her breath varies from person to person. Ideal time per complete breath cycle is 1 minute, where each section of the cycle lasts exactly 15 seconds. This rate of respiration can be achieved by most people within 5 to 6 months for the full 31 minutes with daily discipline. Yogic experiments claim that 90 days of 31 minutes per day using the perfected rate of one breath per minute with 15 seconds per phase will completely eliminate all OC disorders (personal communication, Yogi Bhajan). The hold-out phase is always the most difficult. Starting with 5 seconds for each of the four phases (the inhalation, the hold-in, the exhalation, and the hold-out) is a reasonable beginning for most people after practicing the technique for a while. Then attempt 7.5 seconds per phase with slow graduations. You should not try to make any phase longer than 15 seconds to compensate for the difficulties with the other sections. The balance of the four phases is an important key to this technique.

9. Technique for Meeting Mental Challenges: The "Vic-tor-y Breath"

This technique can be used at any time. It does not require that the practitioner is sitting. It can be employed while driving a car, while participating in a conversation, or taking a test. The eyes can be open or closed depending on the situation. Take a near-full breath through the nose. Hold this breath without straining or tensing the stomach muscles for exactly 3 to 4 seconds and only during this hold phase mentally say to yourself the three separate sounds "vic," "tor," "y," then exhale. Mentally creating the three separated sounds should take 3 to 4 seconds, no longer or less. The entire time of each repetition should take about 8 to 10 seconds. The breath should not be exaggerated to the extent that anyone would even notice that you are taking a deep breath. It can be employed multiple times until you achieve the desired relief. When employed in our therapy sessions, it was usually done for 3 to 5 minutes with the eyes closed and while sitting with a straight spine to maximize the benefits. This technique is very helpful as a "thought stopping" technique for an OCD patient "on the go." There is no upper time limit for its practice. It can be used to help resist obsessive thoughts and as an antidote for compulsive rituals.

10. Technique to Turn Negative Thoughts into Positive Thoughts

This technique should be employed while sitting with a straight spine and with the eyes closed in a peaceful environment. The mantra "Ek Ong Kar Sat Gurprasad Sat Gurprasad Ek Ong Kar" must be repeated a minimum of five times and is best practiced for 5 to 11 minutes, chanting it through rapidly up to five full repetitions of the entire mantra per breath. The "Ek" sound is the same as the "eck" in *neck*. Ong has a long "o" (not "ung"). "Kar" sounds like *car* but with an emphasis on the "k" sound. The "Sat" has a short "a" sound. With *Gurprasad*, the "u" and both "*a*"s are short vowel sounds; the "a" sounds like the "a" in *ah*. Eventually, one no longer thinks about the order of the sounds, they come automatically. The mental focus should be on the vibration created against the upper palate and throughout the cranium. If performed correctly, a very peaceful and "healed" state of mind is achieved.

11. Technique for Tranquilizing an Angry Mind

Sit with a straight spine and close the eyes. Simply chant out loud "Jeeo, Jeeo, Jeeo, Jeeo" continuously and rapidly for 11 minutes without stopping (pronounced like the names for the letters *g* and *o*). Rapid chanting is about 8 to 10 repetitions per 5 seconds. During continuous chanting, you do not stop to take long breaths, but continue with just enough short breaths to keep the sound going. Eleven minutes is all that is needed, no more or less. The effect can last for up to three days. If necessary, it can be chanted for 11 minutes twice a day. This technique is most suitable for treating a "red hot" angry mind.

Case Histories of Treatment

Only selected examples of the 33 patients in the two studies are presented here. Eight people (seven females, one male) volunteered to participate in the first study. They had an average age of 39.4 years (ranging from 29 to 55 years). Twenty-three adults and two adolescents (age 14) volunteered for the second study with an average age for the adults of 39.6 years (ranging from 22 to 67 years). The average age of these two groups was surprisingly similar.

Case History 1

Frank (age 44) was in a stressful marriage with three children and employed as a psychologist. His rituals were primarily mental. His OCD symptoms developed in his teens. He was raised in a dysfunctional family with an alcoholic mother who died when he was 29. Frank is the second oldest of seven children. He tried behavior therapy without success. He was stabilized on 20 mg of fluoxetine for four months prior to the study. He had fears of not saying the right thing, and an obsessive need to know or remember, resulting in rereading, rewriting, and mental repeating and reviewing rituals. Frank was very athletic and he quickly responded to the positive energy of the techniques. He had a healthy body. Early on in the study he left class elated and free of symptoms at least for short periods. These incredible moments of extended relief inspired Frank to apply himself with great vigor to the OCDB technique. He was able to breathe at one breath per minute for the entire 31 minutes after about 4 months of being in the group. This was the shortest time needed by any of the subjects to develop this ability. However, he never managed during the study to achieve the 90 consecutive days that can supposedly eliminate all symptoms. By 5 months, Frank was completely off fluoxetine. After being off it for 3 weeks, he remarked how good it felt not to be experiencing the effects of the drug. Frank remarked that he had forgotten what it was like to physically feel that good. His Y-BOCS score went from a 28 to 11, a 61% improvement. He was initially experiencing his OCD symptoms for 3 to 4 hours per day, which placed him in the severe category. This time was reduced for most of the last 6 months of therapy to 15 to 40 minutes on an average day, a mild category, and less than the 1-hour margin used for the standard psychiatric classification of OCD. When on vacation, his symptoms were completely gone. But Frank's stressful work and home life added a major strain that exacerbated his symptoms.

Case History 2

Dorothy was a homemaker (age 34) with children. In addition to OCD, she also suffered from seasonal affective disorder (SAD). Her OCD symptoms developed in early childhood "as far back as I can remember." Dorothy is the youngest of four children, with a 15-month-older brother, and with two sisters that were 12 and 17 years older and living on their own when Dorothy was seven. Dorothy always "wished that her parents had been younger while she was growing up, and had trouble relating to them." She "never felt like they connected." There was a definite emotional gap between her and her parents that developed early on due to their lack of bonding. Dorothy had been taking fluoxetine for 3 years prior to the start of the study and she was stabilized on 40 mg for one year prior to the start of the study but only for her SAD, as it never helped with her OCD symptoms. She could not tolerate 60 mg. After 4 months in the study she had reduced it to 20 mg, but when trying to discontinue completely she had subtle signs of increased depression that also affected her OCD. She also had severe night sweats during her attempt to go to zero medication. This caused her great alarm, fatigue, and frustration, and the need to change her nightgown and bed sheets on a near-nightly basis. This was probably a side effect from being on the medication for such an extended period and attempting to reduce too quickly. Therefore she resumed the 40 mg dosage after two attempts to reduce medication completely, but required 40 mg for only about 7 to 10 days until reducing again to 20 mg. She had reduced it to 20 mg for at least 2 months prior to the end of the study. This patient had a childhood history of aggressive, contamination, and religious obsessions. At the start of this study, Dorothy experienced obsessions for symmetry and exactness, a need to know, and fear of not saying the right things, with rereading and rewriting compulsions and touching rituals that required her response (to touch back) only when she was touched on the left side of her body, but not on the right. Dorothy's Y-BOCS scores went from a 19 (moderate symptoms) to a 4 (79% improvement) on compulsions (almost none existent), with a 0 on her obsessions. She had mastered the OCDB by six months.

Case History 3

Catherine (age 38) was a teacher who married during the study. Her first symptoms developed at age 18, when she experienced a panic attack while encountering a tour group of lesbians. In her early family life with three older brothers, she was constantly forced to observe her father photograph nude women. Her father was addicted to alcohol, food, sex, and cigarettes. Catherine had constant concerns about "perverse sex." Her parent's relationship was "marred with physical and emotional abuse and extramarital affairs." She had a "traumatic and unhappy childhood and dealt with her emotional problems by internalizing them," by withdrawing, bed-wetting, thumb-sucking, head-banging, and rocking, overeating, and reading all the time. In her teen years she used alcohol and drugs "heavily." She had a series of physically and emotionally abusive relationships with men. She had 3 years of psychoanalytic therapy that helped provide her insight and increased self-esteem, but which was of no benefit with her OCD. Four months of BT helped her with rituals, but not her obsessive thoughts. She also tried BuSpar. Catherine initially had aggressive, sexual (the fear that she was a lesbian), religious, somatic, checking, repeating, and four other miscellaneous compulsions and obsessions. Catherine was stabilized on 40 mg of fluoxetine for at least 3 months prior to the start of the study. Her Y-BOCS score went from 18 to a 3 at the end of the study (83% improvement) with a 0 for her compulsions. She had mastered the OCDB by 7.5 months. Eight months after the study was over, she called and said that she had had a difficult time with her OCD while on vacation. She had gone to Hawaii and people who were dressed somewhat immodestly there acted as a trigger for her OCD symptoms. When questioned more closely about her 10-day stay in Hawaii, she responded that she only had her OCD for three of those days and for no more than 3 minutes each day. This meant that she averaged 1 minute per day! From a clinical perspective she was cured. However, she never wanted to have these thoughts again, even in the form of memories. This is analogous to having a patient with a severe case of acne achieve clear skin and then have a very small pimple return for a short period of time. Everything must be kept in perspective.

Case History 4

Freda (age 55) was a homemaker with three children. She had trichotillomania between ages 14 and 51. She was the oldest of six children. Her father was "an exceedingly compulsive and restless man." The family moved an average of twice a year. She had approximately 25 school changes before completing college, and approximately 15 more moves once she left her nuclear family. These disruptions created a lot of difficulties. She was sure that this had a "profound impact on her and explains much about her insecurities." She had 2.5 years of counseling and some BT. Freda tried clomipramine (25 mg) and fluoxetine (up to 75 mg). She was stabilized on 20 mg of fluoxetine for at least 3 months prior to the start of the study. During the time of the study, her husband had terminal cancer. Freda had obsessions of symmetry and exactness with magical thinking, fear of losing things, intrusive (nonviolent) images, concern with illness, and checking, reading, and rewriting compulsions, as well as repeating rituals, ordering and mental rituals, and the need to tell, ask, and confess since early childhood. After 6 months she chose to leave the study because of her subjective sense of a successful result and increasing back pain resulting from an earlier car accident that made it difficult for her to sit still and comply with the therapy. Freda's Y-BOCS scores improved 65%, from a 17 total to 6 with a 0 on compulsions. She discontinued her fluoxetine after 4 months in the study. One year later she was still off fluoxetine.

Case History 5

Terry was a 38-year-old single mother and grandmother with limited part-time employment. She developed severe trichotillomania at age seven during turbulent years living with her alcoholic, adulterous, gambling father. She was taken to the adulterous interludes by the father and kept outside, and upon returning home to her angered mother, she felt responsible and had internalized the blame. Terry and her brothers were verbally abused by the father, and her brothers were also physically abused. She came close to being shot one night when her father was in a dispute. The fear of being shot through her bedroom window during her sleep remained for years. She had aggressive, somatic, and miscellaneous obsessions, with checking and other compulsions. Terry tried clomipramine with intolerable side effects. Her mother was a compulsive cleaner and was suspected of having OCD. Terry's Y-BOCS scores went from a 24 (moderate to severe rating) to a 5 at

3 months, a 4 at 6 months, a 2 at 9 months, and a 1 at 12 months (with a 0 on obsessions for the 6-, 9-, and 12-month tests). Terry's extraordinary commitment to discipline helped her to manage her own cure. She practiced almost every day since the very beginning of the study and was capable of doing the OCDB at one breath per minute for 31 minutes after 10 months.

Case History 6

Carl was a single male (age 36) with two years of college. He never married. He was born and raised on military bases. Carl, his older brother, and mother had been psychologically and physically abused by the alcoholic father. During the father's binges he would regularly terrorize and occasionally physically abuse them. Also, from the ages of 8 to 19 the father "would come to our room, it would be lights on, stand at attention, room inspection, maybe a few war stories or lessons on how to fight or even kill." They looked forward to their "breaks" when the father went overseas. By the time Carl had finished high school he had moved nine times and attended 12 different schools. He "could never quite relax because he would either be moving or his dad would be on a rampage, or, as the dad called it, his kill program, burn the town and kill the people." Carl's OCD symptoms started at age 13 on the occasion of moving to a new school. He became terrified by some of the "punks" in his remedial math class who verbally abused him right in front of the "neurotic lady teacher who had absolutely no control over them." In order to escape this, he had to enter a higher-level class. Although he had excellent grades in the new class, he lived with the constant fear of falling back. Good grades were "the condition of his freedom." In the new class he developed OC symptoms. For a short time his symptoms diminished, until an incident when his father took him drinking at age 15 and to a house of prostitution. In his later teen years and into his early thirties he used alcohol and illicit drugs extensively "in part to try and fix his head." His early attempts with medication (Nardil, Zoloft) failed and included numerous side effects. Carl's Y-BOCS scores went from a 27 to a 12 over the 12 months, a 56% improvement. His group attendance was poor and his commitment outside was less than moderate.

Case History 7

Don was a single male (age 46) living on Social Security disability. His father was in the military. He was constantly changing schools, lived in a war zone, "all causing a lot of anxiety and insecurity." Don lived in an emotionally and physically abusive family. The father was an alcoholic (suspected of having OCD); his mother, who was angered by this, was "over controlling and demanding." Don's parents were both "withdrawn, depressive people and emotionally distant." He never felt that he bonded with his father or that he belonged in the family. His younger brother became an alcoholic and drug abuser. Don also suffered from chronic fatigue syndrome, attention deficit disorder, learning disabilities, social phobias, and depression exacerbated by seasonal changes. His OCD symptoms started during his preteen years. At the start of the study, his obsessions included: fear of harming himself, violent and horrific images coming up in his mind, fear of blurting out obscenities, concern with dirt, germs, bodily waste, environmental pollution, animal waste, sticky substances, illness due to contamination and getting others ill, perverse sexual thoughts, also including children, hoarding, religious obsessions, a need to know and remember, fear of not saying the right things, losing things, being bothered by certain sounds and words, somatic concern with illness and body parts. His compulsions included: excessive hand washing and showering, measures to prevent contamination, checking locks and appliances, checking tied to somatic obsessions, rereading and rewriting rituals, hoarding, list making, a need to tell, measures to prevent harm to others, and ritualized eating behaviors. Prior to the study, Don tried fluoxetine, sertraline, and clormipramine, three 11-week sessions of ERP, and biofeedback. Don entered the study stabilized on 10 mg of paroxetine, the most that he could tolerate. He was completely off paroxetine by 8.5 months. He had a Y-BOCS score of 27 (near-severe rating) that went to an 11 (mild) at the end of the study, a 59% improvement. Don was also practicing the yoga set (see Chapter 6) specific for treating chronic fatigue syndrome during the same 12-month period of the OCD study to help with this other disabling disorder. By the end of the study, he was able to walk for several hours without incurring any significant fatigue. He now had the energy and vitality of an average man his age. His extraordinary commitment to the therapies got him out of two vicious crises that definitely compounded each other. Two years after the trial, I ran into him on the street and asked him how he was doing. He said he no longer had OCD, ADD, depression, social phobias, learning disabilities, or CFS, but he still has a case of neurally mediated hypotension. I asked, "Do you still do Kundalini yoga?" He replied, "Yes, but only once a week, just to keep toned."

Case History 8

Gwen was a married female (age 40), who was employed as a systems analyst. She had one sister 15 years older and "grew up basically as an only child." When she was 4 years old, her sister married and left the house. Gwen's sister was the primary caregiver prior to leaving. Her parents both worked. Her vivid memories of her parents "were that they drank and fought a lot." "I was afraid and in emotional pain most of the time and I felt obligated to try to make things better. My job was to keep my dad from getting drunk. I never succeeded. I also tried to defend my dad from my mother's vicious words." Her mother had a preoccupation with getting killed and a fear of fire because her own mother (Gwen's grandmother) had died in a fire when she was 13. Gwen's mother was also very concerned about hurting others. "I (Gwen) was in pain (from fear of hurting others) even though I was careful and determined not to do or say anything wrong." Gwen's mother was always depressed (and possibly had OCD), and her father was an alcoholic. Between the ages of 17 and 31 Gwen abused drugs and alcohol, and at age 31 she checked herself into a 30-day drug and alcohol rehabilitation program. Her OCD may have started in childhood, and definitely by the age of 14, and was exacerbated by her depression. She also had BDD. She had been prescribed Elavil, Desyrel, Tofranil, Sinequan, Nardil, Xanax, Parnate, Librium, Tranxene, Zoloft, and eventually got relief from her depression—but not her OCD symptoms—with 80 mg of fluoxetine. At the start of the trial, she had been on fluoxetine for 7 years. Gwen's obsessions included: a fear of doing something embarrassing, harming others, something terrible happening, getting ill due to contaminants and spreading illness to others, a need to know, and excessive concern with body parts. Gwen's compulsions included: checking appliances, and that something bad did not happen, checking that she did not make mistakes, and rereading and rewriting rituals. Gwen's Y-BOCS score was a 21 when she began Kundalini yoga therapy and a 0 at 9 and 12 months.

Case History 9

Doreen was an unemployed married female (age 49) with two children living away from home. She had marital difficulties, and was "a constant worrier and procrastinator" with chronic insomnia. She was prescribed Klonopin after a one-night sleep-clinic evaluation due to suspected myoclonus. Doreen was not warned of the addictive properties and withdrawal symptoms of this drug and had a difficult time getting off the drug, with numerous side effects, including persistent sleep problems during the time of the study. She was the youngest of three children. Her father was ill most of her life and died when she was 13, and her mother had to struggle to support the family. Doreen had a lonely and unhappy childhood. Her OCD began in her adolescence. Doreen's obsessions included: a fear of doing something embarrassing; concern with dirt, environmental contaminants, household cleaners, animals, illness due to contaminants, and spreading illness; fears of sexual activities; hoarding; excessive concern with morality; a need to know; fear of saying certain things, losing things, being bothered by certain sounds; and an excessive concern with illness and body parts. Doreen's compulsions included: measures to prevent contact with contaminants, a range of checking activities, repeating rituals, hoarding, excessive list making, and a need to tell and confess. Her Y-BOCS score was 19 when she entered the study and a 0 at 9 and 12 months.

Case History 10

Danny was a married employed male (age 29) with two children. He came from a "chaotic and dysfunctional family" with an alcoholic father who had OCD. His alcoholic brother was hyperactive and possibly had OCD. His paternal grandfather was an alcoholic and his paternal grandmother was depressed. His OCD started when he was 5 years old. He tried clomipramine and fluoxetine and both exacerbated his OCD. At the age of 20 he attempted suicide as a result of his depression, poor grades, and drug abuse. Between the ages of 18 and 24 he drank heavily. He used cocaine and amphetamines between ages 20 and 23. Danny's obsessions included: violent and horrific images; concern with dirt and germs, sticky substances, and illness due to contamination; hoarding; symmetry and exactness with magical thinking; a need to know; a fear of saying certain things, losing things, intrusive nonviolent images and sounds; and obsessions with lucky and unlucky numbers. Danny's compulsions included: excessive hand washing, cleaning household items, checking locks, rereading and rewriting rituals, and repeating doorway entries/exits, counting, ordering, arranging, hoarding, excessive list making, mental rituals, and blinking rituals. When Danny entered the group, his Y-BOCS score was 25 and it dropped to 5 with a 0 on obsessions by the end of the study. He was a great champion of the "Vic-tor-y Breath" technique, performed extremely well in class with the entire protocol, and was nearly perfect in the group with the OCDB, but had very little discipline at home. He feared that his wife and daughters would object to his meditation practice due to their religious affiliation and views on yoga.

Case History 11

Jackie was a single female (age 26) on Social Security disability. She was raised in a dysfunctional family and abused and beaten by a sister, and raped at 14. Jackie also had anorexia nervosa and bulimia. Her OCD began at age 19. She tried the RRMM group for 2 of the first 3 weeks and quit because she was not getting any relief. She later joined the Kundalini yoga group after the groups merged and attended two of the first four meetings accompanied by a driver (who also brought her to the RRMM group). After two meetings, the driver was no longer able to bring her to therapy, and the attempt to drive herself was too difficult. Jackie also found that practicing at home by herself was too difficult. She frequently suffered OCD symptoms to the extent that she could not get out of her bedroom. Her obsessions included a fear of not saying the right thing and excessive concern with bodily appearance, and her greatest difficulty was with watching the time and scheduling. She could not change her routines or alter her driving patterns. "I can only drive where I have before without suffering great stress." This made it impossible for her to drive to therapy. She had ritualized showering routines, checking time, and eating behaviors. She wanted an education but was unable to attend school due to the driving-related obsessions and those related to time and scheduling. When she entered the Kundalini yoga group, her Y-BOCS score was 38. Jackie was the most extreme case to enter our study.

Case History 12

Dominique was in her second marriage (age 66) with one child and one stepchild, with part-time self-employment. She was "raised in an impoverished home." Her mother was "emotionally abusive to her, was never willing to help her, showed her no affection, and denied sex to the father." Dominique's mother was continuously insulting toward her, "like her worst enemy." The mother had OC symptoms of cleaning and hoarding and eating rituals. When Dominique and her younger brother would leave for school in the morning, the mother would regularly say, "You should get killed by a car," "You shouldn't live to come home." Her brother died of polio at age 19. Dominique eloped at 16, got pregnant, and was intentionally kicked in the stomach by her mother when her mother discovered her pregnancy. Her memories of her OCD symptoms go back to when she first moved out of the house, when she began to acquire things of her own to hoard. Hoarding was her only obsession and compulsion. Dominique's initial score was a 19 and at 3 months a 3; and for the 6-, 9-, and 12-month tests her score was a 0. She brought extraordinary commitment to her practice and stated at the end, "In this year I have seen myself and others transformed in life."

Case History 13

Mendy was a single female (age 30) attending college. Her parents were age 16 when she was born. They immediately placed her into foster care, where she lived in a series of homes until she was adopted at age 6 months. Mendy suffered mental, emotional, and physical abuse from her adoptive parents. She "always felt that something was wrong." Mendy hated herself by age 5, and at age 12 had the fear of hurting herself that would continue. She had been in and out of depression her entire life. Mendy's OCD symptoms "go back as far as I can remember." She tried fluoxetine, sertraline, and clormipramine. She was taking 375 mg of Effexor for 5 months prior to and during the study for her depression. Mendy's obsessions included: fear of harming self and others, violent and horrific images, acting on unwanted impulses, and that she would harm others because she was not careful; excessive contamination concerns with household items, animal matter, getting ill and others ill due to spreading contaminants; hoarding; symmetry and exactness with magical thinking; a need to know and remember; losing things; and obsessions with disease and body parts. Mendy's compulsions included: checking to not harm herself or others and that nothing terrible happened, rereading and rewriting rituals, hoarding, excessive list making, a need to tell, ask, and confess, and measures to prevent harm to herself, others, and terrible consequences. Mendy attended three of the first 10 sessions of the Kundalini yoga therapy and decided to drop out because she "did not believe that it could work for her." She was reluctant to practice at home out of "fear that her roommates would not approve of her odd practices [the yoga]." Her initial Y-BOCS score was a 27, a near-severe rating. When the study was over, she called to learn about the results and at that point remarked that she was very sorry that she had dropped out.

Case History 14

Ralph was a male adolescent (age 14). His parents divorced when he was 18 months and he was separated from his father except for monthly visitations, as the father lived at a significant distance. Ralph developed both OCD and Tourette's symptoms at age 11. He remained living with his mother until he was almost 14, where-upon he moved in with his father and stepmother after his mother no longer wanted him. Ralph had one older normal brother, the model son he could never be. His mother psychologically abused him with increasing negativity, criticism, and unusually high expectations, which Ralph was not capable of fulfilling. Ralph believed his OCD started when his mother forced him to wear used clothes from garage sales, even though they were wealthy. He was attending a special school for students with learning disabilities at the time of the study. Ralph was also diagnosed with attention-deficit/hyperactivity disorder and depression. His Tourette's syndrome included snorting, face touching, heel-to-buttocks kicking, and head-to-shoulder touching for which he was taking Haldol (2 mg), with minimal relief. His past medications included imipramine, Ritalin, and Anaphranil (125 mg) for 2 years for his OCD without satisfactory relief. He was stabilized on 40 mg of fluoxetine for 9 months prior to the study. Ralph's obsessions included: violent and horrific images; the fear of doing something embarrassing; a fear he would harm others if he was not careful and being responsible for something terrible happening; concerns with dirt and germs, household items, animal matter, sticky substances and illness due to contaminants; hoarding; symmetry and exactness; a need to know; a fear of not saying the right thing; intrusive nonviolent images and sounds; being bothered by certain sounds and numbers; superstitious fears; concern with illness and body dysmorphophobia. His compulsions included: excessive hand washing; showering and measures to prevent contact with contaminants; checking that he did not make a mistake; rituals of rereading, rewriting, counting, and hoarding; excessive list making; a need to tell or ask; and superstitious and self-damaging behaviors. After one session, Ralph told his stepmother he no longer wanted to participate in the group because he did not believe that the therapy would work, even though he had waited patiently for 4 months until he was old enough to enter this study (the minimum age requirement was 14). Ralph joined when the groups merged and the other female adolescent had already dropped out. She lasted 7 weeks until she realized she had extra homework to do (the meditation protocol) if she really wanted lasting results. She was beginning to benefit during the group practice even though she usually rebelled by coming to class with a sugar-loaded chocolate shake. She asked her parents (her father was a therapist and her mother a housewife) if she could leave the group. They said staying in the group was her choice. She opted to leave. As the only adolescent in the group at that time, Ralph felt very self-conscious, especially because of his Tourette's symptoms. His initial Y-BOCS score was a 32 (a severe rating).

This 11-part Kundalini yoga protocol for treating OCD can easily be taught to patients suffering from trichotillomania, BDD, or any other OC spectrum disorder, as well as generalized or acute anxiety, phobias, and the impulse-control and addictive disorders (eating and binging disorders, smoking, substance-abuse disorders, sexual obsessions). The patients in both trials also reported a parallel reduction or elimination of the OC spectrum disorders, in addition to anxiety, depression, and all other factors measured by the SCL-90-R and POMS. However, while this protocol would likely demonstrate efficacy with these disorders in independent trials, less complex, easier, and more disorder-specific protocols and techniques are likely to achieve greater compliance and perhaps greater success.

Treating GAD, ASD, Panic Disorders, and Phobias

While anxiety is a normal emotion, it is considered abnormal (sometimes called pathological or morbid anxiety) when it is either excessive for the current stressor, present in the absence of a stressor (free-floating anxiety), or leads to significant distress or disability (Nutt, 2005). In addition to OCD, the anxiety disorders include five main diagnostic subtypes: GAD, ASD, panic disorders, phobias, and PTSD. Included here are techniques and protocols for treating all five subtypes with the exception of PTSD, which is covered in Chapter 8.

Let's start here with the simplest approach to treating any of the anxiety disorders, with a technique that can be used "on the run" to help curb a mildly anxious mind resulting from a mental challenge the patient knows she will soon face. This may be a phone call, a meeting, a stage performance, or any other numerous possibilities that can provoke anxiety. In these situations, the individual would like to have a slight boost of mental energy and inner calm and clarity to better endure the coming moment. Here is where the technique called the "Vic-tor-y Breath" can be of use, and it was frequently the technique of choice employed successfully by my OCD patients. One of these OCD patients was a female executive who frequently had to give 6- to-8-minute talks to the public and she routinely relied on this technique for 2 to 3 minutes while sitting and waiting to face the crowd of several hundred people on each occasion. The "Vic-tor-y Breath" technique is described above in detail (see technique 9, page 78) as part of the 11-part OCD protocol. This technique was originally taught by Yogi Bhajan for "facing mental challenges." It seems too simple to be effective, but just a few breaths using this technique can sometimes be all that is required, and 3 to 5 minutes of proper use can yield a perfect result. It can be practiced anywhere and at anytime, and when a person has experience with it she can employ it without anyone else noticing. Its use does not require a slow deep breath, but can be employed by taking a short breath, filling the lungs about half full, and holding the breath for 3 to 4 seconds, and then exhaling and repeating. The eyes can remain open or closed.

All of the techniques described in this book, with the exception of the "Vic-tor-y Breath," are to be practiced after "tuning in," and this technique is described above (see technique 1, page 71). In addition, techniques 2 and 3 in the OCD protocol, called "spine flexes" and "shoulder shrugs," respectively, are excellent precursors to all of the other techniques listed below. Spine flexes and shoulder shrugs help to energize and improve one's attitude and ability to practice the other techniques. Usually when a patient is feeling highly anxious and needs to practice a technique for any of the anxiety disorders, she is least likely to be in a mood or mindset to practice, and these three precursors are very conducive to producing an enhanced mood and state of mind to engage any of the other techniques. They also help to amplify the benefits.

Treating Generalized Anxiety Disorder, or GAD

When seeing a client that comes without a specific disorder, the meditation technique that I most frequently teach is "When You Do Not Know What to Do" (Shannahoff-Khalsa, 2003; see page 102). The reason it is called this is because this technique can help prevent any anxiety-related disorder by helping the client induce a very quiet, still, peaceful, clear, and stable mind. This is an excellent technique that can be used for prevention or simply to reduce daily mental and emotional stress and strain. This is a relatively easy technique to learn. Eleven minutes of practice is a good starting time, and 31 minutes is the maximum amount of time for practice during one sitting. This technique will help a patient learn what it means to have a *very* quiet, clear, peaceful, and stable mind, a mind with very little chatter. The more the patient engages this state, the more they realize how much more quiet and peaceful and clear they can become. It is a progressive state that only improves with practice. A mind without chatter is a very useful mind. "When You Do Not Know What to Do" is an excellent and effective remedy for GAD, and can quickly help break the cycle of the "persistent and excessive anxiety and worry occurring more days than not for a period of at least 6 months," which is the definition of this disorder according to the American Psychiatric Association (1994). Not only will this technique quiet the mind, but the entire body will become deeply relaxed. If you want to "unwind," this technique is quick and has lasting effects. See the description of the technique below in the 6-Part Protocol for Acute Stress Disorder.

Treating Acute Stress Disorder, or ASD

According to the American Psychiatric Association, ASD is defined as "the development of characteristic anxiety, dissociative, and other symptoms that occurs within 1 month after exposure to an extreme traumatic stressor." Also, "either while experiencing the traumatic event or after the event, the individual has at least three of the following dissociative symptoms: a subjective sense of numbing, detachment, or absences of emotional responsiveness, a reduction in awareness of his or her surroundings, derealization, depersonalization, or dissociative amnesia." While ASD is very similar to PTSD, the key to the definition of ASD is the word "acute," and here the "disturbance lasts for at least 2 days and does not persist beyond 4 weeks after the traumatic event." In its early stages, ASD cannot be differentiated from PTSD, which lasts for longer periods, and frequently for life.

The treatment of ASD can be enhanced by any of the meditation techniques for anxiety. However, there is one called "Gan

Puttee Kriya" that is especially warranted due to the factors of numbing, derealization, dissociation, and so on, that require much deeper work on the subconscious mind. Gan Puttee Kriya is the first of seven techniques in a "7-part protocol for psycho-oncology" (Shannahoff-Khalsa, 2005). This technique (see the description on page 100 and in Chapter 8 for the 8-Part Protocol for PTSD) is also called the "Kriya to Make the Impossible Possible" (Bhajan, 1998b). Gan Puttee Kriya was known to yogis for eliminating the blocks formed in the subconscious mind that stifle growth and frequently lead to destructive, neurotic, and self-defeating patterns of mental activity. Yogis view the subconscious mind as the primary determinant for what habits are developed and how we react to the environment. More often than not, an "extreme traumatic event" is not fully processed in the conscious mind, and it leaves a lasting residue in the subconscious mind resulting in latent fears and anxiety.

Any of the meditation techniques in this book can be enhanced by first using a simple 3-minute technique called "Ganesha Meditation," which is useful for helping to focus the mind, enhance clarity, understanding, and intuition (Shannahoff-Khalsa, 2003).

The 6-Part Protocol for Treating Acute Stress Disorder[*]

Many of these techniques are also presented in the 11-part protocol on pages 71–80. I have repeated them here under the 6-part protocol for ease of reading.

1. Technique to Induce a Meditative State: "Tuning In"

Sit with a straight spine and with the feet flat on the floor, if sitting in a chair (see Figure 2.1). Put the hands together at the chest in prayer pose—the palms are pressed together with 10 to 15 pounds

[*] Copyright © David Shannahoff-Khalsa, 2005. No portion of this protocol may be reproduced without the express written permission of the author.

of pressure between the hands (this is only a mild to medium pressure; it is not intense). The sides of the thumbs touch and should rest on the sternum with the thumbs pointing up (along the sternum), and the fingers together and pointing up and out with a 60-degree angle to the ground. The eyes are closed and focused at the "third eye" (imagine a sun rising on the horizon or the equivalent of the point between the eyebrows at the origin of the nose). A mantra is chanted out loud in a 1½ breath cycle. Inhale first through the nose and chant "Ong Namo" with an equal emphasis on the "Ong" and the "Namo." Then immediately follow with a half-breath inhalation through the mouth and chant "Guru Dev Namo" with approximately equal emphasis on each word. The "o" in Ong and Namo are each a long "o" sound. "Dev" sounds like the name "Dave," with a long "a" sound. The practitioner should focus on the experience of the vibrations that these sounds create on the upper palate and throughout the cranium, while letting the mind be carried by the sounds into a new and pleasant mental space. This should be repeated a minimum of three times.

2. Spine-Flexing Technique for Vitality

This technique can be practiced while sitting either in a chair or on the floor in a cross-legged position. If you are in a chair, hold the knees with both hands for support and leverage. If you are sitting cross-legged, grasp the ankles in front with both hands. Begin by pulling the chest up and slightly forward, inhaling deeply at the same time. Then exhale as you relax the spine down into a slouching position. Keep the head up straight, as if you were looking forward, without allowing it to move much with the flexing action of the spine. This will help prevent a whip action of the cervical vertebrae. All breathing should only be through the nose for both the inhalation and exhalation. The eyes are closed as if you were looking at a central point on the horizon, the "third eye." Your mental focus is kept on the sound of the breath while listening to the fluid movement of the inhalation and exhalation. Begin the technique slowly while loosening up the spine. Eventually, a very rapid movement can be achieved with practice, reaching a rate of one to two times per second for the entire movement. A few minutes are adequate in the beginning. Later, there is no time limit. Food should be avoided just prior to this exercise. Be careful and flex the spine slowly in the beginning. Relax for 1 minute when finished.

3. Shoulder-Shrug Technique for Vitality

While keeping the spine straight, rest the hands on the knees if sitting in a cross-legged position, or with hands on the thighs if in a chair. Inhale and raise the shoulders toward the ears, then exhale, relaxing them down. All breathing is only through the nose. Eyes should be kept closed and focused at the "third eye." Mentally focus on the sound of the inhalation and exhalation. Continue this action rapidly, building to three times persecond for a maximum time of 2 minutes. This technique should not be practiced by individuals who are hyperactive.

4. Ganesha Meditation for Focus and Clarity*

Sit with a straight spine, with the eyes closed (see Figure 2.4). The left thumb and little finger are sticking out from the hand. The other fingers are curled into a fist with fingertips on the moon mound (the root of the thumb area that extends down to the wrist). The left hand and elbow are parallel to the floor, with the pad of the tip of the left thumb pressing on the curved notch of the nose between the eyes. The little finger is sticking out. With right hand and elbow parallel to the floor, grasp the left little finger with the right hand and close the right hand into a fist around it, so that both hands now extend straight out from your head. Push the notch with the tip of the left thumb to the extent that you feel some soreness as you breathe long and deep. After continued practice, this soreness reduces. Do this for 3 minutes and no longer. To

* This short, 3-minute technique was previously published in Shannahoff-Khalsa, 2003.

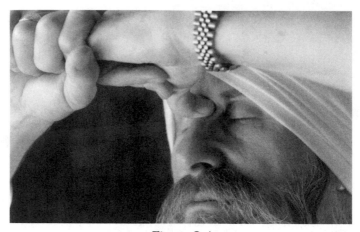

Figure 2.4
Ganesha Meditation

finish, keeping the posture with eyes closed, inhale. Push a little more and pull the naval point in by tightening the abdominal muscles for 10 seconds, then exhale. Repeat one more time.

5. Gan Puttee Kriya

Sit with a straight spine, either on the floor or in a chair. The back of your hands are resting on your knees with the palms facing upwards. The eyes are nine-tenths closed (one-tenth open, but looking straight ahead into the darkness, not the light below), focused at the "third eye." Chant from your heart in a natural, relaxed manner, or chant in a steady relaxed monotone. Chant out loud the sound "Sa" (the *a* sounds like "ah") and touch your thumb tips and index-finger tips together quickly and simultaneously with about 2 pounds of pressure. Then chant "Ta" and touch the thumb tips to the middle-finger tips. Then chant "Na" and touch the thumb tips to the ring-finger tips. Chant "Ma" and touch the thumb tips to the little-finger tips. Chant "Ra" and touch your thumb tips and index-finger tips. Chant "Ma" and touch the thumb tips to the middle-finger tips. Chant "Da" and touch the thumb tips to the ring-finger tips. Chant "Sa" and touch the thumb tips to the little-finger tips. Chant "Sa" and touch your thumb tips and index-finger tips. Chant "Say" (sounds like the word *say* with a long "a") and touch the thumb tips to the middle-finger tips. Chant "So" and touch the thumb tips to the ring-finger tips. Chant "Hung" and touch the thumb tips to the little-finger tips.

Chant at a rate of one sound per second. The thumb tip and finger tips touch with a very light, two to three pounds of pressure with each connection. This helps to consolidate the circuit created by each thumb-finger link. Start with 11 minutes and slowly work up to 31 minutes of practice. To finish, remain in the sitting posture and inhale, holding the breath for 20 to 30 seconds while you shake and move every part of your body. With the arms, stretch up over the head and especially allow the fingers to shake loose. Exhale and repeat this two more times to circulate the energy and to break the pattern of tapping, which effects the brain. Then immediately proceed without rest to technique 6, "When You Do Not Know What to Do."

The sounds used in this meditation are each unique, and they have a powerful effect on the mind, both the conscious and subconscious mind. The sound "Sa" gives the mind the ability to expand to the infinite. "Ta" gives the mind the ability to experience the totality of life. "Na" gives the mind the ability to conquer death. "Ma" gives the mind the ability to resurrect. "Ra" gives the mind the ability to expand in radiance (this sound purifies and ener-gizes). "Da" gives the mind the ability to establish security on the earth plane, provinding a ground for action. "Say" gives the totality of experience. "So" is the personal sense of identity, and "Hung" is the infinite as a vibrating and real force. Together, *So Hung* means "I am Thou." The unique qualities of this 12-syllable mantra help cleanse and restructure the subconscious mind and help heal the conscious mind to ultimately experience the superconsious mind. Thus, all the blocks that result from an extreme traumatic event are eliminated over time with the practice of Gan Puttee Kryia.

6. When You Do Not Know What to Do*

Sit straight, rest the back of one hand in the palm of the other with the thumbs crossing each other in one palm (see Figure 2.5). If the right hand rests in the palm of the left hand, the left thumb rests in the right palm and the right thumb then crosses over the back of the left thumb. Either this hand orientation is acceptable or the reverse, with the left hand resting in the palm of the right hand and then the right thumb is in the left palm covered by the left thumb. The hands are placed at heart-center level, about 2 inches in front of the chest, but the hands do not touch the chest, and the elbows are resting against the ribs. The eyes are open but focused on the tip of the nose (which you cannot actually see). The breathing pattern has four parts that repeat in sequence, first inhale and exhale slowly through the nose only, then inhale through the mouth with the lips puckered as if to kiss or make a whistle. After the inhalation, relax the lips and exhale through the mouth slowly, then inhale through the nose and exhale through the mouth. The last breath pattern is inhaling through the puckered lips and exhaling through the nose. Continue this 4-part cycle for 11 to 31 minutes.

If Gan Puttee Kriya is practiced without following with technique 6, the very last part requires a 1-minute focus with the eyes open and gazing on the tip of the nose, with slow, deep breathing. When practiced here followed immediately with "When You Do Not Know What to Do," this step can be eliminated, since this breath technique employs the use of the eyes open and focused on the tip of the nose.

Treating Panic Attacks

The simplest and most immediate solution to minimize or stop a panic attack is to employ the "Vic-tor-y Breath" described above.

* This technique was previously published in Bhajan, 1980; Shannahoff-Khalsa, 2003; and Shannahoff-Khalsa, 2004.

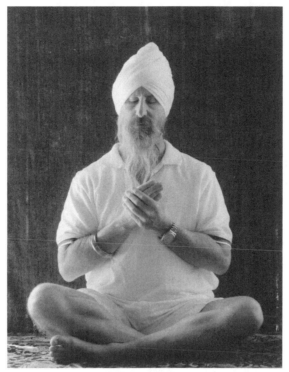

Figure 2.5
"When You Do Not Know What to Do"

All of the other techniques in this chapter will also help to curb the attack. However, the most effective strategy that I have found employs a technique that rebuilds what yogis call the "arcline," or what is also called the halo and relates to functions of the brain involving the frontal lobes and other regions. When a person's arcline is strong, they are much more resilient to trauma. In images of saints we see the halo highlighted by brightness. The halo is in effect a shield for the psyche. The stronger and brighter the shield, the better. When the arcline is weak, either through trauma, abuse, substance abuse, or other destructive habits, the mind can become subject to any kind of fear that can lead to a panic attack. The majority of people who I have treated for panic attacks complain about the loss of their ability to drive on the freeway. I have found the following meditation technique to be very useful for people suffering from either frequent panic attacks or intermittent attacks that are only induced by well-defined circumstantial events.

A Meditation to Rebuild the Arcline to Help Treat Panic Attacks

This technique has also been referred to as the "eight-stroke breath meditation" and was taught as a therapy to strengthen and rebuild the arcline (Bhajan, 1981).

Sit with a straight spine (see Figure 2.6). Extend the elbows out toward the sides and place the hands a few inches in front of the heart-center area of the chest. The two palms are about 4 inches apart, parallel to the ground. The left hand is on top and faces down, and the right hand is directly underneath the left hand, with the right palm facing up. The eyes are open and focused on the tip of the nose (the end you cannot see). Inhale only through the nose in eight equal strokes and exhale only through the nose in eight equal strokes. This means the breath is broken into 16 parts for one cycle, eight equal steps for the inhale and eight for the exhale. To help clarify this procedure, imagine taking in about one-eighth volume of the lungs for each step, consecutively adding one more eighth with each stroke of inhalation or exhalation. Try to start with small volumes so that you can reach eight strokes in and eight strokes out without filling the lungs prematurely. There is no pause once the inhale or exhale is complete. Simply continue breathing eight strokes in and eight strokes out. When breathing, do not count the steps (parts) but mentally employ the use of the mantra "Sa Ta Na Ma" twice for the inhale and twice for the exhale. That is, for each segment of the breath, mentally hear with your "inner ear" one of the four sounds in sequence, for example, "sa" with the first step, "ta" with the second, and so on, so that you go through two cycles of the mantra for the inhale and two cycles for the exhale. The time for this technique is only 11 minutes, no more or less. When finished, inhale deeply and hold the breath for 35 seconds while maintaining the hand posture, then exhale and relax. This technique can be practiced more than once a day and is best practiced everyday until the

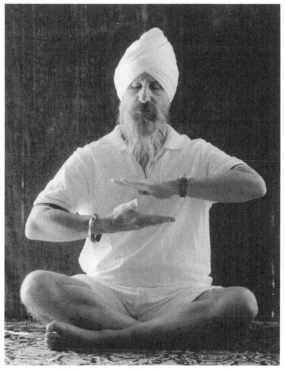

Figure 2.6
Rebuilding the Arcline

panic attacks have subsided. Most of my patients completely over-come their panic attacks within 3 to 5 weeks with daily practice. Some patients have also included the Ganesha Meditation (see above for the 6-Part Protocol for Treating Acute Stress Disorder). A few have also included Gan Puttee Kriya, as well as technique 7 in the OCD protocol to help manage fears (see page 76). Usually the more techniques the patient includes, the quicker the results.

Treating Phobias

Social phobias are now also called "social anxiety disorders" and are believed to have a lifetime prevalence rate of 14% in the United

States (Kessler, Stein, & Bergland, 1998). They begin early in life and rarely remit (Davidson, Hughes, George, & Blazer, et al., 1993) and consist of the generalized and nongeneralized social phobias, where the generalized form is considered more severe (Brown, Heimberg, & Justa, 1995). A study of the generalized social phobia in an HMO showed an 8% prevalence rate (Katzelnick, Kobak, DeLeire, Henk, Greist, et al., 2001). Social phobias are difficult to treat but are responsive to both medication and CBT. A recent 14-week placebo-controlled RCT comparing fluoxetine and CBT, or both, in 295 patients randomized to one of five groups (drug, CBT, drug and CBT, CBT and placebo, or placebo) showed that all active treatments were superior to placebo, but combined treatment did not add any further advantage, and many patients remained symptomatic after the 14 weeks of therapy with fluoxetine ranging in doses from 40 mg to 60 mg, and CBT administered weekly in groups that combined in vivo exposure, cognitive restructuring, and social skills training (Davidson, Foa, Huppert, Keefe, Franklin, et al., 2004). This study may represent the state of the art for conventional therapies. They report the following improvement rates for one of their primary outcome measures (Clinical Global Impression Scale): for drug alone 50.9%, CBT 51.7%, drug + CBT 54.2%, CBT + placebo 50.8%, and for placebo alone 31.7% (Davidson et al., 2004).

Two Kundalini medication techniques are included here for the treatment of phobias. The first is a relatively simple one and can be learned and practiced quickly, and it is very useful for social phobias that have resulted in part from an interaction with another person. The second is difficult but can work for all phobias. Note, the technique for treating addictions in Chapter 4 is also applicable to phobias. In addition, there is a technique in the OCD protocol to help manage fears that would also be applicable. The idea here is not just to reduce the momentary anxiety, but to eliminate the causal underlying factors that are rooted in the psyche.

A Meditation for Removing Haunting Thoughts

"This meditation can cure phobias, fears, and neuroses. It can remove unsettling thoughts from the past that surface into the present. And it can take difficult situations in the present and release them. All of this can be done in forty seconds!" (Yogi Bhajan, personal communication). This technique was first published in 2004 (Shannahoff-Khalsa, 2004). In addition, it is very useful for patients with PTSD who have been the victim of rape, incest, or physical torment. There are 10 steps:

1. Lower the eyelids until the eyes are only open one tenth. Start by mentally concentrating on the tip of the nose. Then silently say "Wha Hay Guru" in the following manner: "Wha" while mentally focusing on the right eye; "Hay" while mentally focusing on the left eye; "Guru" while mentally focusing on the tip of the nose.
2. Remember the encounter or incident that happened to you.
3. Mentally say "Wha Hay Guru" as in number 1.
4. Visualize and personify the actual feelings of the encounter.
5. Again repeat "Wha Hay Guru" as in number 1.
6. Reverse the roles in the encounter you are remembering. Become the other person and experience that perspective.
7. Again repeat "Wha Hay Guru" as in number 1.
8. Forgive the other person and forgive yourself.
9. Repeat "Wha Hay Guru" as in number 1.
10. Let go of the incident and release it to the universe. These are 10 steps to peace.

"Tershula Kriya": An Advanced Technique for Overcoming Phobias

Yogis taught this technique in ancient times for "achieving self-mastery and learning to heal others at a distance" (Shannahoff-Khalsa, 2004), and it is one of the most advanced techniques in the system of Kundalini yoga. It was first taught by Yogi Bhajan in August 1989. "Tershula Kriya can make you into a perfect master" (Bhajan, personal communication). While it presents a challenge for learning, its benefits go far beyond the amelioration of phobias.

Sit in an easy pose (see Figures 2.7 and 2.8). Bring your elbows next to the ribs, forearms extended in front of you, with the hands in front of the heart, right over left, palms up. The hands are approximately 10 degrees higher than the elbows. There is no bend in the wrists; fingertips to elbows forms a straight line. The thumbs are extended out to the side of the hands, the fingertips and palms do not exactly line up but are slightly offset. The eyes are closed looking at the backs of the eyelids. For the inhale, pull back on the navel and inhale through the nostrils and hold. Mentally repeat the mantra "Har Har Wha Hay Guru" as long as you are able to retain the breath. While you are doing this, visualize your hands surrounded by white light. For the exhale, exhale through the nostrils and as you exhale, visualize lightning shooting out from your finger tips. When you have fully exhaled, pull in *mulbhand* (tightening the muscles in the area of the rectum, sex organs, and navel), and hold for as long as you can, again mentally repeating the mantra "Har Har Wha Hay Guru." The maximum time for this technique is 62 minutes.

It has been suggested that this meditation be done in a cool room or at night when the temperature is cooler, because it stimulates the Kundalini directly and generates a great deal of heat in the body. The word *Tershula* relates to the thunderbolt of Shiva, the ultimate deliverer. "Tershula can heal everything. It is a self-healing process. This meditation is for the gunas. It brings the three nervous systems together. It also gives you the ability to heal at a distance, through your touch or through your projection. Many psychological disorders or imbalances in the personality can be cured through practice of this meditation. It is very helpful in getting rid of phobias and especially the 'father phobia'" (Bhajan & Khalsa, 1998; Shannahoff–Khalsa, 2004).

The 20-year-old woman described in "Other Disorders Commonly Occurring with OCD" had a social anxiety disorder, BDD, and OCD for which she used the 11-part OCD protocol. Her self-report describes how she achieved rapid short-term relief and long-term benefit for her social phobia (Shannahoff-Khalsa,

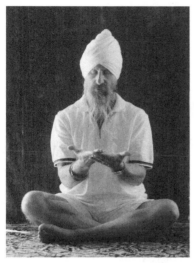
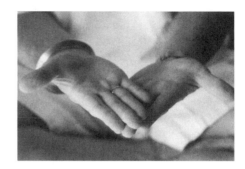

Figures 2.7 and 2.8
"Tershula Kriya"

2003). There are indeed a variety of techniques and protocols that could be constructed to treat social phobias, and frequently, patients present with depression and/or other disorders. Most likely, each individual will benefit more from one combination of techniques than another individual. Much also depends on the severity of symptoms, the patient's will to commit, and his or her physical ability to work for long-term benefits. The techniques presented in this chapter have the potential to yield highly effective and rapid results.

If there is any question about a need for newer, fast acting, and more effective approaches for treating the anxiety disorders without side effects, the following "Editor's Desk" quote from the editor in chief of *CNS Spectrums*, Jack M. Gorman, MD, typifies much of how conventional medical care is practiced in Western countries today.

A friend of mine recently told me a telling analogy concerning benzodiazepines (BZs). I am not sure if he wants to be publicly acknowledged for his quip. He said, "Prescribing benzodiazepines is like watching pornography. If you ask a person at random if he watches pornography, he will vehemently deny it, but someone must be because it is a billion dollar a year business. Similarly, if you ask a physician if he prescribes Valium or Xanax or Ativan [forgive my uncharacteristic use of brand names, but the story loses its impact otherwise], he or she will say of course not, what sensible doctor would prescribe those addicting drugs. Yet, like pornography, benzodiazepine prescriptions generate billions of dollars of revenue around the world, so somebody must be prescribing them. (Gorman, 2005).

Ator noted, "BZs went from safe and effective to addicting and dangerous" (2005). Now many physicians prescribe the serotonin reuptake inhibitors in place of the BZs for the anxiety disorders, though they lack the fast-acting benefits of the BZs (Gorman, 2005).

THREE

Treating the Major Depressive Disorders, Grief, and Bipolar Disorders

A "major depressive disorder (MDD) is characterized by one or more major depressive episodes (that is, at least two weeks of depressed mood or loss of interest accompanied by at least four additional symptoms of depression)" (APA, 1994). And the "additional symptoms of depression can include changes in appetite or weight, sleep, and psychomotor activity; decreased energy; feelings of worthlessness or guilt; difficulty thinking, concentrating, or making decisions; or recurrent thoughts of death or suicidal ideation, plans, or attempts" (APA, 1994). And the major depressive episode must be "accompanied by clinically significant distress or impairment in social, occupational, or other important areas of functioning" (APA, 1994).

The importance of the age of onset, and thus when care may be most appropriate, is clearly the pre-adulthood stage, with the major peaks of onset across the lifetime occurring at 13 to 18 years of age (Zisook, Rush, Albala, Alpent, Balasubramani, et al., 2004). One study looking at "nonpsychotic MDD suggests that MDD that begins before age 18 has a distinct set of demographic (female gender) and clinical correlates (longer duration of illness; longer current episodes; more episodes; more suicidality; greater symptom severity; more psychiatric symptoms associated with

Axis I comorbidity; and more sadness, irritability, agitation, and atypical symptom features), and it appears associated with significant psychosocial consequences (lower educational attainment and marriage rates). Thus, pre-adulthood onset MDD is a particularly severe and chronic condition" (Zisook et al., 2004).

When ranking depression in general, it is considered to be the world's fourth most prevalent health problem (Schulberg, Katon, Simon, & Rush, et al., 1999), and according to the World Health Organization, the leading causes of years of life lived with disability in all ages (WHO, 2001). MDD affects more than 16% of adults in the United States during their lifetime (Kessler, Berglund, Demler, Jin, Koreta, et al., 2003) and costs the U.S. anywhere between $30 to $50 billion in lost productivity and direct medical costs each year (Greenberg, Finkelstein, & Berndt, et al., 1995; Rice & Miller, 1998; Robinson, Geske, Prest, & Barnacle, 2005). Depressed people miss work at twice the rate of the general population (Von Korff, Katon, Unutzer, Wells, & Wagner, et al., 2001), and they also use nonspecialized medical care 50% to 100% more often (Henk, Katzelnick, Kobak, Greist, & Jefferson, et al., 1996). It is also known that primary-care providers are the sole contacts for more than 50% of patients with mental illness and have thus been described as the de facto system of treatment for mental health in this country (Regier, Goldberg, & Taube, et al., 1978; Robinson et al., 2005). Family Medicine and General Internal Medicine physicians recommend treatment for depression with pharmacotherapy as the most widely used intervention (51.9%) and psychotherapy as the least frequently used approach at 4%, and the combination at 27.3%, with counselor-recommended pharmacotherapy at 9.2% and "other" at 7.0% (Robinson et al., 2005).

Now the most common pharmacological approach includes the second-generation antidepressants (primarily the selective serotonin and selective norepinephrine reuptake inhibitors). A very recent meta-analysis of 46 head-to-head RCTs concludes that "88% of comparative efficacy studies reported no statistically significant differences in any outcome measure at the end of the study, but the adverse event profiles differed among drugs; however, the degree and quality of adverse events varied and only 13% of trials used a standardized scale to assess adverse events" (Hansen, Gartlehner, Lohr, Gaynes, & Carey, et al., 2005). They further conclude, "Overall, second-generation antidepressants probably do not differ substantially for the treatment of MDD and choosing the agent that is most appropriate for a given patient is difficult" (Hansen et al., 2005). This same meta-analysis states that the clinical response occurred 4 to 6 weeks after the start of therapy and most trials reported no difference among SSRIs in the speed of patient response.

In addition, according to a 2000 Cochrane Database Systematic Review of 98 studies of the efficacy of SSRIs and related drugs with comparator antidepressants with 5,044 patients treated with an SSRI or related drug, and 4,510 treated with an alternative antidepressant, "There are no clinically significant differences in effectiveness between SSRIs and tricyclic antidepressants. Treatment decisions need to be based on considerations of relative patient acceptability, toxicity and cost" (Geddes, Freemantle, Mason, Eccles, & Boynton, 2000). Another systematic review of medication treatment for MDD concludes "newer antidepressants are clearly effective in treating depressive disorders in diverse settings. Because of similar efficacy, both newer and older antidepressants should be considered when making treatment decisions. Better information is urgently needed on the efficacy of newer antidepressants in patients with nonmajor depression and in special populations, including adolescents" (Williams, Mulrow, Chiquette, Noel, Aguilar, et al., 2000). In respect to efficacy, this same review concludes, "Overall, 51% of patients randomly assigned to active treatment and 32% of those who received placebo experienced at least a 50% improvement in depressive symptoms" and "comparisons within individual classes of newer and older antidepressants showed no significant differences" (Williams et al., 2000). However, when treatment response is defined as a 50% improvement on a depression scale, and this definition of improvement has been the subject of increasing discussion, "there is a problem with definition in that treatment responders may still be considerably ill at the end of treatment, in fact treatment responders might still meet the criteria for the treatment trial in which they were judged to be responders" (Zimmerman, Chelminski, & Posternak, 2004).

In a recent review of five RCTs that utilized different forms of yoga intervention, where the severity of the condition ranged from mild to severe, all trials reported positive results but methodological details such as method of randomization, compliance, and attrition rates were missing (Pilkington, Kirkwood, Rampes, & Richardson, 2005).

There are a number of simple and useful Kundalini yoga meditation techniques to treat the occasional episodes of depression that we all eventually encounter in our lives. Some of these same techniques can be used to help prevent the onset of depression, or the possible downward spiral that frequently leads to MDD. If early warning signs are recognized, prevention with these techniques is the most effective strategy and the most rewarding, since the benefits of these techniques not only ameliorate the symptoms when used but also lead to a highly clear, functional, and focused state of mind. Here I present a protocol that I have used with many patients presenting with depression.

The 6-Part Protocol for Treating Major Depressive Disorders[*]

1. Technique to Induce a Meditative State: "Tuning In"

Sit with a straight spine and with the feet flat on the floor if sitting in a chair (see Figure 2.1, page 72). Put the hands together at the chest in "prayer pose"—the palms are pressed together with 10

---

[*] Copyright © David Shannahoff-Khalsa, 2005. No portion of this protocol may be reproduced without the express written permission of the author.

to 15 pounds of pressure between the hands (a mild to medium pressure, nothing too intense). The area where the sides of the thumbs touch rests on the sternum with the thumbs pointing up (along the sternum), and the fingers are together and point up and out at a 60-degree angle to the ground. The eyes are closed and focused on the third eye (imagine a sun rising on the horizon, or the equivalent of the point between the eyebrows at the origin of the nose). A mantra is chanted out loud in a 1½-breath cycle. Inhale first through the nose and chant "Ong Namo" with an equal emphasis on the Ong and the Namo. Then immediately follow with a half-breath inhalation through the mouth and chant "Guru Dev Namo" with approximately equal emphasis on each word. (The O in *Ong* and *Namo* are each a long "o" sound; *Dev* sounds like *Dave*, with a long "a" sound.) The practitioner should focus on the experience of the vibrations these sounds create on the upper palate and throughout the cranium while letting the mind be carried by the sounds into a new and pleasant mental space. This should be repeated a minimum of three times. We employed it in our group about 10–12 times. This technique helps to create a "meditative state of mind" and is *always* used as a precursor to the other techniques.

2. Spine-Flexing Technique for Vitality

This technique can be practiced while sitting either in a chair or on the floor in a cross-legged position. If you are in a chair, hold the knees with both hands for support and leverage. If you are sitting cross-legged, grasp the ankles in front with both hands. Begin by pulling the chest up and slightly forward, inhaling deeply through the nose at the same time. Then exhale as you relax the spine down into a slouching position. Keep the head up straight, as if you were looking forward, without allowing it to move much while flexing the spine. This will help prevent a whip effect in the cervical verte-brae. All breathing should only be through the nose for both the inhalation and exhalation. The eyes are closed as if you were looking at a central point on the horizon, the third eye. Your mental focus is kept on the sound of the breath while listening to the fluid movement of the inhalation and exhalation. Begin the technique slowly while loosening up the spine. Eventually, a very rapid movement can be achieved with practice, reaching a rate of one to two times per second for the entire movement. A few minutes are adequate in the beginning. Later, there is no time limit. Food should be avoided just prior to this exercise. Be careful and flex the spine slowly in the beginning. Relax for 1 minute when finished.

3. Shoulder-Shrug Technique for Vitality

While keeping the spine straight, rest the hands on the knees if sitting in a cross-legged position or with hands on the thighs if sitting in a chair. Inhale and raise the shoulders toward the ears, then exhale, relaxing them down. All breathing is done only through the nose. Eyes should be kept closed and focused on the third eye. Mentally focus on the sound of the inhalation and exhalation. Continue this action rapidly, building to three times per second for a *maximum* of 2 minutes. This technique should not be practiced by individuals who are hyperactive.

4. Ganesha Meditation for Focus and Clarity

Sit with a straight spine, with the eyes closed (see Figure 2.4, page 106). The left thumb and little finger are sticking out from the hand. The other fingers are curled into a fist with fingertips on the moon mound (the root of the thumb area that extends down to the wrist). The left hand and elbow are parallel to the floor, with the pad of the tip of the left thumb pressing on the curved notch of the nose between the eyes. The little finger is sticking out. With right hand and elbow parallel to the floor, grasp the left little finger with the right hand and close the right hand into a fist around it, so that both hands now extend straight out from your head. Push the notch with the tip of the left thumb to the extent that you feel some soreness as you breathe long and deep. After continued practice, this soreness reduces. Do this for 3 minutes and no longer. To finish, keeping the posture with eyes closed, inhale. Push for about 10 seconds and pull the naval point in by tightening the abdominal muscles, then exhale. Repeat one more time.

5. Technique for Fighting Brain Fatigue

This technique was originally taught by Yogi Bhajan on March 27, 1995 (Bhajan, 2000), and was later published in the scientific literature (Shannahoff-Khalsa, 2004). This technique has been used to help prevent depression and to treat depression. When practiced correctly, it can be a powerful antidote to this disorder, especially if combined with the three previous techniques and the one following in the protocol.

Part 1. Sit with a straight spine either in a chair or on the floor with your elbows bent and your upper arms near your rib cage (see Figure 3.1). Your forearms point straight out in front of your body, parallel to the floor. The right palm faces downward and the left palm faces upward. Breathing through your nose, inhale and exhale in eight equal parts. On each part or stroke of the breath, alternate moving either hand up and down, one hand moving up as the other moves down. The movement of the hands is slight, approximately 6 to 8 inches, as if you are bouncing a ball. Breathe powerfully. Continue for 3 minutes and then change the hand position so that the left palm faces downward and the right palm faces upward. Continue for another 3 minutes and then change the hand position again so that the right palm faces downward and the left palm faces upward for the last 3 minutes. (The total time is 9 minutes.)

Part 2. Begin slow and deep breathing (again only through the nose), stopping the movement and relaxing the hands in the lap. Close your eyes and visually focus your eyes on the center point of the chin. This requires pulling the eyes downward. Keep the body perfectly still and set the intention that the body should heal itself. Keep the mind quiet, stilling all thoughts. (The total time for this part is 5.5 minutes.)

To finish, inhale deeply, then hold your breath, making your hands into fists and pressing the fists strongly against the chest for 15 seconds. Exhale. Inhale deeply again and hold your breath, this time pressing both fists against the navel point for 15 seconds. Exhale. Inhale again then hold the breath. Bend your elbows and bring your fists near your shoulders, pressing your arms strongly against your rib cage for 15 seconds. Exhale as if you are using the upper arms to crush the chest. Now relax. "This exercise balances the diaphragm and fights brain fatigue. It renews the blood supply to the brain and moves the serum in the spine. It also benefits the liver, navel point, spleen, and lymphatic system" (Bhajan, 2000).

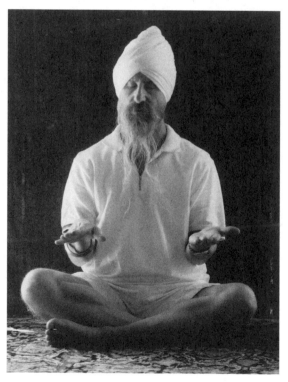

Figure 3.1
Technique for Fighting Brain Fatigue

6. Meditation to Balance the Jupiter and Saturn Energies:
A Technique Useful for Treating Depression, Focusing the Mind,
and Eliminating Self-Destructive Behavior*

Sit with a straight spine either in a chair or on the floor (see Figure 3.2). The hands are facing forward with the ends of the Jupiter (index) and Saturn (middle) fingers pointing straight up near the sides of the body at the level of the earlobes. The elbows are relaxed down by the sides and the hands are near the shoulders. Close the ring and little fingers down into the palm using the thumbs and keep them there against the palm during the meditation. The Jupiter (index) finger and the Saturn (middle) finger are spread open in a V shape (or closed). The eyes are closed. For 8 minutes open and close the Jupiter and Saturn fingers about once or twice per second. Make sure they spread completely open and close completely during the exercise. Simultaneously imagine the planets of Jupiter and Saturn coming together in front of you and then again going apart in synch with the finger movement—the planets should appear to go back and forth along a straight line in and out to the sides in front of you. It does not matter whether you have Jupiter or Saturn on the left or right side. Continue this imagery movement for 8 minutes along with the fingers opening and closing. (In the beginning, the imaging is difficult to do but this should not slow down the pace of the fingers, which play a more important role here.) After 8 minutes, while continuing the same exercise, now begin to inhale and exhale through the nose only with the movement (inhale as the fingers are spread, exhale as the fingers close). Continue with the planets. Continue this part for 2 additional minutes. Then, for the last minute, spread the two fingers wide and hold them wide apart (now they do not open and close, they remain in the fixed V shape), keeping them very stiff

---

* This technique was previously published as an individual technique for treating depression (Shannahoff-Khalsa, 2003, 2004), and was originally taught by Yogi Bhajan in a lecture on December 12, 1995.

(which requires considerable effort) while also keeping the mouth in an O, or ring, shape. Breathe in and out of the mouth using only the diaphragm (not the wall of the upper chest) with a rate of one to three breaths per second. After 1 minute, inhale, hold the breath in, and tense every muscle tightly (including the hands, fingers, with the "v" kept rigid, arms, back, stomach) in the body for 10 seconds. Exhale and repeat twice for 10 seconds. Then relax.

Yogi Bhajan said that "this meditation will help increase a person's ability to focus and concentrate and also increase the IQ of an individual over several months of practice. The mind becomes very focused and clear, the brain becomes very energized.

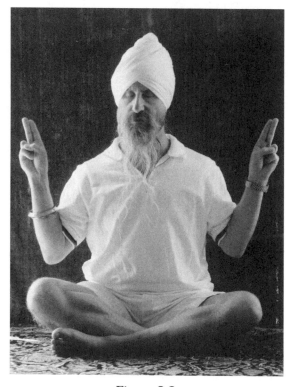

Figure 3.2
Meditation to Balance the Jupiter and Saturn Energies:
A Technique to Reduce Depression and Self-Destructive Behavior

This technique will also help eliminate depression. This technique can also enhance math skills for those who have difficulties with math. The Jupiter and Saturn energies become balanced (the brain is balanced) and this allows one to overcome any challenge, including mastery of the self. This technique also helps to eliminate self-destructive behavior and undesirable (acting out) behavior toward others. In addition, during the beginning of the technique, around the 4- to 8-minute mark, a person can feel very irritable and sometimes it can bring out deep-seated anger" (Bhajan, 1995). Note: If a person feels dizzy during the meditation, they should stop and try it again on another occasion.

I have used this same protocol with many patients who complain of depression, and when they do the whole protocol, or even the first five parts or less, many quickly develop a big smile on their faces and a sincere look of appreciation.

The following is a single but representative case study of a woman patient using this 6-part protocol. Rajinder, age 26, came to me complaining of depression. She was visiting from Europe and working on her doctoral dissertation. She said, "I can't focus my mind, I am finding it nearly impossible to motivate myself to work, and I have a deadline in 2 months to finish this work before returning to Europe. I am also having problems sleeping and I am going to bed at 3 to 4 A.M. and getting up at noon. I am accomplishing almost nothing in the office. Most of the time I just sit at my desk and ruminate. On top of that, my energy sucks and even coffee isn't helping much. This sluggish nature and my depressed mood leave me with thoughts of suicide." Rajinder had an 8-year intermittent history of MDD on and off medication(s), a brother who committed suicide, and a family that could not accept her views on how to live her life. Both parents frequently told her to give up her education and get married and have children. This parental aggravation was the major reason she came to the U.S. The first time I taught her this 40-minute protocol, she realized that she did not have to surrender to her depression and that her life could have meaning and purpose again. She regained the hope of completing her work on time. Her mind was clear, focused, and she felt energetic, positive, and normal again, claiming, "I can't remember the last time I felt this good." In follow-up, she found it necessary to practice at least once every other day or she would regress. However, her rut was never as deep again. She knew she had a solution. Rajinder's condition was a case of moderately severe MDD, and the circumstances of her life are not atypical among young adults today. She remains a member of the working world and now continues both her own practice once or twice a week and attends weekly yoga classes. She says she feels now that her circumstances and challenges in life are not too complicated. She is gainfully employed and living independently. (Other cases of depression, along with other axis I and II disorders, are presented in later chapters.)

Treating Grief

Many individuals suffer from grief. Yogis claim that grief, anger, and anxiety are major factors in the onset of a wide range of diseases (Shannahoff-Khalsa, 2004). The technique described here is effective by itself, but will yield even more effective results when practiced with techniques 2 through 4 listed in the 6-Part Protocol for Treating Major Depressive Disorders. The first technique, called "Tuning In," is essential here.

Meditation for Treating Grief*

There are three separate parts to this technique to maximize overall benefits; however, part 1 can be done alone. The suggested music for each part is optional, though the benefits of the music will only add to the therapeutic value.

* This technique was previously published in Shannahoff-Khalsa, 2004.

Part 1: Siddh Shiva. "Whenever you have grief, do this exercise. It gets rid of centuries-old grief" (Bhajan, 1990). In position A (Figure 3.3), sit with a straight spine in a cross-legged position. The eyes are wide open (do not meditate). The elbows are bent by the sides, and the upper arms are kept by the sides. The forearms are parallel to the ground just above each leg, with the palms open and facing up and placed about 6 inches above the knees.

In position B (see Figure 3.4), raise the arms up so the hands quickly bounce up to the shoulders. As you do this, the tongue sticks out as far as possible (this is important because it affects the subconscious mind and helps get rid of the grief). Then return to position A. The tongue goes back into the mouth, the mouth closes, and the arms go back down to the position above the legs. Do this powerfully with the breath. Inhale through the nose as you go into position A and exhale through the mouth as you go into position B. Breathe heavily and practice this movement at a rate of two times per second. Listen to the song "Se Saraswati" by Nirinjan Kaur and Guru Prem Singh (available at the Ancient Healing Ways web site, www.a-healing.com). Do this technique for 7 minutes total. To end, inhale and hold the breath in and press the tongue against the upper palate as hard as you can for 20 seconds. Exhale. Repeat this tongue process two more times (three times total), then relax for 3 minutes.

Part 2. A second technique here is optional (taught as a companion technique by Yogi Bhajan on May 17, 1990). This exercise helps to create an inner balance that then helps to further induce healing.

Stretch the arms up over the head, elbows straight, palms very flat and stiff, facing forward with the fingers together and the thumbs extended stiffly to the sides of the hands. Begin moving the left arm in a clockwise circle overhead and over the left side of the body. Move the right arm in a counterclockwise direction overhead and over the right side of the body. The movements of the two arms do not seem to be related in any fashion. One arm gets into a certain rhythm of a circular movement while the other arm does the same.

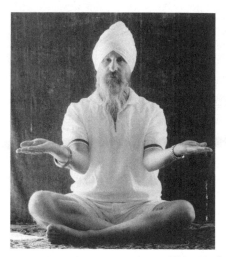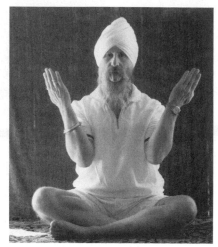

Figures 3.3 and 3.4
Meditation for Treating Grief

(Note: You can reverse directions if you wish.) The song "Heal Me" by Nirinjan Kaur is played (available at the Ancient Healing Ways web site, www.a-healing.com). Do this for 11 minutes and then rest for 5 minutes. Bhajan said, "The idea of the movement is that the armpits get stimulated, so make the movement of the arms just an extension of the movement of the armpits and the sides of the rib cage. Usually we condemn ourselves and we have to feel guilty to be happy. This completely breaks through that" (1990).

Part 3. The third part of this exercise is to combine the breath of life (prana) and to help balance the ida and pingala, the major left and right meridians of the body, respectively. Begin by inhaling through the left nostril by blocking the right nostril with the right thumb, then exhale only through the right nostril by blocking the left nostril with the right index finger, continuing with this pattern for 3 minutes (do not reverse nostrils). Then, firmly grasp the knees by placing the palms flat down on top of them. Begin swaying your body forward approximately one foot and then backward approximately one foot in a rhythmic fashion. The grip of the hands should be so firm that it keeps you from tilting over when you go backward. Keep your spine "tight" while doing the exercise.

Play the song "Humee Hum Tumee Tum" by Livtar Singh (available at the Ancient Healing Ways web site, www.a-healing.com). Do this technique for 3 minutes. To end, inhale deeply and tighten the whole body, then shake the body as much as possible. Do this five times total, holding the breath approximately 20 seconds the first time and 15 seconds the other four times. "It is said that this posture increases the circulation in the area of the breasts for females so they will not develop breast cancer. It will develop your automatic concentration, so you can concentrate whenever you want. It will also help expel the dead cells out of the physical body" (Bhajan, 1990).

Treating Bipolar Disorders

There are two major types of bipolar disorders, where type I is characterized by one or more manic or mixed episodes usually accompanied by a major depressive episode, and type II is characterized by one or more major depressive episodes accompanied by at least one hypomanic episode (APA, 1994). The type I form affects at least 1% of the U.S. adult population (Regier, Farmer, Rae, Locke, Keith, Judd, et al., 1990), and is considered to be among the world's greatest public health problems (Murray & Lopez, 1996a). The *Diagnostic and Statistical Manual of Mental Disorders*, fourth edition (*DSM-IV*), defines a manic episode as a persistently elevated, expansive, or irritable mood, plus at least four characteristic signs and symptoms (racing thoughts, diminished need for sleep, grandiose or overvalued ideas, and poor judgment), that last for at least 1 week (APA, 1994).

The first episode of bipolar disorder occurs early in life for the majority of patients, usually before the age of 30 (Goodwin & Jamison, 1990). The younger the patient at the first onset of the manic episode, the more severe the illness tends to be throughout life, and the greater the chance of psychotic features and the poorer the response to therapy (Goodwin & Jamison, 1990).

However, the depressive phase is the most vexing phase of the disorder for patients and clinicians alike. Three different studies have recently documented that depression is by far the more problematic state and that people with bipolar disorder spend up to 33% of their adult lives depressed (Judd, Akiskal, Schettler, Endicott, Maser, et al., 2002; Kupfer, Frank, Grochocinski, Cluss, Houck, et al., 2002; Hirschfeld, Calabrese, Weissman, Reed, Davies, et al., 2003). While Kraepelin once described manic depressive insanity to be a "good prognosis" illness (1921), today we know the majority of people with bipolar disorders struggle with a highly recurrent and potentially disabling condition (Sachs & Thase, 2000). In addition, it is well known that bipolar disorder patients have a 60% lifetime prevalence risk of co-morbid substance abuse disorders (Regier et al., 1990), which lead to a higher risk of suicide and other problems (Dalton, Cate-Carter, Mundo, Parikh, & Kennedy, 2003). The reason that substance abuse and substance dependence occur more frequently with bipolar patients has been the substance of debate. Some evidence suggests the reason for this highly linked condition is that a subgroup of patients in whom substance abuse occurred prior to the bipolar condition results in the disorder due to behavioral sensitization and/or kindling mechanisms (Sonne, Brady, & Morton, 1994). And indeed, clinical data suggest that this subgroup is relatively common and that many patients abuse substances before the onset of affective illness (Tsai, Chen, Kuo, Lee, Lee, et al., 2001). It also turns out that bipolar patients with co-occurring substance abuse may have lower family rates of mood disorders (DelBello, Strakowski, Sax, McElroy, Keck, et al., 1999), which suggests that perhaps substance abuse does help precipitate bipolar disorder in those individuals (Winokur, Coryell, Maser, Keller, et al., 1995).

Bipolar disorders are one of the most problematic psychiatric disorders to treat. The difficulty is that bipolar patients easily switch between extremes of manic-activity to severe depression, thus complicating treatment and leading to potentially dangerous results with drugs that can induce the polar state in an attempt to ameliorate either the manic or depressive condition. In fact, the rate of switching varies widely, from periods lasting from weeks to months in duration with one mood (a condition more frequent with adults), commonly called *episodes*, to switching occurring every few days, daily, or even with four events or more per day, now called *ultradian cycling* (Tillman & Geller, 2003). Thus, these variations have now led to suggestions for new definitions, where *episodes* can now be defined by "(a) the duration from onset to offset of a period of at least 2 weeks in length during which only one mood state persists or (b) the duration from onset to offset of a period of ultra rapid or ultradian cycling for at least 2 weeks. And cycles can be defined by mood switches occurring daily or every few days during an episode" (Tillman & Geller, 2003).

It may be that the ultradian rhythm of alternating cerebral hemispheric activity (Werntz et al., 1983; Shannahoff-Khalsa, 1991a; Shannahoff-Khalsa, 1993) and its coupled relationship to the basic rest activity cycle through lateralized rhythms of the ANS plays a role in switching, where the left hemisphere and right-nostril-dominant mode prevail during the manic phase and the right hemisphere and left-nostril-dominant mode prevail during the depressed phase. This could easily account for many facets of the mental and physical activity states of the multiple daily ultradian events, and it may be that there is a bias toward one side of this natural "pendulum," where one hemisphere tends to dominate for prolonged periods in the episodes without complete transitions to the alternate mode. This would help account for a mechanism that underlies the switching that can occur within minutes, whether it happens once in several months or multiple times per day.

A similar near-instantaneous transition of personalities has been observed in two case studies of multiple personality disorder (MPD), with this lateralized CNS-ANS relationship explained as the possible mechanism (Shannahoff-Khalsa, 1991a). In 1955, Ischlondsky reported significant lateralized findings during a neurological examination of two different patients with similar personality traits where each patient had "two diametrically-opposed personality types. One was an impulsive, irresponsible, mischievous, and vindictive personality, full of rebellion against authority and of hate toward the people around her, the patient in this phase was extremely aggressive, using abusive language and scaring other patients with lurid tales of state hospitals, sex relations, etc.; in the opposed behavioral pattern to which the first personality would suddenly switch, the patient appeared dependent, submissive, shy, self-effacing, affectionate, and obedient. In a very timid way she expressed friendliness, sought affection, acceptance, and approval from the same personnel she had reviled and abused. There was no trace left of any inappropriate word or expression, no manifestation of hostility to her surroundings, and not the slightest reference to sex. In fact, any sex thought or word would induce in her extreme fears of perdition, feelings of guilt and anxiety, depression, and shame" (Ischlondsky, 1955).

In each of these two opposed mental states, there was amnesia to the other, which is characteristic of MPDs (now referred to as *dissociative identity disorders*), although "a strong stimulus was capable of evoking the antipode of the existing mental condition" (Ischlondsky, 1955). During the aggressive or active phase of the patient's behavior

> examination revealed that the left and right sides of her body responded differently to sensory stimulus; while the right side was hypo-sensitive the left side displayed hyper-sensitivity. Thus, vision and hearing were unclear and far away on the right side but very clear and close on the left side. Her response to touch and pain showed a high threshold on the right, and a low threshold on the left side. Characteristically, with regard to the olfactory sense the patient in this mental state manifested a diametrically opposed attitude: she was hyper-sensitive to smell on the right side and her *right nostril was clear* (my emphasis), while on the left side her sense of smell was absent and the *nostril congested and closed* (my emphasis). With regard to the other neurological signs such as the

size of pupils, reflexes, salivation, and sweating, there was a similar difference in the response of the two sides of the body: the aggressive personality type displayed on the right side—with a small pupil, a hypo-secretion of saliva, an absence of sweating on sole, palm, and the lack of abdominal reflexes—while on the left side there was a large pupil, hyper-secretion of saliva, very strong sweating on sole and palm and extremely strong abdominal reflexes. (Ischlondsky, 1955)

(It is difficult to account for the observation of pupil size, etc., inconsistent with nasal congestion.) And just as fast as the psyche switched to the shy, passive, and permissive personality, all neurological manifestations also switched to reverse dominance, where the "olfactory sense proved now to be very sharp on the left side while completely absent and with *nostril congested and closed on the right side*" (Ichlondsky, 1955). This extraordinary case study showing that lateralized ANS phenomena switch instantaneously with the psyche in two patients suggests that right-nostril dominance or sympathetic dominance on the right side of the body correlates with the active phase of the BRAC and the fight-or-flight response pattern (Shannahoff-Khalsa, 1991a). Needless to say, it would be very interesting to at least measure the nasal cycle and perhaps other ANS features that are known to exhibit ultradian dynamics and how they may vary in bipolar patients. This may tell us something more about neural mechanisms supporting switching in bipolar patients and other mood disorders. For example, are MDD patients relatively more left-nostril dominant during phases of depression?

Included below is a protocol that includes three Kundalini yoga meditation techniques specific for the treatment of bipolar disorders. Two are phase-specific meditations—one for the depressed phase and one for the manic phase. The third is phase-independent and can be used to help resolve the condition when the patient is not depressed or manic as well as during either the manic or depressed phase. However, when the patient is clearly manic, the manic-specific technique is recommended, and of course the one specific for the depressed phase is only recommended for times when the patient is clearly depressed. The technique that is phase-independent is more difficult than the other two, and is also less likely to be employed when a patient is suffering in deep depression. In fact, most patients find it requires significant rigor, but in time they develop the skill for the full practice time of 31 minutes, even if this takes several months. While the phase-appropriate techniques can be employed independently of the suggested protocol, there is one addition here (Gan Puttee Kriya), along with the required tuning in, which I have used to help patients who want to resolve the condition in general. Here Gan Puttee Kriya is employed as the technique immediately before the phase-independent technique because it can help clear the mind for the rigor to come. Gan Puttee Kriya is a useful technique here because it leads to mental balance without overstimulation, a concern with bipolar patients whether they are being treated with medications or meditations.

A Meditation Protocol Specific for the Treatment of Bipolar Disorders[*]

1. Technique to Induce a Meditative State: "Tuning In"

This technique is a precursor, as is the case with all other Kundalini yoga protocols or individual techniques in this book or any other book on Kundalini yoga as taught by Yogi Bhajan, and it should be practiced before any of the three disorder-specific techniques here for bipolar disorders, whether they are done independently or in the suggested series for resolving the condition in general. Technique 2 (Gan Puttee Kriya) can be left out, but the patient will receive reduced overall benefits. Technique 2 would also add additional benefits to techniques 4 and 5.

Sit with a straight spine and with the feet flat on the floor if sitting in a chair (see Figure 2.1., p. 71). Put the hands together at the chest in "prayer pose"—the palms are pressed together with 10 to 15 pounds of pressure between the hands (a mild to medium pressure, nothing too intense). The area where the sides of the thumbs touch rests on the sternum with the thumbs pointing up (along the sternum), and the fingers are together and point up and out at a 60-degree angle to the ground. The eyes are closed and focused on the third eye (imagine a sun rising on the horizon, or the equivalent of the point between the eyebrows at the origin of the nose). A mantra is chanted out loud in a 1½-breath cycle. Inhale first through the nose and chant "Ong Namo" with an equal emphasis on the Ong and the Namo. Then immediately follow with a half-breath inhalation through the mouth and chant "Guru Dev Namo" with approximately equal emphasis on each word. (The O in *Ong* and *Namo* are each a long "o" sound; *Dev* sounds like *Dave*, with a long "a" sound.) The practitioner should focus on the experience of the vibrations these sounds create on the upper palate and throughout the cranium while letting the mind be carried by the sounds into a new and pleasant mental space. This should be repeated a minimum of three times. We employed it in our group about 10–12 times. This technique helps to create a "meditative state of mind" and is *always* used as a precursor to the other techniques.

2. Gan Puttee Kriya

Sit with a straight spine, either on the floor or in a chair. The back of your hands are resting on your knees with the palms facing upwards. The eyes are nine-tenths closed (one-tenth open, but looking straight ahead into the darkness at the "third eye" point, not the light below). Chant from your heart in a natural, relaxed manner, or chant in a steady, relaxed monotone. Chant out loud the sound "Sa" (the *a* sounds like "ah"), and touch your thumb tips and index-finger tips together quickly and simultaneously with about 2 pounds of pressure. Then chant "Ta" and touch the thumb tips to the middle-finger tips. Chant "Na" and touch the thumb tips to the ring-finger tips. Chant "Ma" and touch the thumb tips to the little-finger tips. Chant "Ra" and touch your thumb tips and index-finger tips. Chant "Ma" and touch the thumb tips to the middle-finger tips. Chant "Da" and touch the thumb tips to the ring-finger tips. Chant "Sa" and touch the thumb tips to the little-finger tips. Chant "Sa" and touch your thumb tips and index-finger tips. Chant "Say" (sounds like the word *say* with a long "a") and touch the thumb tips to the middle-finger tips. Chant "So" and touch the thumb tips to the ring-finger tips. Chant "Hung" and touch the thumb tips to the little-finger tips.

Chant at a rate of one sound per second. The thumb tip and finger tips touch with a very light, 2 to 3 pounds of pressure with each connection. This helps to consolidate the circuit created by each thumb-finger link. Start with 11 minutes and slowly work up to 31 minutes of practice. To finish, remain in the sitting posture and inhale, holding the breath for 20 to 30 seconds while you shake and move every part of your body, with the hands and arms extended over the head. Exhale and repeat this two more times to circulate the energy and to break the pattern of tapping, which effects the brain.

The sounds used in this meditation are each unique, and they have a powerful effect on the mind, both the conscious and subconscious mind. The sound "Sa" gives the mind the ability to expand to the infinite. "Ta" gives the mind the ability to experience the totality of life. "Na" gives the mind the ability to conquer death. "Ma" gives the mind the ability to resurrect. "Ra" gives the mind the ability to expand in radiance (this sound purifies and energizes). "Da" gives the mind the ability to establish security on the earth plane, providing a ground for action. "Say" gives the totality of experience. "So" is the personal sense of identity, and "Hung" is the infinite as a vibrating and real force. Together, *So Hung* means "I am Thou." The unique qualities of this 12-syllable mantra help cleanse and restructure the subconscious mind and help heal the conscious mind to ultimately experience the superconscious mind. Thus, all the blocks that result from an extreme traumatic event are eliminated over time with the practice of Gan Puttee Kriya.

3. Technique for the Resolution of the Bipolar Condition in General (Phase-Independent)

The posture involves four 90-degree angles (see Figure 3.5). Sit on the floor with both legs extended straight out in front side by side, with the thighs and heels touching. The first 90-degree angle is with the feet slightly pulled back with the toes pointing straight up. The second 90-degree angle is formed with the spine perpendicular to the floor, that is, with the torso and legs at right angles. The third 90-degree angle is formed by the two upper arms extending straight in front of the body parallel to the ground, or at right angles to the torso. The last 90-degree angle is formed with the forearms at 90 degrees to the upper arms. The forearms are side by side. The hands are pressed together with the thumbs side by side and tucked inside the palms up to the first joint (see Figure 3.6). The middle fingers fold over and touch the back of the opposite hand. The remaining three fingers extend up straight. The eyes remain open and focused on the area that is a triangle formed by the two index fingers and tops of the thumbs. Inhale and exhale deeply through the nose (mouth remains closed). During the exhale, mentally hear a deep heart-felt sighing sound. Listen to the sounds of the breath and become lost in it. Practice this technique for 11 to 31 minutes. Then lay down and relax for 5 to 15 minutes.

4. Technique for Treating the Manic Phase of the Disorder

This technique is not recommended to follow directly after technique 3, unless of course the patient feels like he is in a manic phase, which would be very unlikely after practicing the three previous techniques. Note that if the patient is in a manic phase, he should first tune in and then skip to this technique. He can also do it after Gan Puttee Kriya.

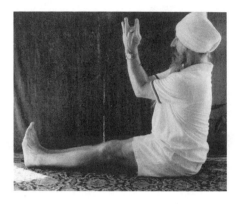

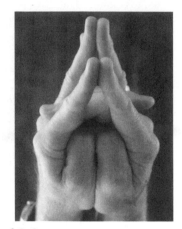

Figures 3.5 and 3.6
Technique for the Resolution of the Bipolar
Condition in General (Phase-Independent)

Squat in "crow pose" and hold the head up straight. During the inhale, the hands are in fists in front of the body, almost touching (see Figure 3.7). Keep the forearms parallel to the ground with the eyes closed. During the exhale, the eyes are opened and the fingers are spread with the hands palm to palm (see Figure 3.8). The fingers point up and out at about a 60-degree angle. Continue the inhale and exhale rhythm with the eyes closed and open respectively for 3 to 11 minutes. Then relax on the back.

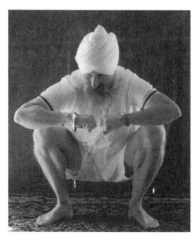

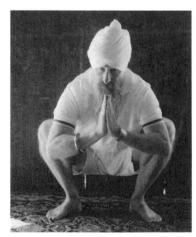

Figures 3.7 and 3.8
Techniques for Treating the Manic Phase of the Disorder

5. Technique for Treating the Depressed Phase of the Disorder

This technique is not recommended to follow directly after technique 3, unless of course the patient feels like he is depressed, which would be very unlikely after practicing the first three techniques. Note that if the patient is in a depressed phase, he should first tune in and then do this technique. He can also do it after Gan Puttee Kriya.

Sit with the buttocks on the ground with the bottoms of both feet touching, pulled close to the body (see Figure 3.9). The thumb tips touch the mounds on the palms just below the little finger on their respective hands throughout the entire exercise. The breathing pattern begins by inhaling through a curled tongue in four equal parts (four counts), holding the breath for four equal counts, then exhaling through the nose in four equal parts and holding the breath out for four counts. The hands are by the ears with the palms facing backwards. The hands are stroked past the ears (6 to 9 inches) in rhythm with the count (so there are 16 strokes of the hands past the ears per breath). The eyes remain closed. Perform this technique for 3 to 11 minutes. Then relax on the back. Note, the hands in Figure 3.9 are shown facing forward so that the view of the thumbtip on the mound of the little finger is clear. However, the hands actually face backwards when practiced.

Case Histories of Two Bipolar Patients

Case History 1: A Mild Case in a High-Functioning Patient

Alberto is a male, aged 30, who was diagnosed with bipolar disorder at age 21, at the time of his first acute manic crisis, which lasted 20 days. He was not hospitalized. Before his first crisis, he had played water polo for a national South American team competing internationally. He excelled in education and was in his fourth year of medical school when he had his first crisis. Several months after this crisis he was able to return to his studies and water polo

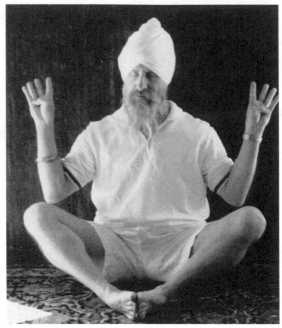

Figure 3.9
Technique for Treating the Depressed Phase

programs. The following year he went to the United States for 5 months, as a college student with a water polo scholarship. He graduated medical school and entered and completed a residency in radiology. He started his career as a radiologist and married a physician. He and his wife left South America for the United States for a year-long research-fellowship program, and there he had his second acute manic crisis. Although it was less severe than the first, he was hospitalized for 5 days.

Alberto commented about his disorder in this way: "I think I was pushing myself very hard to be successful during my medical school, and the atmosphere at the university was competitive and very stressful. Besides, my national water polo team program was very intense, and I did not have any emotional support from my parents to keep playing and studying hard. One week before the first crisis, I had an important disagreement with my father. I believe these events helped lead to the onset of my disorder. For the second crisis, I think the changes of my work routine, the different culture, the language, staying away from my friends and family, and the stress to be successful in my research contributed to the manifestation of the disorder again." He further comments about his background: "My parent's relationship was not good. I found out that my dad had another woman and that was hard on my mom and to me. I was 12 or so. My parents' relationship was bad before I was 10. They are both medical doctors (neuro) and they were always kind of busy. I could never feel love and respect between them. They divorced just 4 years ago, but during my childhood I thought they should be divorced already. I had a lovely grandfather (my mother's father), but he died in 1984 when I was 10 years old. That was hard for me too. Also, my brother was diagnosed at age 27 with mania at the same time that I was. He had seen me in mania and then took on the same state of mind."

Alberto took haloperidol for 2 months and lithium for 2 years after the first crisis. He took risperidone for nine weeks after the second crisis and started lithium again. "I have been doing psychotherapy since my first crisis in 1995. I think it helps me. It makes me feel better and more confident to keep going." He said, "I was always curious about meditation and yoga. I started to read and study it in 2002. A few months after I got married, I started to practice, on my own, for about 20 minutes every morning. I realized that my mind was becoming calmer and more focused. I started to feel more connected, more complete. But after the second crisis I was afraid to meditate. I thought it could push me to another crisis. At that time I did research on the Internet on bipolar disorder and meditation and found some articles by David Shannahoff-Khalsa. I contacted him. A few days later he taught me a Kundalini yoga protocol to revert the bipolar disorder. Since that time, February 2005, I have been practicing at least 40 minutes every day. I am feeling very well, confident, and stable."

Case History 2: A Severe Case in a Hospitalized Patient

Shui-Lian presented at the age of 27 diagnosed with bipolar disorder, borderline personality disorder, and psychosis. She describes her own history: "I was born in Beijing in the winter of 1977, the second and last child in a middle-class family of the intelligentsia. At the age of two, I woke up one morning and found my mother gone without having said good-bye. The nanny told me that she had gone to America. I stared blankly for a moment, then I began to cry with neither feeling nor regret. In the 5 years that she was gone, my father was both father and mother to me. My father is a poet famous in China and other parts of the world for his neoclassical style of poetry. We had just moved into our apartment in the city; I was 5 and we were inseparable. He had let me help him place his valuable stamp collection into albums. Those having an embroidered border were of a particular liking to me. On impulse, I cut off their laced edges to piece them together. When my father saw this, he turned away from me slowly, saying in an almost whisper, "It's over, it's over, it's over." The light went out of my eyes then and I was in the grips of a desperate panic, for I knew not what was going on in his mind. To this day I cannot bear the impact nor taste the chilling beauty of the tragic without wanting to flee from it. At the same time, ironically, I have always sought out the moments of melancholy, such as that of a petal falling by a small bridge over a creek, whose foaming ripples disappear as they flow over the pebbles.

"The first portrait I recall taking is of my father and me at age 4. He was holding me with both hands and he never looked happier. Upon my second time seeing the photograph 20 years later in the Shanghai City Hospital, where I was hospitalized for the very first time at age 24 for my mania, my father's profile seemed severed from me, though we were next to each other. I scratched out his face with a blue pen in all the pictures of the album, and later threw them all away. I myself haven't photographed in years. My father recently asked me about those photographs and I said I had destroyed them, but promised to paint them in acrylics.

"When I was 24 the signs of my depression became indisputable after a major breakdown resulting from the separation from my boyfriend and an ensuing suicide attempt. At this point, my mother took me to a well-known psychiatrist (in the U.S.) who prescribed Celexa, my first antidepressant. Two weeks later, we were back in China in my mother's parents' house in Nanjing. My mother left me for an extended vacation and she returned to the U.S. On the night of my first manic episode, at age 24 (in China), I was about to take a bath when all of a sudden an irresistible urge overtook me and I crawled out of the bathroom licking the dust on the uneven wooden floors. In my mind I was performing some kind of penance to memorialize my grandfather, who had passed away never having approved of my mother's marriage to my father. My relatives decided to let my father take me to Beijing. For the next few days, I went on shopping sprees and was singing Chinese opera that the whole neighborhood could hear.

"At this point, I was taken to the Shanghai City Hospital, where I stayed for 2.5 months. Hypnotherapy attested to the devastation of my last breakup with my boyfriend, while the medications and the electro-acupressure treatments made me docile and passive. But how I felt in my being—enslaved to emotional love and decimated by drug use—had not changed; it was only masked by sedation. My father then took me to Nanjing and left me in the care of my grandmother (mother's side) after I was discharged, and I have not seen him since.

"In Nanjing, my cousin and her mother introduced me to a modern sect of apocalyptic Buddhism. My bias against Western medications was established, and I stopped taking my meds. My hypomania erupted. I began a full-scale rearrangement of the cookware and the cutlery, making a big mess in their new kitchen. They sent me to the Nanjing City Hospital. Another 2.5 months of treatment followed, including more electro-acupuncture. The time would have been extended indefinitely had my mother not come back to China to take me to the States.

"It was during the year after coming back from China that I went to support myself by working in administrative jobs in Los Angeles. I was under the care of the same psychiatrist who saw me before and who had prescribed me Celexa. He followed the guidelines recommended by the Chinese doctors who claimed that I was "cured," and gradually reduced my medications in segments of 3 months at a time. I was 25, and still very heavily in the grips of the psychedelic party culture (carried over from college). I moved to Los Angeles aspiring to become a costume designer. However, daily indulgence in marijuana turned my attention to writing. After a year of working, smoking, and writing poetry, I collapsed under a wave of depression and came back to San Diego. Soon afterward, I started taking group yoga classes from David Shannahoff-Khalsa, but I did not tell him about my psychiatric history. It took me 3 or 4 months of continuous daily practice of Kundalini yoga to distill a state of clear and focused mind. Once again I stopped taking my meds, and as a result I was hospitalized in San Diego five times after getting picked up by the police.

"Because I was no longer able to live on my own, I was living in a rundown boarding care facility near downtown, and my hypomania was hitting at its worst. In December of 2004, I finally saw David Shannahoff-Khalsa in a private session for my bipolar condition, where he taught me the protocol for bipolar disorders. However, I was still sharing a room and fighting with my roommate and could not find the time to practice yoga.

"The last hospitalization, which led to my stay at the long-term locked facility where I am now, was in March of 2005. I was given a medication whose name I do not recall that made me lose my balance in movement. As a result, I had trouble putting on a sweater by myself, and fell down every time I bent down to pick up something, scarring my face. The doctor took me off the medication then, but only reluctantly. Life at this facility is degrading and monotonous. If it was not for my Kundalini yoga practice, my animal side is in constant danger of being absorbed into the mass mentality of the criminally insane. Sixty percent of the patients here were homeless before someone called the police on them for their disturbance, and were consequently put on government support to be treated at this facility.

"My grip on reality has become sure through meditation and yoga. I am able to remain attached to positivism, even when besieged by the predators of the lower human aspects (in other words, the demonic) on all sides. When I first learned the bipolar technique, getting into the pose, I immediately felt strength in my mind and body. But it became increasingly difficult to sustain the posture, and I thought I had to stop after 4 minutes. David encouraged me through the rest of the 7 minutes, which I did not believe I could do. I then successfully practiced this technique on a daily basis, first for 11 minutes for four weeks, extending to 22 minutes for 3.5 weeks, and finally to 31 minutes at a sitting until the present. The first time doing the technique on my own, I felt like I was back in my college years, years before my illness broke out. It was the most difficult thing I had ever done, and it continues to be difficult. The cycles of mania-depression, major depression, and rapid cycling that reside in the depth of my psyche are one by one brought out during this exercise and are "resolved" without them having a chance to take me into their grips. Instead I experience the disruptions of these ups and downs as physical and emotional pain, through which the rigid posture of the technique pulls me. I have been stable since May 2005, however my meds have not been brought down due to my inappropriate behavior at the facility. Living with 43 other patients in close quarters sometimes brings out my negative aspect in violent ways. One day in May, after a 2.5 hour session that ended with 31 minutes of Sat Kriya, one of the other exercises I learned in David's classes, I experienced a state of total lucidity unrivaled by any experience in my life. I knew that there had to be an end to any other religious rituals. I had been until then converting to the Catholic faith, which I attempted to incorporate into my yoga practice. But the rigid mindset of the church did not allow me being there. On that day in May I officially ended my conversion."

I conducted one therapy session with Shui-Lian in December 2004, have kept up regular phone calls, and on occasion I receive an e-mail message, to which I reply. During her hospitalization, she has discontinued smoking cigarettes after years of consumption. She spent 9 months in a psychiatric hospital and was released to a half-way house in December 2005 with plans to soon live again by herself.

Shui-Lian's case is all too common today. This complex case history may suggest that this disorder-specific protocol would have benefits for other patients suffering from bipolar and co-morbid disorders. I have seen her case go from long periods of outrageous and uncontrolled language and behavior, when she was often incoherent, to her current status of lucidity. She has finally realized that she has to take responsibility for her own behavior and plans to apply to graduate school. My e-mail contact with her has almost solely focused on her need to change her language and behavior toward others, including her mother, the person to whom she has directed her worst belligerence and occasional physical aggression. The yoga without counseling would not be sufficient in her case. Fortunately, she now listens to my advice and recognizes what she has to change in order to have a chance at living a normal life.

FOUR

Treating the Addictive, Impulse Control, and Eating Disorders

After phobias, the substance-abuse disorders, which include alcohol and prescription and illicit drugs, rank as the number-two most prevalent category for psychiatric disorders (Rasmussen & Eisen, 1990). This ranking does not include the impulse-control and behavioral disorders—eating disorders, paraphilias, conduct disorders, antisocial personality disorders, intermittent explosive disorders, kleptomania, pyromania, pathological gambling, and trichotillomania. "The essential feature of an impulse control disorder (ICD) is the failure to resist an impulse, drive, or temptation to perform an act that is harmful to the person or to others" (APA, 1994). This chapter is intended to be helpful for treating all of the above disorders.

In defining the ICDs (and this also holds true for the substance-abuse and eating disorders), the APA states "the individual feels an increasing sense of tension or arousal before committing the act and then experiences pleasure, gratification, or relief at the time of committing the act; and following the act there may or may not be regret, self-reproach, or guilt" (APA, 1994). The ICDs, substance-abuse disorders, and eating disorders involve behaviors that could be grouped under the umbrella of "self-destructive" behaviors, which may then constitute the largest single "psychiatric problem." Last, but not least, let's not fail to include smoking, the leading preventable cause of death in the United States, as an addictive behavior (General, 1994). A very recent U.S. figure for smoking rates for individuals that do not have a concurrent mental illness is 22.5% (Lasser, Boyd, Woolhandler, Himmelstein, McCormick, et al., 2000). Therefore, the number of individuals afflicted with at least one addictive self-destructive behavior must be staggering. If we consider overeating as a "soft" addiction, 66% of the U.S. is now considered overweight, 30% obese, and 8% morbidly obese (100 pounds overweight). In fact, for the first time in history, greater than 50% of people worldwide are considered overweight. The U.S. figures do not include the statistics for the food-related problems of anorexia nervosa, bulimia nervosa, and binge eating without purging and laxatives that may all be increasing in parallel with the growing obesity in this nation. Anorexia nervosa is considered to be the most deadly psychiatric disorder, with a near 20% mortality rate over a lifetime, and a prevalence rate among adolescent and early-adulthood females of 0.5% to 1.0% (APA, 1994). The prevalence rate for bulimia nervosa, again for the adolescent and early adulthood females, is thought to be 1% to 3%, with the rate of occurrence in males of about 10% of that in females (APA, 1994).

With respect to alcohol, the National Institute on Alcohol Abuse and Alcoholism currently provides a chilling summary of the problem, using less than current data: "Alcohol-related problems have a significant impact on the nation's health and welfare." Economic estimates of this impact indicate that alcoholism and alcohol abuse cost about $100 billion annually (Rice, 1993). Approximately 14 million Americans—about 7% of the adult population—meet the diagnostic criteria for alcohol abuse and/or alcoholism (Grant, Harford, Dawson, Chou, Dufour, et al., 1994). About 40% of Americans report having a direct family experience with alcohol abuse or alcoholism (Harford, 1992). More recently (SAMHSA, 2004), the current situation of alcohol dependency can be described where nearly 19 million Americans (8% of the U.S. population) require treatment for an "alcohol problem," and 16 million drink heavily. But only 2.4 million have been diagnosed with alcoholism, and 139,000 receive medication to treat it. Also, one in four children lives with a parent who is dependent on, or abuses, alcohol (Grant, Dawson, Stinson, Chou, Dufour, et al., 2004).

The misuse of alcohol is involved in approximately 30% of suicides (Hayward, Zubrick, & Siburn, et al., 1992), 50% of homicides (Wiezorek, Welte, & Abel,, 1990), 52% of rapes and other sexual assaults, 48% of robberies, 62% of assaults, and 49% of all other violent crimes (Murdock, Phil, & Ross, 1990; Pernanen, 1991). Alcohol is also a factor in 30% of all accidental deaths, including up to 50% of motor vehicle deaths. In fact, more than 100,000 Americans die each year from alcohol-related causes, which, if it were ranked independently, would make alcohol-related problems the third leading cause of death in the United States (NHTSA, 1991; Stinson, Dufour, Staffens, & Debakey, 1993).

When it comes to substance abuse with controlled prescription drugs, a thorough and up-to-date report shockingly concludes: "While America has been congratulating itself in recent years on curbing increases in alcohol and illicit drug abuse and in the decline in teen smoking, the abuse and addiction of controlled prescription drugs—opioids, central nervous system depressants and stimulants—have been stealthily, but sharply, rising. Between 1992 and 2003, while the U.S. population increased 14%, the number of people abusing controlled prescription drugs jumped 94%—twice the increase in the number of people abusing marijuana, five times in the number abusing cocaine, and 60 times the increase in the number abusing heroin. Controlled prescription drugs like OxyContin, Ritalin, and Valium are now the fourth most abused substance in America behind only marijuana, alcohol and tobacco. Particularly alarming is the 212% increase from 1992 to 2003 in the number of 12- to 17-year-olds abusing controlled prescription drugs, and the increasing number of teens trying these drugs for the first time. New abuse of prescription opioids among teens is up an astounding 542%, more than four times the rate of increase among adults. The explosion in the prescription of addictive opioids, depressants, and stimulants has, for many children, made the medicine cabinet a greater temptation and threat than the illegal street drug dealer, as some parents have become unwitting and passive pushers. Teens who abuse controlled prescription drugs are twice as likely to use alcohol, five times likelier to use marijuana, 12 times likelier to use heroin, 15 times likelier to use Ecstasy, and 21 times likelier to use cocaine, compared to teens who do not abuse such drugs" (CASA, 2005).

In respect to illicit drug use, the National Institute on Drug Abuse (NIDA) provided the following fairly recent information: "In 2002, an estimated 19.5 million Americans, or 8.3% of the population aged 12 or older, were current illicit drug users; an estimated 2.0 million persons (0.9%) were current cocaine users, 567,000 of whom used crack; hallucinogens were used by 1.2 million persons, including 676,000 users of Ecstasy, and an estimated 166,000 current heroin users. Among youths aged 12 to 17, 11.6% were current illicit drug users. The rate of use was highest among young adults (18 to 25 years) at 20.2%. Among adults aged 26 or older, 5.8% reported current illicit drug use. Among pregnant women aged 15 to 44 years, 3.3% reported using illicit drugs in the month prior to their interview. This rate was significantly lower than the rate among women aged 15 to 44 who were not pregnant (10.3%). In 2002, an estimated 11.0 million persons reported driving under the influence of an illicit drug during the past year. This corresponds to 4.7% of the population aged 12 or older. The rate was 10% or greater for each age from 17 to 25, with 21 year olds reporting the highest rate of any age (18.0%). Among adults aged 26 or older, the rate was 3.0%." NIDA also provided rates for alcohol and tobacco use: "An estimated 120 million Americans aged 12 or older reported being current drinkers of alcohol in the 2002 survey (51.0%). About 54 million (22.9%) participated in binge drinking at least once in the 30 days prior to the survey, and 15.9 million (6.7%) were heavy drinkers. An estimated 71.5 million Americans (30.4% of the population aged 12 or older) reported current use (past month use) of a tobacco product in 2002. About 61.1 million (26.0%) smoked cigarettes, 12.8 million (5.4%) smoked cigars, 7.8 million (3.3%) used smokeless tobacco, and 1.8 million (0.8%) smoked tobacco in pipes. The percentage of youths aged 12 to 17 who had ever used marijuana declined slightly from 2001 to 2002 (21.9 to 20.6%). Among young adults aged 18 to 25, the rate increased slightly from 53.0% in 2001 to 53.8 % in 2002. The percentage of youths aged 12 to 17 who had ever used cocaine increased slightly from 2001 to 2002 (2.3 to 2.7%). Among young adults aged 18 to 25, the rate increased slightly from 14.9% in 2001 to 15.4% in 2002."

In all fairness, we must discriminate between use and abuse, but clearly, we can conclude that for those living in the U.S., the major "psychiatric problem" may in part be described as an "oral activity" problem! One way to define a yogi is a person who has mastery over the intake and output through the various holes in the body. So what does Kundalini yoga have to offer toward both treatment and prevention when it comes to addictions, ICDs, and eating disorders?

Included in this chapter are two very unique meditation techniques. One that is specific for any form of addiction, called the "Medical Meditation for Habituation" (see technique 6 in this chapter), supposedly can help remedy all of the problems in this chapter, including the addiction to drugs, alcohol, smoking, and the various ICDs. However, also included here is a technique (see technique 7 in this chapter) specific for ICDs. Here I outline a single protocol for substance-abuse disorders, ICDs, and eating disorders, and end with several case histories of treatment.

A 7-Part Meditation Protocol Specific for the Treatment of Addictive, Impulse Control, and Eating Disorders*

1. Technique to Induce a Meditative State: "Tuning In"

Sit with a straight spine and with the feet flat on the floor if sitting in a chair (see Figure 2.1). Put the hands together at the chest in "prayer pose"—the palms are pressed together with 10 to 15 pounds of pressure between the hands (a mild to medium pressure, nothing too intense). The area where the sides of the thumbs touch rests on the sternum with the thumbs pointing up (along the sternum), and the fingers are together and point up and out at a 60-degree angle to the ground. The eyes are closed and focused on the third eye (imagine a sun rising on the horizon, or the equivalent of the point between the eyebrows at the origin of the nose). A mantra is chanted out loud in a 1½-breath cycle. Inhale first through the nose and chant "Ong Namo" with an equal emphasis on the Ong and the Namo. Then immediately follow with a half-breath inhalation through the mouth and chant "Guru Dev Namo" with approximately equal emphasis on each word. (The O in *Ong* and *Namo* are each a long "o" sound; *Dev* sounds like *Dave*, with a long "a" sound.) The practitioner should focus on the experience of the vibrations these sounds create on the upper palate and throughout the cranium while letting the mind be carried by the sounds into a new and pleasant mental space. This should be repeated a minimum of three times. We employed it in our group about 10–12 times. This technique helps to create a "meditative state of mind" and is *always* used as a precursor to the other techniques.

---

* Copyright © David Shannahoff-Khalsa, 2005. No portion of this protocol may be reproduced without the express written permission of the author.

2. Spine-Flexing Technique for Vitality

This technique can be practiced while sitting either in a chair or on the floor in a cross-legged position. If you are in a chair, hold the knees with both hands for support and leverage. If you are sitting cross-legged, grasp the ankles in front with both hands. Begin by pulling the chest up and slightly forward, inhaling deeply through the nose at the same time. Then exhale as you relax the spine down into a slouching position. Keep the head up straight, as if you were looking forward, without allowing it to move much while flexing the spine. This will help prevent a whip effect in the cervical vertebrae. All breathing should only be through the nose for both the inhalation and exhalation. The eyes are closed as if you were looking at a central point on the horizon, the third eye. Your mental focus is kept on the sound of the breath while listening to the fluid movement of the inhalation and exhalation. Begin the technique slowly while loosening up the spine. Eventually, a very rapid movement can be achieved with practice, reaching a rate of one to two times per second for the entire movement. A few minutes are adequate in the beginning. Later, there is no time limit. Food should be avoided just prior to this exercise. Be careful and flex the spine slowly in the beginning. Relax for one minute when finished.

3. Shoulder-Shrugs Technique for Vitality

While keeping the spine straight, rest the hands on the knees if sitting in a cross-legged position or with hands on the thighs if sitting in a chair. Inhale and raise the shoulders toward the ears, then exhale, relaxing them down. All breathing is done only through the nose. Eyes should be kept closed and focused on the third eye. Mentally focus on the sound of the inhalation and exhalation. Continue this action rapidly, building to three times per second for a *maximum* of 2 minutes. This technique should not be practiced by individuals who are hyperactive.

4. Ganesha Meditation for Focus and Clarity*

Sit with a straight spine, with the eyes closed (see Figure 2.4, page 100). The left thumb and little finger are sticking out from the hand. The other fingers are curled into a fist with fingertips on the moon mound (the root of the thumb area that extends down to the wrist). The left hand and elbow are parallel to the floor, with the pad of the tip of the left thumb pressing on the curved notch of the nose between the eyes. The little finger is sticking out. With right hand and elbow parallel to the floor, grasp the left little finger with the right hand and close the right hand into a fist around it, so that both hands now extend straight out from your head. Push the notch with the tip of the left thumb to the extent that you feel some soreness as you breathe long and deep. After continued practice, this soreness reduces. Do this for 3 minutes and no longer. To finish, keeping the posture with eyes closed, inhale. Push a little more and pull the naval point in by tightening the abdominal muscles for 10 seconds, then exhale. Repeat one more time.

* This short 3-minute technique was previously published in Shannahoff-Khalsa, 2003.

5. Gan Puttee Kriya

Sit with a straight spine, either on the floor or in a chair. The back of your hands are resting on your knees with the palms facing upwards. The eyes are nine-tenths closed (one-tenth open, but looking straight ahead into the darkness, not the light below), focused at the "third eye." Chant from your heart in a natural, relaxed manner, or chant in a steady, relaxed monotone. Chant out loud the sound "Sa" (the *a* sounds like "ah") and touch your thumb tips and index-finger tips together quickly and simultaneously with about 2 pounds of pressure. Then chant "Ta" and touch the thumb tips to the middle-finger tips.. Chant "Na" and touch the thumb tips to the ring-finger tips. Chant "Ma" and touch the thumb tips to the little-finger tips. Chant "Ra" and touch your thumb tips and index-finger tips. Chant "Ma" and touch the thumb tips to the middle-finger tips. Chant "Da" and touch the thumb tips to the ring-finger tips. Chant "Sa" and touch the thumb tips to the little-finger tips. Chant "Sa" and touch your thumb tips and index-finger tips. Chant "Say" (sounds like the word *say* with a long "a") and touch the thumb tips to the middle-finger tips. Chant "So" and touch the thumb tips to the ring-finger tips. Chant "Hung" and touch the thumb tips to the little-finger tips.

Chant at a rate of one sound per second. The thumb tip and finger tips touch with a very light, 2 to 3 pounds of pressure with each connection. This helps to consolidate the circuit created by each thumb-finger link. Start with 11 minutes and slowly work up to 31 minutes of practice. To finish, remain in the sitting posture and inhale, holding the breath for 20 to 30 seconds while you shake and move every part of your body, with the arms and hands extended above the head. Exhale and repeat this two more times to circulate the energy and to break the pattern of tapping, which effects the brain. Then immediately proceed with focusing the eyes on the tip of the nose (the end you cannot see) and breathe slowly and deeply for 1 minute.

The sounds used in this meditation are each unique, and they have a powerful effect on the mind, both the conscious and subconscious mind. The sound "Sa" gives the mind the ability to expand to the infinite. "Ta" gives the mind the ability to experience the totality of life. "Na" gives the mind the ability to conquer death. "Ma" gives the mind the ability to resurrect. "Ra" gives the mind the ability to expand in radiance (this sound purifies and energizes). "Da" gives the mind the ability to establish security on the earth plane, providing a ground for action. "Say" gives the totality of experience. "So" is the personal sense of identity, and "Hung" is the infinite as a vibrating and real force. Together, *So Hung* means "I am Thou." The unique qualities of this 12-syllable mantra help cleanse and restructure the subconscious mind and help heal the conscious mind to ultimately experience the superconscious mind.

6. Medical Meditation for Habituation:
A Technique to Cure Any Addiction

Sit either in a chair or on the floor (see Figure 4.1) (Bhajan, 1976; Shannahoff-Khalsa, 2004). Straighten the spine and make sure the first six lower vertebrae are locked forward. This means the lower back is pushed forward as if you are "at attention." Make fists of both hands and extend the thumbs straight. Place the thumbs on the temples and find the niche where the thumbs just fit. (This is the lower anterior portion of the frontal bone above the temporal-sphenoidal suture.) This place is usually sensitive to the touch, so do not apply pressure per se, simply touching is adequate. Lock the back molars together and keep the lips closed. Vibrate the jaw muscles by alternating the pressure on the molars. A muscle will move in rhythm under the thumbs. Feel it message the thumbs. Keep the eyes closed and look at the brow point, or third eye, the point where the top of the nose meets the forehead. Silently vibrate the five primal sounds "Sa Ta Na Ma" at the brow point, applying pressure to the molars with one pressure per sound (the fifth sound here is the sound "ah," which is basic to the other four sounds). The effects of the mantra are the following. The sound "Sa" gives the mind the ability to expand to the infinite; the sound "Ta" gives the mind the ability to experience the totality of life; the sound "Na" gives the mind the ability to conquer death; and the sound "Ma" gives the mind the ability to resurrect under all circumstances. In other words, the mantra puts ones consciousness through the cycle of infinity, life, death, and rebirth. This mantra cleanses and restructures the subconscious mind to help live in a conscious state that is merged with the infinite. Continue 5 to 7 minutes and slowly build the practice to 31 minutes maximum.

Yogi Bhajan comments on this technique in this way: "This meditation is one of a class of meditations that will become well-known to the future medical society. Meditation will be used to alleviate all kinds of mental and physical afflictions, but it may be as many as 500 years before the new medical science will understand the effects of this kind of meditation well enough to delin-

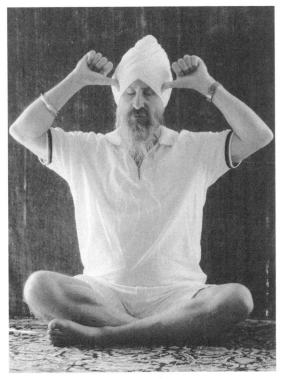

Figure 4.1
Medical Meditation for Habituation:
A Technique to Cure Any Addiction

eate all of its parameters in measurable factors. The pressure exerted by the thumbs triggers a rhythmic reflex current in the central brain. This current activates the brain area directly underneath the stem of the pineal gland. It is an imbalance in this area that makes mental and physical addictions seemingly unbreakable. In modern culture, the imbalance is pandemic. If we are not addicted to smoking, eating, drinking or drugs, then we are addicted subconsciously to acceptance, advancement, rejection, emotional love, etc. All these lead us to insecure and neurotic behavior patterns. The imbalance in this pineal area upsets the radiance of the pineal gland itself. It is this pulsating radiance that regulates the pituitary gland. Since the pituitary regulates the rest of the glandular system, the entire body and mind go out of balance. This meditation corrects the problem. It is excellent for everyone but particularly effective for rehabilitation efforts in drug dependence, mental illness, and phobic conditions" (Bhajan, 1976).

7. Meditation for Treating Impulsive Behavior

Sit with a straight spine and place the left arm in front of the body with the left hand facing straight out in front of the heart center. The left arm and hand are parallel to the ground. The right arm is extended straight out parallel to the left arm and in front of the body, right palm facing up (see Figure 4.2). The eyes are closed. Chant the mantra "Whahay Guru Whahay Guru Whahay Guru Whahay Jeeo," with at least one entire round of the mantra per breath cycle. The sound "Wha" is like "wa" in *water*; and "hay" has a long "a"; and "Jeeo" sounds like the two letters "g" and "o" run together. Practice for 18 minutes maximum,then place both hands on the chest at the heart center. The left hand is touching the chest and the palm of the right hand is on the back of the left hand. Continue chanting the mantra but in a whisper for 2 more minutes, then remain silent for 1 minute with the hands on the chest. To end, inhale deeply and hold the breath, tightening the muscles of the arms, hands (pressing against the chest), and spine. Then exhale out powerfully through the mouth like a cannon, and repeat the inhale, tightening, and exhale sequence two more times.

This meditation will also balance the "earth" and "ether" elements of the psyche, and is a useful meditation for young children who have gone astray in life. It will increase their ability to remain stable and secure and help develop their temperament, tolerance, and restraint.

This 7-part protocol is designed to help overcome any substance-abuse disorder, including smoking; the ICDs, including the paraphilias, conduct disorders, antisocial personality disorders, intermittent explosive disorders, kleptomania, pyromania, pathological gambling, and trichotillomania; and the eating disorders, including anorexia nervosa, bulimia nervosa, binge eating, and "overeating." One difficulty with this protocol is that both tech-

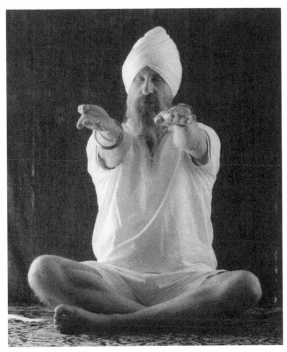

Figure 4.2
Meditation for Treating Impulsive Behavior

niques 6 and 7 require an arm posture that some individuals may find hard to hold for an extended amount of time. However, as with the practice of other difficult techniques, or for beginners in general, the times for these techniques can be reduced in the beginning. In time the practice can be extended to maximum practice times. Usually, patients find that they can quickly lengthen the times for these two techniques if they persevere. For those with a severe weakness in the shoulders, they may choose to initially leave out technique 7 until they are inclined to endure a greater challenge and have built greater strength through the use of technique 6. In fact, the reason that technique 7 is added here is only to expedite the rate of recovery overall. It is likely that all of the disorders in this chapter can be treated successfully with only techniques 1 through 6. Once a patient achieves the ability to practice technique 6 for the full practice time of 31 minutes per day, he has overcome a major hurdle. Maintaining a daily practice with technique 6 at 31 minutes per day will help keep the patient on safe ground, and after 40 days he is likely to remain in remission. Ninety to 120 days would virtually guarantee complete remission. Including technique 7 will further accelerate the patient's overall progress. Both techniques work toward the same goal, however, through different pathways.

One virtue of this entire 7-part protocol is that it can be practiced while sitting in a chair. Sitting erect on the ground adds no significant advantages or additional benefits. The first four techniques are included to help prepare for the use, ease, and maximum benefit of techniques 5 through 7, which are the key components for treating the respective disorders in this chapter. Technique 5 actually helps to set a "mental stage" for attempting the more arduous technique 6. Technique 5 helps to create an inner balance and clear negative thoughts from the subconscious mind that lead to self-defeat. This 7-part protocol is a "catch-all protocol" that provides the greatest assurance and most rapid rate of relief for the entire spectrum of unique disorders in this chapter. However, there are possible substitutions with other meditation techniques that would also benefit these patients. In addition, there are many "on-the-floor" Kundalini yoga exercise sets that would be helpful adjuncts to therapy and recovery.

Case Histories of Treatment

Case History 1: A Couple Addicted to Heroin and Cocaine Seeking Rapid Detoxification

In the early nineties two people who had been arrested for possession of small amounts of heroin and cocaine sought my services knowing that I had a background in teaching Kundalini yoga for drug rehabilitation. When they called me, they had a single intention. They were not looking to kick their habits for good, but simply to be able to appear in court before a judge without being under the influence. Hope was a female, age 24, and Tony a male, age 28. They were not a romantic couple, but friends who were arrested together and partners in crime. Hope had a very successful drug pusher of a boyfriend who provided her with many hundreds of dollars worth of heroin and cocaine everyday, and Tony had access to a reduced rate and was addicted to a lesser amount of both drugs. Hope and Tony had drug histories that started in their early teens, and both had been using both heroin and cocaine sporadically for at least 5 years and continuously for the last 3 years. Both had been through several programs in the past in an attempt to break their habits. Both were from relatively wealthy families, "unemployed," and not living at home with their parents. However, they were successful at managing their respective cash flows and making ends meet. Both had graduated high school, and had attempted education in college, but chose to enter the apparently less arduous and more lucrative world of drug sales as a career. When they called me, I agreed to take them into my home and treat them as if it were a hospital with all the necessary restrictions. I explained in detail what the three days would entail and they agreed to all the terms. They were goal directed—wanting to appear to be clean in court, and thus hoping for a lighter sentence or no time in jail. They timed their visit with me to end on the morning when they had to go to court. We agreed on a starting time of 12 noon, but they arrived late, at 3 P.M. and under the influence, which was expected. They reported to have only taken heroin earlier in the day. They and their light baggage were searched when entering, and they arrived by taxi as agreed. They were not allowed to make phone calls or to have visitors before their departure or to leave the property without being accompanied. They knew they would be under supervision the entire time. The intention was to put them through a yogic detox regime that included frequent freshly juiced vegetables and fruits (equal amounts of carrot, celery, and apple twice a day), a light vegetarian cuisine with only melons in the morning and a sandwich for lunch, and steamed vegetables for dinner, if they had an appetite. Herbal teas were served throughout the day, along with yoga and meditation three times a day, two to three walks throughout the neighborhood for physical exercise, two showers, one in the morning upon wake-up at 6 A.M., and one in the evening before dinner, and lights out at 9 P.M.

When they arrived they were served freshly squeezed juice and we again went over the routine. Within 30 to 40 minutes we started to proceed using the 7-part meditation protocol sitting in chairs. They complied fully up to technique 6, with which they found that 5 minutes was their maximum time limit. They were able to do 11 minutes of Gan Puttee Kriya. They were then given 15 minutes to lay down and relax after the protocol. Clearly they were still under the influence of the heroin and reported feeling very good. However, they noted how peaceful and calm the protocol made them feel. Their apprehension of not having access to drugs soon began to surface, and since they had both been through detox before, they had a sense of what to expect. After the short rest period, we took a 45-minute walk throughout the scenic neighborhood with the intent of keeping their metabolism from crashing and keeping their activity levels high. They were then allowed to lay out and rest again for another 15 to 20 minutes, followed by a shower. During all of the rest periods, peaceful and pleasant Indian-style raga music was played. Dinner was served along with fresh juice, and immediately after, we took another walk before sunset. Upon returning, meditation was again practiced for 45 minutes. At this point they felt exhausted and showed major signs of fatigue. Before going to bed at 9 P.M., they had a mixture of ginger and chamomile tea. They did not leave the bedroom until being awakened in the morning promptly at 6 A.M. They reported that they had hardly slept at all and perspired frequently throughout the night. They took showers, and were again given ginger tea followed later by freshly squeezed juice. Around 7:30 A.M., a shortened version of a yoga exercise set called Nabhi Kriya (Bhajan & Khalsa, 1975) was first taught to help give them strength and the will to continue. A rest of 30 minutes was then provided, followed by the 7-part protocol. Around 9:30 A.M., they were again given a 20-minute rest period and then another walk in the neighborhood was taken for 45 minutes. Upon returning, a light breakfast of fresh fruit was served, followed by another opportunity to relax.

While feeling somewhat miserable, they knew they had little choice but to continue. If not, they realized they were likely to face a rather unpleasant jail sentence. (They had both been arrested at least once before on lesser charges.) Around noon, they again practiced some of the exercises from the set called Nahbi Kriya and the same 7-part meditation protocol, again followed by rest. Juices and herbal teas were furnished throughout. Lunch followed, with another opportunity to relax. Another walk was taken and rest and more juices were provided. The same routine was followed for the next 2 days.

On night two, both Hope and Tony noted that they were able to get some sleep, perhaps several hours. After about 36 hours, they began to feel much better. Hope wanted to leave after 2 days, but Tony knew what would happen if they left early and he encouraged her to stay, and she complied. After the third night, both had what they called a decent night's sleep, and in the morning appeared and reported to be feeling better and able to present in court. They both commented at the end that the amount of pain and discomfort they had to go through was about one-tenth of what they had to endure under other programs. They then took a taxi to court. I never heard from either of them again.

This case is not meant to suggest that miracles can be performed, but to show the potential for the use of Kundalini yoga and a strict health regime in surmounting the most difficult stage of recovery, the detoxification period. Obviously, this regime could be employed in long-term rehabilitation along with a range of other modalities that could include group counseling, acupuncture and/or acupressure therapies, herbal therapies, hydrotherapies, and service through work in any institution set up to facilitate patients through the long-term treatment that is required for full rehabilitation. This sort of routine was employed by a program in Tucson, Arizona, called 3HO SuperHealth, that had full Joint Commission accreditation up until about 1990 when it was closed as a result of changes in insurance coverage policies for substance abuse hospitalization.

Case History 2: A Female with a History of Anorexia Nervosa and Bulimia Nervosa

Beth had rented a room from a friend of mine who taught Kundalini yoga. Beth was originally from England and had been living in the U.S. for about 6 months. She was employed part-time by an elderly couple whom she helped with routine duties around the house, including fixing their meals and driving them to the market and other places to help them maintain their independent lifestyle in an upscale neighborhood. Beth had suffered for years from eating disorders. She was raised in a dysfunctional family with alcoholic and combative parents and reported sexual abuse by her father from ages 7 to 12, which occurred with regularity several times a week during the night when her mother was asleep. When she was 12 years of age, her parents divorced and her mother became the primary parent. However, the stress in the household overall seemed to remain nearly constant compared to the pre-divorce state, due to the mother's increased financial and household responsibilities and her more outward and active bouts of anger. Beth remained living with the mother and rarely saw her father, who had moved to a town nearby. She never told her mother about the sexual abuse, fearing that their already-troubled family would "completely fall apart." She did not want to be blamed for any of the families problems.

At age 12, Beth began to show classic signs of anorexia. She believed she was "too fat" when she had been of normal height and weight. She also believed that she "did not deserve good things in her life." Her school work was always mediocre, and she did not have many friends. Beth was shy, but she would join other girls in her neighborhood for sports. She enjoyed running best, which soon became an obsession with her. For the first 3 years of her "careful dietary habits," her mother paid little or no attention. Finally, by the age of 15, her mother wondered why she lacked the interest in being more social, going out with her girlfriends and taking a normal interest in boys, and why her school performance had declined. At this point, the mother took her to the doctor, and the doctor diagnosed her with depression and prescribed an antidepressant. However, the medication did not help, and she was again prescribed another antidepressant but also with little or no benefits. She remained moody, antisocial, with the exception of her now self-imposed daily running program, which she did every day while her friends only ran three days a week. She continued to lose weight. She graduated from high school and took a full-time job as a nanny with a wealthy family that traveled frequently abroad to the U.S. and to countries throughout Europe. She enjoyed her work and helping with the children and grew much less concerned with her weight problems over time. But when she was sexually molested by a business partner of the father who had employed her, she decided to quit that job and see if she could manage on her own.

During these times she reported feeling very insecure and her mild eating disorder shifted more toward a bulimic condition with an ever greater concern for her health. She continued her running routine and became obsessed with the healthy nature of her diet. She developed an obsession with eating a restricted diet of only raw foods grown organically. However, the binge eating was not restricted, and frequently, eventually nightly, she would consume an entire large bag of low-priced cookies. She had little or no restrictions on her binge-eating routine, but maintained a strict routine for her "normal eating" habits.

When she moved into my friend's house, she began stealing food from the refrigerator that they shared. This usually occurred during the middle of the night, followed by a nearly silent purging in the bathroom. After some time, my friend confronted her, though all was met with denial. After several more weeks, she was again caught in the middle of the night stealing food. She apologized, saying that she had not had a chance to go shopping and that she was extremely hungry and promised to replace the food. While the stealing seemed to be curbed to near-undetectable levels, the binge and purge behavior seemed to increase. After several more weeks, she was confronted about her bathroom exploits, and at this point she was told either to move out or to seek help.

Yoga classes were taught in the house, and she decided that this might be her best solution. She had no health insurance or money to seek professional counseling. Beth started by going to evening yoga classes several times a week and found them to be helpful for reducing her stress and anxiety. Almost immediately, her binging and purging began to reduce in frequency and her nightly assaults on the refrigerator also reduced in number. Once she discovered the benefits of doing yoga, she became more open and willing to discuss her eating habits. She maintained her strict raw-foods diet and running program but noticed how beneficial the yoga classes were for her life. At this point she elected to see me to learn the 7-part protocol that she was told could be of more specific benefit for her eating disorder. She continued to do the group yoga classes, and several times a week she employed the 7-part protocol on her own after seeing me once a week for 3 weeks. She knew she needed help for her disorder, but prior to this time she had not found any effective solutions. She loved the effects of all the techniques she employed. One of her virtues was her strong discipline toward physical activities, which she had developed through running. Fortunately, after only 3 weeks she was able to do technique 6 for the full amount of time, and not long after that had managed also to achieve full time with technique 7. She continued the protocol on a near-daily basis for about a month. After another month, she chose to return to England to be near her family. In the beginning she would send me reports about her continued progress and how much she liked going to regular yoga classes because "they were so much easier than the 7-part protocol." At that point she discontinued the protocol on a regular basis and employed it only when she thought the stress of her life might lead to a return of her eating disorders. Six months after returning to England, she met a man who also practiced Kundalini yoga, and eventually the two were married and had one daughter. (Two other patient case studies that include eating and other disorders are described in Chapter 8.)

The first case history of Hope and Tony and the case of Beth both illustrate how successful this protocol can be when patients are faced with little or no alternative. While I have no information of what eventually happened to Hope and Tony, I am fairly certain that they quickly returned to their drug habits and "lucrative" careers. They did, however, meet their immediate needs of facing the court system while not being under the influence of drugs. The case of Beth is entirely different. She managed to completely overcome her eating disorder and she returned to a happy and productive life. What is clearly needed now is widespread testing of this protocol with or without other complementary yoga sets that could vary based on the patient demographics for the following disorders: substance abuse disorders, ICDs, smoking, and eating disorders. These therapies would be best administered by trained therapists and yoga teachers in institutionalized settings, either in restricted residential programs (prisons and hospitals), or outpatient programs for those with lesser severity.

FIVE

Treating Sleep Disorders

There are at least 88 sleep-wake disorders listed in the International Classification of Sleep Disorders (ICSD, 1990). Sleep disorders in general fall into four categories: (1) the primary sleep disorders defined by the dyssomnias, which include insomnia, characterized by abnormalities in the amount, quality, and timing of sleep, and the parasomnias, characterized by abnormal behavioral or physiological events occurring in association with sleep, specific sleep-stage, or sleep-wake transitions; (2) a sleep disorder related to another psychiatric disorder; (3) a sleep disorder resulting from another medical condition; and (4) a sleep disorder that results from a substance-induced disorder (APA, 1994). Sleep disorders in general are reported by 13% to 49% of the population (Walsh & Ustun, 1999) and are associated with significant medical, psychological, and social disturbances (Vgontzas & Kales, 1999). Insomnia is the most common sleep disorder and affects 3% to 19.4% of the population (Walsh & Ustun, 1999). The percent variation here represents a range of studies over the last 30 years that used various symptom duration criteria and sampling methodologies to assess prevalence. The National Commission on Sleep Disorders Research concluded more than 10 years ago that insomnia "is a silent epidemic of staggering proportions" affecting 30 million American adults intermittently and another 30 million chronically (NCSDR, 1993). One definition of insomnia is a difficulty in falling asleep plus or minus a difficulty in staying asleep or early final awakening (Vgontzas & Kales, 1999). The International Classification of Sleep Disorders (ICSD, 1990) defines insomnia as a "difficulty in initiating and/or maintaining sleep." There is no final consensus on the definition of insomnia (Walsh & Ustun, 1999). The earliest recorded citation for this perennial disorder is a monograph by Aristotle on sleeplessness in 350 B.C. Dement, a pioneer in sleep research, claims that "insomnia affects 20–40% of all adults, especially women and the elderly" (1993). Insomnia also affects as many as one-fifth of all patients who consult a general-practice physician (Kales, Soldatos, & Kales, 1987). The other though less prevalent "primary" sleep disorders are narcolepsy, idiopathic hypersomnia, and the parasomnias—sleepwalking, night terrors, and nightmares.

While insomnia is a heterogeneous complaint with multiple origins, it has been characterized in the ICSD as having primary and secondary subtypes. First, the primary insomnias are (1) psychophysiological, (2) subjective insomnia, and (3) idiopathic insomnia. Psychophysiological insomnia is the most classic form and is a condition where subjective complaints are confirmed by polysomnography. Subjective insomnia, or "sleep state misperception," is when the patient's complaint is not verified by polysomnography, which accounts for 5% to 10% of all insomnias (Coleman, Roffwarg, Kennedy, Guilleminault, Cinque, et al., 1982). Idiopathic insomnia has a childhood onset and is a lifelong inability to obtain adequate sleep (Hauri & Fisher, 1986). It is the most persistent form and does not present with a temporal variation as does psychophysiological insomnia. This form is assumed to be the result of abnormal neurological mechanisms involving the sleep-wake system, and is otherwise not linked with earlier psychological trauma or medical illness (Morin, 1993). The secondary subtypes of insomnia are equivalent to categories 2 through 4 listed above.

Dement states that "Most physicians dread the arrival of a patient with severe chronic insomnia," because "the sense is that nothing can be done, or that achieving a therapeutic improvement is very difficult" (1993). The awareness of sleep disorders has only recently increased, and this is largely due to the recent recognition of breathing disorders (sleep apnea) during sleep as a major health problem. Unfortunately, there is also a tremendous gap between a growing interest in sleep disorders and medical-school training programs. When it comes to medical education, "sleep and sleep medicine are certainly nonexistent in the core of clinical teaching" (Kryger, Lavie, & Rosen, 1999). Thus the number of people who require treatment in the United States far exceeds the handful of specialists currently trained to treat insomnia and/or other sleep disorders. Among the sleep disorders, insomnia "takes the greatest toll . . . represents an immense burden in terms of human suffering, economic cost, and other untoward consequences to society as a whole. Therefore, urgent action is needed to reduce the negative impact of insomnia" (Costa e Silva, 1999).

The consequences of insomnia include association with a greater risk of traffic accidents, health problems, hospitalizations, psychiatric disorders, impaired performance, productivity, mood and increased risk, absenteeism, diminished intellectual and cognitive performance, increased nursing-home stays and utilization of health care resources, greater medical expenses, and a greater predisposition to substance abuse (Kales, Kales, Bixler, Soldatos, Cadieux, et al., 1984; Pollack, Perileck, & Linsner, 1990; Ford & Kamerow, 1989; NCSDR, 1993).

When it comes to the use of medications to treat insomnia, a compelling review article summarizes the status as follows "In the United States, roughly 2/3 of all hypnotic prescriptions go to chronic users, who have taken hypnotics for an average of 5 years or more. Two large prospective epidemiological studies have shown that reported hypnotic use, especially use 30 times per month, is associated with an excess hazard of death. Indeed, use of hypnotics 30 times per month is associated with a similar mortality hazard to smoking 1–2 packs of cigarettes per day. Moreover, the hypnotic user's wish to improve daytime function is usually unfulfilled. The preponderance of evidence is that hypnotics impair performance, cognition and memory, increase the risk of automobile accidents and falls, and promote unfavorable changes in personality. Due to tolerance, the sleep-promoting effects of hypnotics appear to be lost with chronic use. With long-term use, there is little controlled evidence that hypnotics produce benefits of any sort. More study of long-term hypnotic effects by public agencies is needed, but available evidence weighs strongly against long-term prescribing" (Kripke, 2000). In Europe the proportion of chronic users may be even greater than in the U.S. (Ohayon, Caulet, & Lemoine, 1996).

This chapter will focus on category 1, the primary sleep disorders, and will also include a technique specific for nightmares, and another technique for inducing super-efficient sleep that shortens sleep times to 3 to 5 hours while maximizing the functions of sleep and the depth of sleep.

Treating Primary Physiological Insomnia

Two techniques are included here for treating insomnia. One is called Shabd Kriya, and it is specific for treating sleep disorders that exhibit with abnormal rhythmic sleep processes. Shabd Kriya is most useful for treating longstanding and severe cases of insomnia (Shannahoff-Khalsa, 2004). The second technique, called Yuni Kriya, is a meditation technique that can be used to treat less problematic cases of insomnia. It is thought that nearly all primary physiological insomnia cases result from stress or hyperarousal. Years of research support this hypothesis with studies on the autonomic nervous system and functions of the hypothalamic-pituitary-adrenal axis. Therefore, stress is viewed as the leading cause of insomnia for the vast majority of people. When prolonged stress is combined with a poor knowledge of healthy sleep habits, insomnia is a frequent end result.

However, a side effect of using Shabd Kriya is that with initial use it can lead to a mild disruption of sleep processes and excess dreams that sometimes last 3 to 5 weeks prior to obtaining apparent day-to-day improvements. This does not mean that the patient is not benefiting at all from the practice, but only that there is an underlying process of change that can have unpleasant effects. These side effects do not happen in all cases, but in my experience the events happen in a significant number of cases that warrant another possible approach when such disturbances do occur. These same side effects can also occur when Shabd Kriya is practiced by those who do not suffer from insomnia, but simply choose to practice the technique for its restorative effects and for the supposed benefits toward mastery of the mental realm. One claimed benefit of Shabd Kriya is that it can be used to refine rhythmic brain processes and enhance the development of the personality (Bhajan & Khalsa, 1975).

The occasional side effects with Shabd Kriya have led me to first employ Yuni Kriya as a meditation technique for treating patients with less severe cases of shorter duration. Yuni Kriya leads to a very deep state of relaxation, and it is best employed immediately before sleep. However, it can also be used as a technique to reduce stress and anxiety during the day, but ample time (several hours) should be allotted for rest thereafter. Yuni Kriya can lead to a spacey state of mind, but one that is coupled with a deep state of relaxation. Thus this technique is a valuable tool for the early stages of insomnia for many patients. I have had patients that have become annoyed by the side effects of Shabd Kriya in the beginning stages of treatment, and inevitably the switch to practicing Yuni Kriya leads to more satisfying results overall. Some patients are willing to do both, or to start with Shabd Kriya during the day for a while, and then use Shabd Kriya alone before bed. Patients differ in severity, their will and priority to overcome their condition, and in the occurrence of side effects. Many other Kundalini yoga meditation techniques and exercise sets would also be helpful in the treatment of insomnia. However, Shabd Kriya is likely to be the most effective tool for severe cases and when nothing else works. There is no reason not to employ Shabd Kriya first and then to gauge if side effects manifest. If so, the patient may prefer to start with a practice of Yuni Kriya, and then if needed eventually incorporate Shabd Kriya as the primary or single technique for treatment.

As with all other Kundalini yoga meditation techniques or protocols, the first step is to "tune in." If the patient is employing either Shabd Kriya or Yuni Kriya immediately before bed or within several hours beforehand, the other techniques that have been used frequently in this book as precursors, like spine flexes and shoulder shrugs, should be avoided, as they act as stimulants.

1. Technique to Induce a Meditative State: "Tuning In"

Sit with a straight spine and with the feet flat on the floor if sitting in a chair (see Figure 2.1, page 72). Put the hands together at the chest in "prayer pose"—the palms are pressed together with 10 to 15 pounds of pressure between the hands (a mild to medium pressure, nothing too intense). The area where the sides of the thumbs touch rests on the sternum with the thumbs pointing up (along the sternum), and the fingers are together and point up and out at a 60-degree angle to the ground. The eyes are closed and focused on the third eye (imagine a sun rising on the horizon, or the equivalent of the point between the eyebrows at the origin of the nose). A mantra is chanted out loud in a 1½-breath cycle. Inhale first through the nose and chant "Ong Namo" with an equal emphasis on the Ong and the Namo. Then immediately follow with a half-breath inhalation through the mouth and chant "Guru Dev Namo" with approximately equal emphasis on each word. (The O in *Ong* and *Namo* are each a long "o" sound; *Dev* sounds like *Dave*, with a long "a" sound.) The practitioner should focus on the experience of the vibrations these sounds create on the upper palate and throughout the cranium while letting the mind be carried by the sounds into a new and pleasant mental space. This should be repeated a minimum of three times. We employed it in our group about 10–12 times. This technique helps to create a "meditative state of mind" and is *always* used as a precursor to the other techniques.

2. Meditation for Treating Insomnia and Regulating Sleep Stages: Shabd Kriya

This technique was first reported in the scientific literature along with Yuni Kriya in an introduction to Kundalini yoga meditation techniques specific for the treatment of psychiatric disorders (Shannahoff-Khalsa, 2004).

Sit with a straight spine, with both feet flat on the floor if sitting in a chair. Place the hands in the lap, palms up, with the right hand over the left hand (see Figures 5.1 and 5.2). The thumb pads, last joint, are touching together and point forward. Focus the eyes on the tip of the nose with the eyelids half closed. The tip of the nose is the point you cannot actually see, but if you use a finger tip to touch the end of the nose this is where the eyes are focused. This is not an eyes-crossed posture but may seem like it initially. (The sides of the nose will look blurry during the focus, but having the eyes crossed makes the nose appear to balloon up, which is not the correct eye posture.) Inhale through the nose in only four equal parts, mentally vibrating the mantra "Sa Ta Na Ma" (one syllable per part of the four-part inhale). Hold the breath and mentally vibrate the four-syllable mantra a total of four times for a total of 16 "beats," then exhale through the nose in two equal parts, mentally vibrating the mantra "Whahay Guru," one word per part or beat. This equals a 22-part, or 22-beat, cycle. Continue for at least 15 minutes, working up to 62 minutes. When finished, relax completely and go to sleep.

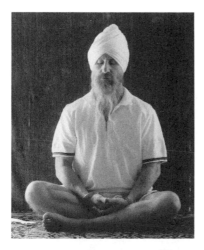
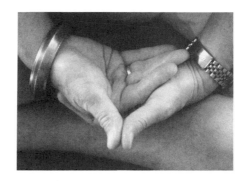

Figures 5.1 and 5.2
Meditation for Treating Insomnia and Regulating
Sleep Stages: Shabd Kriya

3. Meditation for Deep Relaxation: Yuni Kriya

Sit with a straight spine, with both feet flat on the floor if sitting in a chair (see Figure 5.3). The eyes are open and focused on the tip of the nose (to know where this spot is, take the index finger tip and touch the end of the nose, which is not a spot you can actually see, but the point that you attempt to see while keeping the eyes fixed in that position). Only the blurry sides of the nose and anything else that may be in front of you is visible. The elbows are relaxed against the sides. Both hands come up to meet in front of the body at the level of the solar plexus, about one foot in front of the body. The little finger, edges of the hand, and sides of the thumbs are touching. The thumbs are pointing up and the little fingers are pointing away from the body. No other parts of the hands are touching. The three other fingers (index, middle, and ring, grouped together side by side and not touching the little fingers or thumbs) are pointed forward at about a 60-degree angle to each other. In this position, the hands form a cave-like structure pointing away from the body. Inhale through the nose and exhale through the mouth and then inhale through the mouth and exhale through the nose, and so on, continuing the cycle for 11 minutes. When inhaling through the mouth, the lips are puckered as if one is about to whistle or kiss. When exhaling through the mouth, the lips are relaxed. In the beginning the hand posture is a little difficult to hold correctly for many people, but in time it becomes very easy to perform. This breath can take you into a very deep state of relaxation and should only be practiced right before going to bed or if you have nothing to do for several hours afterward. This technique should not be practiced for more than 11 minutes.

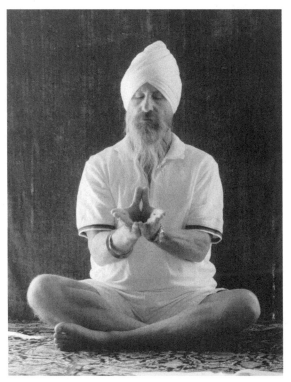

Figure 5.3
Meditation for Deep Relaxation: Yuni Kriya

4. Meditation Breath to Prevent Nightmares

Sit with a straight spine and do a breath equal to a panic breath, that is, very quickly open the mouth, the navel point jerks like it is getting pulled in, the tailbone gets pulled up, the tongue comes just to the point of beginning to come out of the mouth, and the diaphragm is jerked to exchange oxygen maximally. This breath technique is to be practiced 20 times a day, one after the other in succession, to help prevent nightmares. It is also supposedly good for hysteria and paranoia.

5. Meditation Technique to Deepen, Shorten, and Induce Super-Efficient Sleep

Sit with a straight spine with the lower back pushed forward to attain a very alert posture (see Figure 5.4). The hands are in ghyan mudra (index finger tip touching the thumb tip, not the index nail touching the pad of the thumb tip). The palms face up (see Figure 5.5). The tips of the Mercury (little), Sun (ring), and Saturn (middle) fingers touch their respective counterparts on the opposite hand. The Mercury fingers are closest to the face, and you can see the six fingers grouped in their respective postures back to back. The Mercury fingers meet along their respective back-sides, and the Sun and Saturn fingers only touch near the sides of their nails at the ends of the fingers. The six fingers point up and out at a 60-degree angle away from the body and are held at the heart-center level, with the elbows touching the ribs at the sides. The hands are about 9 to 12 inches in front of the body. The eyes are open and they focus down the nose tip, looking directly at the meeting point where the six finger tips meet. There is no breathing pattern. The breath will slowly adjust and should not be consciously regulated. No mantras are to be used. The entire mental and visual focus is on the ends of the six finger tips as a group. The time should be 11 to 15 minutes and no more per sitting. This meditation can make a person sleepy and should be done immediately before bed for best results. The side effect of this meditation is that it can create bizarre dreams and disrupt sleep patterns for the first 1 to 3 weeks. Also, visual hallucinations can occur while looking at the finger tips during the practice of this technique. These hallucinations should be ignored and the practitioner should continue with the practice, allowing the extraneous visual images to disappear. Optimal results are achieved by practicing this technique every night for 15 minutes maximum for 90 to 180 nights in succession. This technique induces such a deep and efficient sleep that sleep time can be reduced down to 2 to 4 hours for most healthy young people.

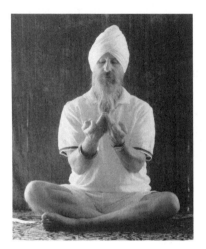
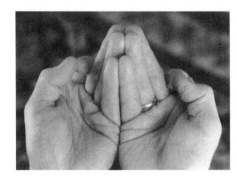

Figures 5.4 and 5.5
Meditation Technique to Deepen, Shorten, and
Induce Super-Efficient Sleep

This technique was the very first Kundalini yoga meditation technique that I practiced on a regular daily basis with an intent to explore its long-term effects. At that time I was 26 years of age. After 90 days of perfect night-to-night practice for 15 minutes immediately before bed, I was sleeping from only 11 P.M. to 2 A.M. At this point I would get up and practice other techniques for two hours. However, after the 90 days, I quit the practice of this specific technique and eventually my sleep increased in length to 4 to 5 hours per night. Prior to the practice of this technique, I routinely slept for 6 to 7 hours per night. At the age of 52, I again practiced the technique but found that I was only able to reduce my sleep to 3.5 to 4 hours per night and I practiced for 120 nights. No doubt the ultimate utility of this technique is dependent on one's age, health status, lifestyle, and how long one wants to employ it. It is claimed that this technique can increase the initial times spent in stage 4 non-rapid eye movement (NREM) sleep and adjust the CNS to support a more efficient, deeper, and restorative sleep (Yogi Bhajan, personal communication). When I practiced this technique, I found that my dreams increased for several weeks. I also had the same experience with Shabd Kriya.

A Sleeping Position to Help Induce Sleep

In my nonstatistical analysis of individuals in groups attending my lectures, I find that about 80% of people attempt to fall asleep while lying on their right side. This position helps induce left-nostril airflow dominance, which is coupled with right brain hemisphere dominance and stage 4 NREM sleep (Shannahoff-Khalsa et al., 2001). Most individuals do not easily fall asleep if they are right-nostril dominant. If they do, it does not quickly lead to the deeper stage 4 NREM sleep, but rather to REM sleep, the more active form of sleep. Some people have physically obstructed or partial occlusions of one nostril and when this is permanent on the left side, these individuals find it difficult or nearly impossible to fall asleep while lying on their right side. This occurs because the left side may not allow for sufficient airflow for normal healthy sleep due to the initial partial or complete occlusion. So the take-home lesson for those without complicated nasal passages is to attempt to induce a deep state of sleep by first reclining on the right side. While lateral pressure has been studied extensively as a means to alter nasal dominance (Rao & Potdar, 1970; Cole & Haight, 1986), nasal airflow patterns do not always quickly change.

Much depends on the state of stress and relaxation prior to a sleep effort. The patterns of the nasal cycle are more a marker for the rhythmic activity of the CNS-ANS pendulum that helps to define rest and activity states (Shannahoff-Khalsa, 1991a; Shannahoff-Khalsa, 1991b). Thus it may be that many people suffering from insomnia are not quickly engaging a state of left-nostril and right-hemispheric dominance. Right-nostril dominance is more related to a stressed state. The practice of Yuni Kriya or other techniques may help reduce and eliminate all of the effects of stress prior to a sleep effort and thus help minimize the time prior to sleep onset.

There are many factors that can determine how quickly an individual will fall asleep and how deep and stable the sleep will be. I have found that it is not unusual for patients to be unaware of how heavy foods prior to sleep can disturb sleep, and how caffeine or sugar, even in the form of fruits or fruit juices, can lengthen the time before sleep onset. Many factors are important for healthy sleep hygiene and they have been studied and reported at length along with a discussion of cognitive behavioral therapies (Morin, 1993).

Case History of Treatment

Nancy presented with a severe case of insomnia. She was 44 years old, a gainfully employed psychotherapist, divorced for 10 years with two children living at home, and was apparently healthy. She complained about her inability to sleep, daily fatigue, and her temperament. She felt like she had become "overly touchy" and noted how this was affecting her personal life and career. In the past she had enjoyed being around people but had developed a preference for being alone. Nancy said that she felt like she "almost never slept" and this had continued for almost 3 years. She had tried hypnotics but noted feeling worse the next day with less clarity. She reported that she had a 20-year strict practice of daily meditation consisting of a silent mantra routine. In my experience, practitioners of this common technique frequently find themselves preferring the comfort that they enjoy with the silent and calm space produced only during their practice. Normal worldly activities in time tend to present too much stress, which conflicts with the experience of their silent meditative space. I have noticed how many of these practitioners tend to withdraw from the harsher challenges and realities of daily life, and thus prefer a more secluded life. This simple technique tends to lead to a cycle where one practices to achieve calm and peace, then experience the discomfort of the outer world, practices again, and so on. I explained my view about how her practice might be leading to her withdrawal and increased temperament, and that perhaps it raised her sensitivity to a level where she was too easily disturbed to sleep deeply. Reluctantly, she understood my rationale. It was also clear that her meditation practice was not solving her sleep disorder. She elected to end this 20-year practice. I knew there was a high probability that Shabd Kriya might lead to an initial worsening of sleep, if hers could get worse, and also a likelihood of disturbed dreams. I taught her Yuni Kriya. She immediately felt very relaxed. I suggested that she use it every night after tuning in and to make sure that she sat perfectly straight, which was not a requirement of her silent-mantra meditation practice. After about 2 or 3 days, she noted that her inability to sleep had improved. The next week, she said she actually felt like she was sleeping again. She continued to use Yuni Kriya at night for 2 weeks, and reported how much more refreshed she felt "but wanted to feel even more energetic during the day, like her old self." I taught her Shabd Kriya, which I recommended she practice only during the day while continuing with Yuni Kriya at bedtime. After one month, she added Shabd Kriya to her nightly routine for 11 minutes. Once she got to 31 minutes of Shabd Kriya, she continued with this technique alone. She reported feeling much more refreshed from her sleep and that she now thought she was sleeping almost straight through for 5 to 6 hours.

In sum, we know from Kripke's seminal review paper on chronic hypnotic use that medications to date have severe limitations for long-term use. He ends his review with the following: "The risk/benefit ratio of chronic hypnotic use is highly unfavorable. Death is a serious risk. Moreover, epidemiologic evidence and studies of short-term administration indicate that hypnotics impair function. On the other hand, there is essentially no controlled evidence for any benefit when use of hypnotics becomes chronic. For the chronic user, even the belief that the hypnotics slightly augment sleep is probably incorrect. The public will want more convincing information to overcome more than a century of widespread habituation and dependence. While we await definitive long-term clinical trials, chronic hypnotic use should be discouraged" (Kripke, 2000). He further lists three practice points: (1) Prescriptions for hypnotics should not be renewed for long-term use. (2) Chronic users of hypnotics should be gradually withdrawn, combined with possible provision of cognitive-behavioral therapy. (3) Cognitive-behavioral therapies are the best-supported treatment for chronic insomnia. Through the year 2000, little progress was made for treating insomnia through medication alone. There is a clear need to investigate other forms of treatment for insomnia and other sleep disorders.

To date, only one study has been published that has employed Kundalini yoga meditation techniques for the treatment of any sleep disorder (Khalsa, 2004). This 8-week study with 20 participants used Shabd Kriya and several other techniques for the treatment of "chronic insomnia patients consisting of sleep-onset and/or sleep-maintenance insomnia and primary or secondary insomnia." Measurements included sleep efficiency, total sleep time, total wake time, sleep onset latency, wake time after sleep onset, and number of awakenings. Personal diaries were the only source of data, and no polysomnographic measures were included for this intervention. Statistically significant improvements were observed with all parameters. However, the study was not a controlled trial and comparisons were made solely from pre- and post-treatment self-report measures. Patients were allowed to use hypnotic medications, presumably only in doses comparable to that of the 2-week baseline recording period. Without polysomnographic measures, the accuracy of the reported data is in question. In addition, the lack of a control group leaves the possibility that the effects are due to placebo expectations or to an additional relaxation period prior to the sleep effort.

SIX

Treating Chronic Fatigue Syndrome

A year 2000 State-of-the-Science Conference Report on chronic fatigue syndrome (CFS), published by the National Institutes of Health (Cassell, Demitrack, Engel, Mayberg, McCully, et al., 2000), opened with a 1994 statement to define the status and conundrum facing the CFS research and patient communities: "The CFS is a clinically defined condition characterized by severe disabling fatigue and a combination of symptoms that prominently features self-reported impairments in concentration and short-term memory, sleep disturbances, and musculoskeletal pain. Diagnosis of the CFS can be made only after alternative medical and psychiatric causes of chronic fatiguing illness have been excluded. No pathognomic signs or diagnostic tests for this condition have been validated in scientific studies; moreover, no definitive treatments exist." Recent longitudinal studies suggest that some persons affected by the CFS improve with time but that most remain functionally impaired for several years (Fukuda, Straus, Hickie, Sharpe, Dobbins, et al., 1994). The NIH report added, "A key addition to the quote from the 1994 CFS definition is that the duration of symptoms is not limited to 'several years,' but for most patients remains a lifelong issue" (Cassell et al., 2000).

The NIH report further summarized efforts: "The U.S. and other countries have pursued several possible etiologies and markers for CFS. No pathogen nor consistent primary immunologic abnormality has emerged. A variety of treatments have been tried, with many studies involving small case series or anecdotal reports. Cognitive behavioral therapy, cognitive behavioral stress management, graded exercise, and antidepressant medications have benefited some patients, but their overall efficacies remain to be established. Of the true clinical trials that have been undertaken, benefits have typically been limited to subsets of patients" (Cassell et al., 2000).

The Centers for Disease Control and Prevention (CDC) stated in 2005: "In order to receive a diagnosis of CFS, a patient must satisfy two criteria: (1) Have severe chronic fatigue of 6 months or longer duration with other known medical conditions excluded by clinical diagnosis, and (2) concurrently have four or more of the following symptoms: substantial impairment in short-term memory or concentration, sore throat, tender lymph nodes, muscle pain, multi-joint pain without swelling or redness, headaches of a new type, pattern or severity, unrefreshing sleep, and post-exertional malaise lasting more than 24 hours. And the symptoms must have persisted or recurred during 6 or more consecutive months of illness and must not have predated the fatigue" (Wagner, Nisenbaum, Heim, Jones, Unger, et al., 2005). The CDC further added, "A variety of therapeutic approaches have been described as benefiting patients with CFS. Since no cause for CFS has been identified and the pathophysiology remains unknown, treatment programs are directed at relief of symptoms, with the goal of the patient regaining some level of pre-existing function and well-being. Although desirable, a rapid return to pre-illness health may not be realistic, and patients who expect this prompt recovery and do not experience it may exacerbate their symptoms because of overexertion, become frustrated, and may become more refractory to rehabilitation" (Wagner et al., 2005).

A recent report prepared for the Agency of Healthcare Research and Quality concluded: "Existing case definitions for CFS appear to characterize a group of people with prolonged fatigue and impaired ability to function. The validity and superiority of any particular case definition are not well established. Surveys suggest that the prevalence of CFS in community populations is less than 1%. Precise estimates of rates of recovery, improvement, and/or relapse from CFS are not available. Although several therapies have been studied, potential benefits as well as harms of most therapies are not well established. Behavioral interventions that emphasize increasing activity levels may improve quality of life and function in some people with CFS" (Mulrow, Ramirez, Cornell & Allsip, 2001).

CFS occurs in men and women of all age groups, including children as young as 5 years of age and older adults in all ethnic, racial, and socioeconomic groups (Komaroff & Buchwald, 1998). In clinical settings, the typical patient is a middle-class white woman in her thirties (Komaroff & Buchwald, 1998). In the community at large, approximately 1 in 1,000 U.S. adults meet the CDC criteria for the syndrome (Buchwald, Umali, Umali, Kith, Pearlman, et al., 1995) and among patients seeking primary medical care for any reason, CFS occurs in approximately 1 in 100 adults (Bates, Schmitt, et al., 1993). One community-based study in the U.S. cites a prevalence rate in women of 0.52% and 0.29% in men (Jason, Richman, Rademaker, Jordan, Plioplys, et al., 1999). And in addition to the listed "definitive" symptoms, many patients with CFS also frequently report anorexia, nausea, drenching night sweats, intolerance of alcohol and pharmaceuticals that affect the central nervous system, and dizziness (Komaroff, Fagioli, Geiger, Doolittle, Lee, et al., 1996).

Today CFS is recognized as a complex and multisystemic, multifactorial illness (Cassell et al., 2000). However, syndromes of debilitating fatigue and other associated symptoms have engaged the attention of physicians for more than a century and have been called neurasthenia, Icelandic Disease, and myalgic encephalomyelitis (Komaroff & Buchwald, 1998). Clearly, like all the other disorders in this book, CFS is not a new illness. This disorder was recognized thousands of years ago by yogis. What follows is a 9-part, 37-minute Kundalini yoga protocol specific for the treatment of CFS that includes 27 minutes of work and 10 minutes of rest. Several case histories of treatment and their results using this protocol will follow.

A 9-Part Kundalini Yoga Protocol for Treating Chronic Fatigue Syndrome[*]

1. Technique to Induce a Meditative State: "Tuning In"

Sit with a straight spine and with the feet flat on the floor if sitting in a chair (see Figure 2.1, page 72). Put the hands together at the chest in "prayer pose"—the palms are pressed together with 10 to 15 pounds of pressure between the hands (a mild to medium pressure, nothing too intense). The area where the sides of the thumbs touch rests on the sternum with the thumbs pointing up (along the sternum), and the fingers are together and point up and out at a 60-degree angle to the ground. The eyes are closed and focused on the third eye (imagine a sun rising on the horizon, or the equivalent of the point between the eyebrows at the origin of the nose). A mantra is chanted out loud in a 1½-breath cycle. Inhale first through the nose and chant "Ong Namo" with an equal emphasis on the Ong and the Namo. Then immediately follow with a half-breath inhalation through the mouth and chant "Guru Dev Namo" with approximately equal emphasis on each word. (The O in *Ong* and *Namo* are each a long "o" sound; *Dev* sounds like *Dave*, with a long "a" sound.) The practitioner should focus on the experience of the vibrations these sounds create on the upper palate and throughout the cranium while letting the mind be carried by the

* Copyright © David Shannahoff-Khalsa, 2000. No portion of this protocol may be reproduced without the express written permission of the author.

sounds into a new and pleasant mental space. This should be repeated a minimum of three times. We employed it in our group about 10–12 times. There is no upper time limit for this technique, the longer the better. However, one must keep in mind that the other techniques will also induce profound changes.

2. Rotating the Spine While Maintaining the Hips in a Steady Position

Sit in an easy pose (a cross-legged posture with knees relaxed down toward the floor as much as possible). Hold the knees with both hands and rotate the torso for 1 minute first in a clockwise direction and then again for 1 minute in a counterclockwise direction, with long, deep breathing through the nose only. (If this sitting posture is not comfortable, practice this technique while sitting in a chair.) Keep the head erect, focusing on the movement of the torso. Keep the eyes closed and focus on the sound of the breath as you inhale and exhale. Make one inhale and exhale for each rotation of the spine and torso. This exercise helps to loosen the spine and you may feel like you are "grinding" the spine. However, it should not feel uncomfortable.

3. Spine-Flexing Technique in Rock Pose for Vitality

This technique increases metabolism, uplifts the spirit, and induces the healthy glandular changes that give an experience of vitality. For this technique, sit on the heels ("rock pose") with the knees coming together in front of the body and the hands resting on the thighs. (If this exercise position is difficult, the patient can substitute spine flexing while sitting in a chair, as taught in Chapter 2, pages 72–73.) Begin by pulling the chest up and slightly forward, inhaling deeply at the same time. Then exhale and relax the spine down into a slouching position. Keep the head up straight, as if looking forward, without allowing it to move much with the flexing action of the spine. This will help prevent a whip action of the cervical vertebrae. All breathing should only be through the nose for both the inhala-

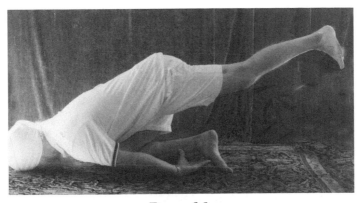

Figure 6.1
Third Exercise for the CFS Protocol

tion and exhalation. The eyes are closed and focused at a central point on the horizon, which is equivalent to the third eye, a point where the nose and eyebrows meet. The mental focus is kept on the sound of the breath while listening to the fluid movement of the inhalation and exhalation. Begin the technique slowly while loosening up the spine. Eventually a very rapid movement can be achieved with practice, reaching a rate of one to two times per second for the entire movement. Two minutes is adequate in the beginning. Later, there is no upper time limit. Food should be avoided just prior to this exercise. Be careful and flex the spine slowly in the beginning. Relax for 1 to 2 minutes when finished.

4. Third Exercise for the CFS Protocol

Place the chin on the floor, use both hands to hold the right ankle (the right knee is under the chest) and balance on the arms with the left leg extended out behind keeping the left foot at 90 degrees to the left leg (retracted in) (see Figure 6.1). The eyes are closed and focused at the crown of the head. Breathe slowly and deeply for 1 minute (building to three minutes over time), then relax on your back for 1 minute, and then repeat by reversing the exercise with the right leg up, and so on, for 1 to 3 minutes, followed again by 1 minute relaxing on your back.

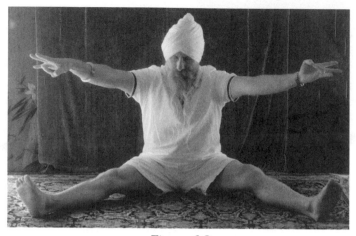

Figure 6.2
Fifth Exercise for the CFS Protocol

5. Fourth Exercise for the CFS Protocol

Lay on the back and bring the knees up to the chest with the hands in venus lock (interlock the fingers) held over the legs. The head is held up with the nose between the knees. Breathe slowly and deeply for 1 minute, and relax on the back for 1 minute. Repeat this exercise for 1 minute, and again follow with 1 minute of rest on the back.

6. Fifth Exercise for the CFS Protocol

Sit with the legs spread halfway out to the sides (45 degrees), bend forward 30 degrees (60 degrees up from the ground) (see Figure 6.2). Keep the spine straight and head in line with the spine. The arms are out to the sides, parallel to ground. The left hand has the palm facing up and the right hand has the palm facing down. With both hands, touch the tip of the ring finger to the tip of the thumb (sun mudra). When in this posture, breathe only through the nose, inhaling in four parts and exhaling in four parts for 3 to 5 minutes.

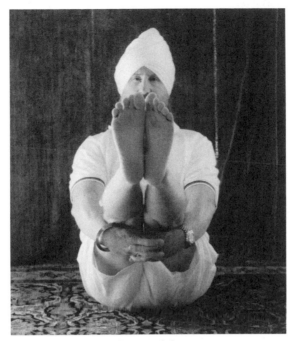

Figure 6.3
Sixth Exercise for the CFS Protocol

7. *Sixth Exercise for the CFS Protocol*

Balance on the buttocks with the hands in venus lock (interlaced fingers) held under the legs at the knees with the legs held up and heels together about 30 to 45 degrees above the ground (see Figure 6.3). Lean back and create approximately a 120-degree angle between the legs and the torso. The head is held in line with the torso. Focus the eyes on the two big toes. Do slow deep breathing through the nose only for 2 minutes. Then relax flat on the back for 1 minute. If there is trouble holding this position, place a pillow behind the back, but maintain the angle; the posture is the important element in this exercise.

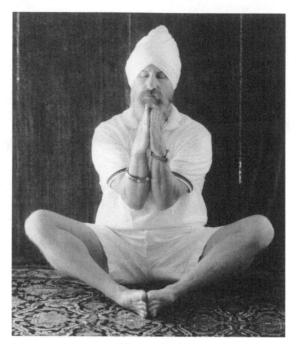

Figure 6.4
Seventh Exercise for the CFS Protocol

8. Seventh Exercise for the CFS Protocol

Sit with the soles of the feet touching together in front of the body (see Figure 6.4). The feet are as close to the groin as possible. The forearms are together side by side in front of the body with the elbows touching at the solar plexus. Both of the palms are flat, touching together with the fingers pointing up. The eyes are open and focused on the tip of the nose (the end you cannot see). Breathe slowly and deeply, with four parts segmented for the inhale and one part for the exhale, for 3 minutes. Then relax on the stomach for 2 minutes.

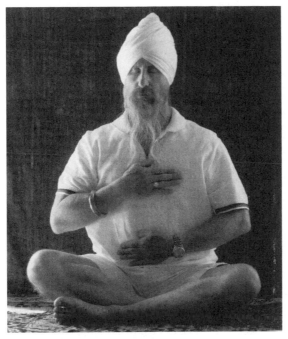

Figure 6.5
A Specific Meditation to Follow the Exercise Set for the CFS Protocol

9. A Specific Meditation to Follow the Exercise Set for the CFS Protocol

This meditation is for passing energy around the blocked solar plexus (part of the condition for CFS patients). Sit in an easy pose (or in a chair if necessary) (see Figure 6.5). The left palm is on the navel point (left fingers point right) and the right palm is on the heart center (right fingers point to the left). The eyes are closed, and the patient breathes slowly and deeply, but inhales through a curled tongue and exhales through puckered lips, making a whistle. This is continued for 11 minutes (if the patient cannot make the actual sound of the whistle, it is okay, but the effort should be made to exhale through puckered lips).

This series works on the orbit of the lower triangle of the chakras (chakras one through three) and the related glands and organs. The final meditation bypasses the solar plexus as the energy is moved from the lower triangle into the heart center. The glands and organs primarily affected in the exercise set are the adrenals, kidneys, liver, gall bladder, and spleen. The meditation (technique 9) also affects the thyroid, parathyroid, and pituitary. The 4-part breath orders and organizes the glands (guardians of the body) to create a balanced blood chemistry. This protocol is the most efficient and direct Kundalini yoga routine for treating CFS.

Case Histories of Treatment

Case History 1: An OCD Patient with CFS

Don (see case history 7 in Chapter 2, page 86) was a single Caucasian male (age 46) living on Social Security disability and undergoing treatment for his severe OCD when he started treatment for his CFS. He initially scored a 30 on his Y-BOCS. Not only did he have CFS and OCD, but he also had seasonal affective disorder, attention deficit disorder, low testosterone levels, and social phobia. He said to me, "Because my life has had so many ups and downs, it is impossible for me to analyze what caused what."

Don was born in England at his grandmother's house, while his father was a soldier away in Germany at the time. At age 9 months he moved with his mother to Germany to live with his father. He told me, "I don't think there was a real bond between my father and me. My father was very distant, and my mother was over-controlling and demanding. I never felt that I belonged in my family, and I do not miss any of them now." His father was an alcoholic, depressed, and had OCD. His mother was depressed, and a brother 2 years younger eventually became depressed as well as an alcoholic and drug abuser. Prior to moving to the U.S., Don had lived in England, Germany, and Cyprus (which was a war zone at the time). "My home life was emotionally and physically abusive.

Constant moves and difficult schools as well as living in a war zone caused a lot of anxiety and insecurity." His OCD symptoms started during his preteen years as a child. He was also dyslexic and was often shamed by teachers and other students because of his learning disabilities. In his youth, upon returning from sunny Cyprus to England, he developed seasonal affective disorder. As an adult he later experienced depression at ages 26, 29, 34, and 38. It took him 11 years to graduate college. He had "been lonely and unsuccessful in forming close friendships or intimate relationships." He had many periods of unemployment, part-time employment, and a variety of jobs ranging from a janitor to teaching and being a counselor. "All of my mental and physical problems have gotten worse, progressively culminating in being unable to work at age 43," at which time he was diagnosed with CFS. Don felt like a "victim." His life was one of "many disappointments and substantial stress that did not include the nurturing and care that would otherwise perhaps have helped to weather the circumstances." He had a "diminished will to live, but also a will to be healthy."

Don's ability to uplift himself given the right yogic formulas for combating the awesome combination of CFS and OCD is testimony to his will to be healthy. Don's CFS was nearly completely eliminated by the end of the OCD trial, when he claimed that he could go for a 2-hour walk before feeling really tired. He practiced the protocol three to four times a week during a 12-month period. This was a great feat, as prior to his initiation with the protocol, just walking from the parking lot to the class was a major fatiguing activity. He claimed that at that point he was unable even to walk a quarter of a mile.

Case History 2: A Highly Accomplished Female Physician

Joanne was 42 and a highly accomplished physician who had passed her boards in both psychiatry and neurology and was in private practice when she developed CFS. Two weeks prior to her onset she was faced with a surprise divorce from her second husband.

Joanne was raised in the South, where she lived on a farm with two older brothers. From the ages of 8 to 11 she was routinely raped by male family members. Her father was an alcoholic and her mother died shortly after her birth. At the age of 12, she went to live with her maternal grandparents. Her grandfather was a university professor and they lived in a prominent university community in the Northeast. She excelled in education, "feeling like she had a new lease on life and finally things were going her way." She was the valedictorian for her high school class and editor for the high school newspaper, and finally had a successful social life with other students. Suddenly, at the end of her senior year, her grandmother was diagnosed with pancreatic cancer and died within 2 months. During that summer, she "felt like the world had dropped out from underneath her" and she developed a case of severe depression that waxed and waned for 2 years. She had entered college, and in her second year met the man who became her first husband. This marriage lasted less than a year. The romance and marriage had been an upswing for her emotionally, until she discovered her husband's infidelity with one of her close friends. Her mood plummeted again, however this time, the depression was treated with antidepressants and she managed to get back into the swing of life. She graduated college and was accepted to medical school. Her dream, and the dream of her grandparents, would be fulfilled. She excelled throughout medical school. During her residency, she met husband number two, and after several years of courtship they were married and eventually moved to the West Coast, where they both found positions. Their careers were flourishing, his was academic and hers was in a private-practice clinic. She reluctantly elected to forgo motherhood, primarily because he never showed any enthusiasm to become a father. As their careers moved along, they spent less time at home and less time with each other. When her husband announced his choice of a divorce, she was completely surprised and asked why. He said, "I am in love with another woman." Joanne felt devastated. He moved out. She attempted to recover from the news, and in several weeks, when the shock and instant anger wore off, she entered a state of depression. However, this time she developed severe fatigue and she began to show signs of CFS, with frequent headaches, a vaginal yeast infection, an unremitting sore throat, lower back pain, and painful joints. After 2 months off from work, with no benefits from two antidepressants, she was finally diagnosed with a probable case of CFS. Her blood panels showed no signs of Epstein Bar Virus. However, after 2 months she developed a case of the shingles on her left back and left abdomen, leading to further incapacity. After her shingles resolved, a colleague suggested she try something nontraditional for her CFS, and he referred her to me. Perhaps I could somehow help her, at least with her mood. She was desperate and realized she had little choice. When she came to see me, I explained that I had been successful in several cases with CFS in the past and one much more complicated than her own. She said, "What do I have to lose?" I taught her the entire protocol the first time I saw her and made house calls once a week for the next 6 weeks. She finally started to show significant signs of recovery after 4 weeks. She usually practiced the protocol two to three times per week independently. After 3 months of practice, she was able to go back to work part-time, and after 4 months of practice she resumed a nearly full-time schedule. Her other somatic symptoms seemed to disappear in parallel with her fatigue. The last time I saw her, she smiled and said, "I have recovered once again," implying that her life had been a series of unexpected traumatic events that left her all too often feeling like an undeserving victim. During our weekly discussions, she occasional remarked that she did not understand why these kinds of things always seemed to happen to her.

SEVEN

Treating Attention Deficit Hyperactivity and Co-morbid Disorders

Attention deficit hyperactivity disorder (ADHD) is "arguably the most common of childhood mental disorders and it comprises the lion's share of economic cost and human suffering caused by childhood mental disorders" (Richters, Arnold, Jensen, Abikoff, Conners, et al., 1995). If not treated effectively, difficulties experienced by children with ADHD may continue or even increase into adulthood, resulting in problems with the justice system, substance abuse (Kupfer, Baltimore, Berry, et al., 2000), increased rates of child abuse, adult mental illness, and accidents with severe injuries (Fischer, Barkley, Fletcher, & Patel, 2001; Knapp, 1997). ADHD accounts for one-third to one-half of all referrals for child mental health services (Popper, 1988). "Children with ADHD usually have functional impairment across multiple settings including home, school, and peer relationships with long-term adverse effects on academic performance, vocational success, and social-emotional development" (Richters et al., 1995).

A 1982 listing of the core clinical features of ADHD includes developmentally inappropriate activity levels, low frustration tolerance, impulsivity, poor organization of behavior, distractibility, and an inability to sustain attention and concentration (Pelham,

1982). More recently, the *Diagnostic and Statistical Manual of Mental Disorders* (DSM-IV) defines three subtypes of ADHD, based on degrees of inattention and hyperactivity. The first and most common variant is "ADHD Combined," where six or more of nine symptoms of inattention and six or more of nine symptoms of hyperactivity-impulsivity have persisted for at least 6 months. Second is the "ADHD Predominantly Inattention Type," where there are six or more symptoms of inattention, but fewer than six of the hyperactivity-impulsivity type that have persisted for 6 months. Third is the "ADHD Predominantly Hyperactivity-Impulsivity Type," where there are six or more symptoms of the hyperactivity-impulsivity type, but fewer than six of the inattention type that have persisted for 6 months (APA, 1994). The APA's list of the nine inattention symptoms include: "(1) often fails to give close attention to details or makes careless mistakes in schoolwork, work, or other activities, (2) often has difficulty sustaining attention in tasks of play or activities, (3) often does not seem to listen when spoken to directly, (4) often does not follow through on instructions and fails to finish schoolwork, chores, or duties in the workplace, (5) often has difficulty organizing tasks and activities, (6) often avoids, dislikes, or is reluctant to engage in tasks that require sustained mental effort, (7) often loses things necessary for tasks or activities, (8) is often distracted by extraneous stimuli, and (9) is often forgetful in daily activities" (APA, 1994). The APA's list of the nine hyperactivity-impulsivity types include: "(1) often fidgets with hands or feet or squirms in seat, (2) often leaves seat in classroom or in other situations in which remaining seated is expected, (3) often runs about or climbs excessively in situations in which it is inappropriate, (4) often has difficulty playing or engaging in leisure activities quietly, (5) is often on the go or often acts as if driven by a motor, (6) often talks excessively." The last three symptoms are "impulsivity" based: "(7) often blurts out answers before questions have been completed, (8) often has difficulty awaiting turn, (9) often interrupts or intrudes on others" (APA, 1994). In addition, the APA definition requires that some impairment is present in two or more settings (e.g., at school, work, or home), with significant impairment in social, academic, or occupational functioning, and finally, that some symptoms should be apparent before age 7. However, this last criterion has been the subject of considerable controversy, since determining whether a patient meets a specific behavioral criterion (e.g., "often has difficulty organizing tasks and activities") depends on the observer's interpretation of terms such as "often," "difficulty," and "organizing" (Voeller, 2004). "Nearly all youths who met symptom criteria for the predominantly hyperactive-impulsive subtype also met the *DSM-IV* age of onset of impairment criterion, but 18% of youths who met symptom criteria for the combined type, and 43% of youths who met symptom criteria for the predominantly inattentive type, did not manifest impairment before seven years" (Applegate, Lahey, Hart, Biederman, Hynd, et al., 1997). Therefore, for the "combined" and "inattentive-subtype" using the onset cutoff age of 7 years reduced the accuracy of identification of currently impaired cases of ADHD (Applegate et al., 1997). This same finding was also noted in another large epidemiologic sample, with 25% of the youths with inattentive symptoms reporting onset after age 7 years, and this differs significantly to the 13% of the combined subtype or 8% of the hyperactive-impulsive subtype reporting onset after age 7 (Willoughby, Curran, Costello, & Angold, 2000).

The U.S. prevalence rate is also somewhat controversial. The 1994 *DSM-IV* estimates 3% to 5% (APA, 1994). One report is consistent with that, and claims ADHD affects an estimated 4.1% of youths ages 9 to 17 in a 6-month period (Shaffer, Fisher, Dulcan, Davies, Piacentini, et al., 1996). Most recently, ADHD has been called "a relatively common brain disorder, affecting as many as 10% of school-aged children" (Voeller, 2004). Another recent report states that ADHD "is a worldwide and highly prevalent disorder, estimated to affect 5%–10% of children (Faraone, Sergeant, Gillberg, & Biederman, 2003). And yet another report claims ADHD affects 8% to 12% of children worldwide and states that the rate of ADHD falls with age, but at least half of children with the disorder will have impairing symptoms in adulthood (Biederman & Faraone, 2005).

In surveys dealing with children referred to clinics, the ratio of boys to girls varies from 6:1 to 12:1, but in epidemiologic samples, the male-to-female prevalence ratio is much lower, 3:1 (Voeller, 2004). Girls with ADHD have half of the rates of conduct disorder (CD) and oppositional defiant disorder (ODD), but are much more likely to have significant social problems, manifest more emotional distress, have higher rates of depression and anxiety, be highly vulnerable to stress, and have poor self-esteem and a limited sense of control (Greene, Biederman, Faraone, Monuteaux, Mick, et al., 2001).

According to Voeller, "It is rare to encounter a child with "pure" ADHD without other emotional or learning problems because ADHD is associated with an extremely high rate of co-morbid psychiatric disorders and is usually accompanied by a learning disability" (2004). CD, ODD, antisocial behavior, dyslexia, MDD, bipolar disorder, anxiety disorders, including OCD and Tourette's syndrome are all common co-morbidities. If left untreated, pure ADHD alone can have long-term effects on a child's ability to make friends or do well at school or work, and this disorder frequently persists into adolescence and occasionally into adulthood. However, ADHD is not always associated with long-term impairment. Using indices of emotional, educational, and social adjustments, results indicate that "20% of children functioned poorly at follow-up in all three domains; 20% did well in all three domains; and 60% had intermediate outcomes" (Biederman, Mick, Faraone, 1998).

However, the costs to adults with ADHD alone are staggering. A recent Reuters Health Information report on Medscape quotes one of the world's leading ADHD experts, Joseph Biederman, MD, speaking at an American Medical Association briefing in New York, saying, "ADHD costs adult Americans with the condition about $77 billion in lost income a year, more than the total costs of drug abuse or depression. It has been shocking to me when we calculate the economic impact of this condition. ADHD is one of the costliest medical conditions that we have. By comparison, the direct and indirect costs of drug abuse are estimated at $58.3 billion a year, depression about $43.7 billion, and alcohol abuse about $85.8 billion" (Aubin, 2004).

One survey showed that adults with ADHD are three times more likely to have a stress disorder, depression, or other emotional problems; 24% reported that they were unable to participate in normal activities (an average of 11 days a month) because of poor mental or physical health, compared with only 9% of adults without ADHD (Shire, 2004). "Also, only 40% of adults with ADHD, versus 67% of adults without ADHD, 'strongly agree' that their future is bright. Only half of the ADHD adults reported that they liked and accepted themselves for who they are, compared with 76% of the adults without ADHD" (Shire, 2004). In addition, more than 60% of the adults in this survey have been addicted to tobacco; 52% have used drugs recreationally; and they were twice as likely to have been arrested compared to those without ADHD, with 37% acknowledging a prior arrest. They were twice as likely to be divorced or separated, and fewer than half of those surveyed who were currently in a relationship said they were "completely satisfied" with their significant other, compared with 58% of those without ADHD. Seventeen percent did not graduate from high school and only 18% graduated from college, compared with 7% and 26%, respectively, of those without ADHD. They held an average of 5.4 jobs in a 10-year period, compared with an average of 3.4 jobs for those without ADHD; 52% were currently employed at the time of the survey, compared with 72% of adults without ADHD; and of those currently employed who had more than one job in the past 10 years, 43% reported that they left or lost one or more of those jobs in part because of their ADHD symptoms (Shire, 2004).

In a recent 5-year follow-up of girls in the U.S. with ADHD with a mean age of 16.7, the Massachusetts General Hospital

Group noted high rates of co-morbidities (Monuteaux, 2005). The 1-year prevalence at follow-up was 36% for anxiety disorders, 23% for MDD, 3% for bipolar disorder, 34% for ODD, 11% for CD, 8% for antisocial personality disorder (ASPD), and 5% for psychosis. All these rates were significantly higher in the girls with ADHD than controls, except for psychosis. Substance-use disorders likewise occurred at higher rates in the ADHD girls: nicotine 38% versus 12% in controls; drug abuse 13% versus 3%; and alcohol 4% versus 0%. There was also a trend toward higher rates of bulimia in girls with ADHD, with an onset of symptoms at age 12 years.

In a 10-year follow-up of boys with ADHD (mean age 22 years), many still met criteria for ADHD (Spencer, 2005). Higher rates of all co-morbid disorders persisted in the males with ADHD and most co-morbidities had peaked during an earlier 4-year follow-up. However, there were a few exceptions. The incidence of bipolar disorder was 35% in young men with ADHD versus 4% in men without ADHD. Nicotine use, CD, and ASPD also increased from year 4 to year 10, with rates for nicotine at 45% for those with ADHD versus 21% for non-ADHD controls; CD 49% versus 6%; and ASPD 29% versus 10% (Spencer, 2005).

Clearly, the addition of severe, moderate, or even mild CD or the lesser problematic behavioral disorder of ODD, as opposed to ADHD alone, adds significant complication to the treatment of ADHD, and thus presents a major challenge to both the family and physician. The APA describes CD as having three subtypes, the "childhood-onset type," the "adolescent-onset type," and the "unspecified onset" type when the age of onset is unknown. The first subtype usually leads to more severe problems over time (APA, 1994). "For males under age 18 rates of CD range from 6% to 16%, and for females rates range from 2% to 9%," making CD "one of the most frequently diagnosed conditions in outpatient and inpatient mental health facilities" (APA, 1994). CD is defined as problems with aggression to people and animals, destruction of property, deceitfulness or theft, and serious violation of rules

(APA, 1994). The prevalence rate for ODD according to the APA is from 2% to 16% and is described as having "a pattern of negativistic, hostile, disobedient, and defiant behavior lasting at least 6 months, and it causes clinically significant impairment in social, academic, or occupational functioning, and the behavior is not the result of a psychotic or mood disorder, and the patient does not meet the criteria for CD, and if the patient is older than 18, they do not meet the criteria of antisocial personality disorder" (APA, 1994).

Treatment has largely consisted of the use of stimulant medications (methylphenidate, dextroamphetamine, and amphetamine) and/or behavioral therapies for helping children with ADHD gain some control for their activity levels, impulsiveness, and attention on tasks. Like all medications, those used to treat ADHD do have side effects and need to be closely monitored. According to a 2001 APA Fact Sheet, "Medications can be extremely helpful for many children with ADHD. Research indicates that between 70% and 80% of children with ADHD respond to medication. But medication alone is rarely an appropriate treatment for complex child psychiatric disorders such as ADHD. It should only be used as a component of a comprehensive treatment plan." However, "it is worth noting that in some US schools, as many as 30–40% of a class may be receiving treatment with methylphenidate" (Ghodse, 1999). In comparison, "patients with ADHD in the USA consumed a total of 330,000,000 defined daily doses (DDD) compared with a total of about 65,000,000 DDDs for patients in all other parts of the world," according to the International Narcotic Controls Board Report (RINCB, 1998). In addition to this alarming increase in prescribed treatment in the U.S., another note of caution is due. A recent uncontrolled trial was conducted on 12 children (mean age 8.5 +/- 3.5 years) assessing the potential mutagenicity or carcinogenicity effects of methylphenidate at therapeutic doses. "In all participants, treatment induced a significant 3, 4.3, and 2.4-fold increase in chromosome aberrations, sister chromatid exchanges, and micronuclei frequencies, respectively (P=0.000 in all cases)." The authors concluded, "These findings warrant further investigations of the possible health effects of methylphenidate in humans, especially in view of the well-documented relationship between elevated frequencies of chromosome aberrations and increased cancer risk" (El-Zein, Abdel-Rahman, Hay, Lopez, Bondy, et al., 2005).

A 1992 Multimodal Treatment Study of Children with ADHD was cosponsored by the National Institute of Mental Health and the U.S. Department of Education (Group, 1999). This study was conducted at six different sites in the U.S. and involved 579 boys and girls who met the *DSM-IV* criteria for ADHD "combined type." The children were randomly assigned to four different treatment conditions: medication only, medication plus behavioral treatment, behavioral treatment only, and "community care" (i.e., after the initial evaluation, families were provided with a report summarizing the assessment results and a list of mental health resources in their community and were then followed as part of the study). Daily records of behavior and side effects were kept, and the optimal dose was selected after the records were reviewed blindly by experienced clinicians at a different site. Of the 289 subjects who entered this segment of the study, 256 completed it. After the optimal dose was determined, the children were seen at monthly visits, and the response to the treatment and side effects were monitored. No side effects were reported in 35.9%, mild side effects in 49.8%, moderate side effects in 11.4%, and severe side effects in 2.9% (Group, 1999).

A recent report using the same 579 children from this multimodal four-arm treatment study looked at the cost-effectiveness of ADHD treatments and concluded: "Treatment costs varied fourfold, with medication management being the least expensive, followed by behavioral treatment, and then combined treatment. Lower costs of medication treatment were found in the community care group, reflecting the less intensive (and less effective) nature of community-delivered treatment. Medical management was more effective but more costly than community care and more cost-effective than combination treatment and behavioral treatment alone. Under some conditions, combination treatment (medical management and psychotherapy) were somewhat more cost-effective, as demonstrated by lower costs per additional child 'normalized' among children with multiple co-morbid disorders" (Jensen, Garcia, Glied, Cowe, Foster, et al., 2005). They concluded, "Medical management treatment, although not as effective as combined medical management and behavioral treatment, is likely to be more cost effective in routine treatment for children with ADHD, particularly those without co-morbid disorders. For some children with co-morbid disorders, it may be cost-effective to provide combination treatment" (Jensen et al., 2005).

I am aware of only two trials using either meditation or yoga to treat ADHD. One uncontrolled trial used what is called "Sahaja Yoga Meditation" in a 6-week program of twice-weekly sessions with the parents playing an active role in guiding children at home through their meditation practice. The authors did not publish the actual details of the technique but stated, "The meditation process involved practicing techniques whereby participants were helped to achieve a state of thoughtless awareness. Instructors directed participants to become aware of this state within themselves by becoming silent and focusing their attention inside" (Harrison, Manocha, & Rubiez, 2004). Forty-eight children (41 boys, 7 girls) met the criteria for inclusion in the study and 31 were receiving medication (e.g., ritalin, dexamphetamine), 14 were not medicated, and medication information was not provided for the other 3 children. The primary assessment tool was the Conners Parent–Teacher Questionnaire (CPTQ) where parents are rating their own children. Twenty-six children with pre- and post-treatment data showed a marked improvement in ADHD symptoms as measured on the CPTQ. "Mean scores decreased from Mpre = 22.54, SD = 4.61, to Mpost = 14.62, SD = 5.15. The average mean decrease in reported ADHD symptoms was 7.91 points (SD = 4.91, range 0–19), which represented an improvement rate of 35%. Statistical analysis using paired samples t-test showed that the difference in pre- and post-treatment scores was highly signif-icant (t = 8.23, p < .001)" (Harrison et al., 2004). In addition, no differences in improvement rates were found between medicated and unmedicated patients.

Another study with boys only (Jensen & Kenny, 2004) combined four basic elements in treatment, (1) "respiratory training," where boys were taught to "breathe naturally through both nares in a regulated rhythmical manner," (2) "postural training that included stretching; load bearing; backward, forward, and lateral flexion; and extensions and inversions performed in sitting, standing, supine, and prone positions combined with respiratory exercises in static and dynamic positions," (3) "relaxation training," described as "becoming progressively aware of and relaxing body parts and tensing and relaxing muscles," and (4) "concentration training," where participants focused on a word or shape followed by seeing the image with eyes closed and continuing to see the image on a blank piece of paper. They were stabilized on medica-tion and randomly assigned to a 20-session yoga group (n = 11) or a control group (cooperative activities; n = 8). Boys were assessed pre- and post-intervention using the long version of the Conner's Parent and Conner's Teacher Rating Scales-Revised (CPRS-R:L and CTRS-R:L), and with the Test of Variables of Attention (TOVA). There were no significant differences observed for either the yoga or control groups by teachers. However, significant improvements from pre-test to post-test were found for the yoga, but not for the control group, on five subscales of the CPRS: Oppositional, Global Index Emotional Lability, Global Index Total, Global Index Restless/Impulsive, and ADHD Index. Signifi-cant improvements from pre-test to post-test were found for the control group, but not the yoga group, on three CPRS subscales: hyperactivity, anxious/shy, and social problems. Both groups improved significantly on CPRS Perfectionism, DSM-IV Hyperac-tive/Impulsive, and DSM-IV Total. Those in the yoga group who engaged in more home practice showed a significant improvement on TOVA Response Time Variability with a trend on the ADHD score, and greater improvements on the CTRS Global Emotional Lability subscale. The authors concluded, "Although these data do not provide strong support for the use of yoga for ADHD, partly because the study was under-powered, they do suggest that yoga may have merit as a complementary treatment for boys with ADHD already stabilized on medication, particularly for its evening effect when medication effects are absent" (Jensen & Kenny, 2004).

11-Part Kundalini Yoga Protocol for Attention-Deficit/ Hyperactivity Disorder and Co-morbid Disorders[*]

This 11-part protocol has been designed and tested for use with children, adolescents, and adults with ADHD and any combination of co-morbid disorders, including CD, ODD, depression, anxiety, and some learning disorders.

1. Technique to Induce a Meditative State: "Tuning In"

Sit with a straight spine and with the feet flat on the floor if sitting in a chair (see Figure 2.1). Put the hands together at the chest in "prayer pose"—the palms are pressed together with 10 to 15 pounds of pressure between the hands (a mild to medium pressure, nothing too intense). The area where the sides of the thumbs touch rests on the sternum with the thumbs pointing up (along the sternum), and the fingers are together and point up and out at a 60-degree angle to the ground. The eyes are closed and focused on the third eye (imagine a sun rising on the horizon, or the equivalent of the point between the eyebrows at the origin of the nose). A mantra is chanted out loud in a 1½-breath cycle. Inhale first through the nose and chant "Ong Namo" with an equal emphasis on the Ong and the Namo. Then immediately follow with a half-breath inhalation through the mouth and chant "Guru Dev Namo" with approximately equal emphasis on each word. (The O in *Ong* and *Namo* are each a long "o' sound; *Dev* sounds like *Dave*, with a long "a" sound.) The practitioner should focus on the experience of the vibrations these sounds create on the upper palate and throughout the cranium while letting the mind be carried by the sounds into a new and pleasant mental space. This should be repeated a minimum of three times. We employed it in our group about 10–12 times. This technique helps to create a "meditative state of mind" and is always used as a precursor to the other techniques. There is no upper time limit for this technique; the longer the better. However, one must keep in mind that the other techniques will also induce profound changes.

2. Spine-Flexing Technique for Vitality

This technique increases the patient's metabolism, uplifts the spirit, and helps induce healthy glandular changes that give the energetic experience of vitality. This is a very helpful precursor to the other techniques, because it helps set the mood and energy.

This technique can be practiced while sitting either in a chair or on the floor in a cross-legged position. If you are in a chair, hold the knees with both hands for support and leverage. If you are sitting cross-legged, grasp the ankles in front with both hands. Begin by pulling the chest up and slightly forward, inhaling deeply through the nose at the same time. Then exhale as you relax the spine down into a slouching position. Keep the head up straight, as if you were looking forward, without allowing it to move much while flexing the spine. This will help prevent a whip effect in the cervical vertebrae. All breathing should only be through the nose for both the inhalation and exhalation. The eyes are closed as if you were looking at a central point on the horizon, the third eye. Your mental focus is kept on the sound of the breath while listening to the fluid movement of the inhalation and exhalation. Begin the technique slowly while loosening up the spine. Eventually, a very rapid movement can be achieved with practice, reaching a rate of one to two times per second for the entire movement. A few minutes are adequate in the beginning. Later, there is no time limit. Food should be avoided just prior to this exercise. Be careful and flex the spine slowly in the beginning. Relax for 1 minute when finished.

3. Spine Twists for Reducing Tension

This technique helps to reduce stress and tension and induce a change of mood by bringing a balance to the nervous system and electromagnetic field. Place the hands on the shoulders, right hand on the right shoulder, left hand on the left shoulder, with the fingers in the front and the thumbs behind pointing toward the back. Keep both elbows up and out toward the sides. Inhale and twist the spine-torso-head to the left, exhale and twist to the right. Inhale and exhale only through the nose. Continue this motion while slowly warming up the spine and then picking up the pace for 1 minute. Keep the eyes closed and focused on the third eye to help prevent the possibility of becoming dizzy. When finished, inhale with eyes closed, sitting forward with the arms remaining up, and exhale. Relax for 30 seconds.

4. Ganesha Meditation for Focus and Clarity

Sit with a straight spine, with the eyes closed (see Figure 2.4, page 100). The left thumb and little finger are sticking out from the hand. The other fingers are curled into a fist with fingertips on the moon mound (the root of the thumb area that extends down to the wrist). The left hand and elbow are parallel to the floor, with the pad of the tip of the left thumb pressing on the curved notch of the nose between the eyes. The little finger is sticking out. With right hand and elbow parallel to the floor, grasp the left little finger with the right hand and close the right hand into a fist around it, so that both hands now extend straight out from your head. Push the notch with the tip of the left thumb to the extent that you feel some soreness as you breathe long and deep. After continued practice, this soreness reduces. Do this for 3 minutes and no longer. To finish, keeping the posture with eyes closed, inhale. Push a little more and pull the naval point in by tightening the abdominal muscles for 10 seconds, then exhale. Repeat one more time.

5. Meditation for Learning Disabilities, ADD, and ADHD

Sit with a straight spine, either in a chair or on the floor with the lower spine pushed forward, as if "standing at attention." The eyes are closed and focused at the third eye, the point where the nose emerges from the forehead. Use the thumb tip of the right hand (or a nasal plug) to block the right nostril and begin breathing only through the left nostril. The pattern of the breath is as follows: inhale slowly for the count of 10, hold the breath for the count of 10, and exhale slowly for the count of 10. The "count of 10" can approximate 10 seconds once the practitioner has had some experience with this meditation, and eventually can reach 20 seconds. The time should be increased to a maximum time of 31 minutes, and a good starting time is 11 minutes. Eventually build the practice to do it perfectly for 31 minutes for 120 days in a row. However, when combined here with the other techniques, 11 to 15 minutes is adequate.

When the ability to do this technique for the full time of 31 minutes is reached, the patient should begin to notice that their receptive qualities (the ability to listen, the ability to retain what they hear, and the ability not to be reactive to what they hear and see) are much improved. This technique is also excellent for the condition where "things go in one ear and right out the other." The effects of this technique can help relax an individual both physically and mentally. When practicing this technique, always do it for at least three to five minutes; doing it for a minute or two can actually make the patient slightly more active for a few minutes. However, most people would not notice the difference if they started while already feeling agitated or overstimulated and had already practiced techniques 1 through 4.

6. Meditation to Balance and Synchronize
the Cerebral Hemispheres

Sit with a straight spine. The eyes are open and focused on the tip of the nose (the very end, which is not visible to the patient). Both hands are at the shoulder level with palms facing forward and the hands loosely open, the fingers spread pointing up and not straight, as if holding a heavy ball in each hand (see Figure 7.1). Chant out loud "Har Har Gur Gur," and with each sound ("Har" or "Gur"), rotate the hands to where the palms face toward the back (see Figure 7.2) and then quickly return them to face the forward position. The left palm rotates in the clockwise direction and the right hand rotates in the counterclockwise direction (the only natural direction for rotation of each hand when starting with the palms facing forward). Make sure that the tongue quickly touches (flicks) the upper palate on "Har" and the lower palate on "Gur." Also pump the navel point lightly with each "Har" or "Gur." The rate of chanting for the entire mantra and rotating the hands reaches 2 seconds per round of the mantra. The time for practice is 11 minutes. The effects are that the frontal lobes and other paired regions of the hemispheres are synchronized to bring clarity, peace, vitality, and intuition.

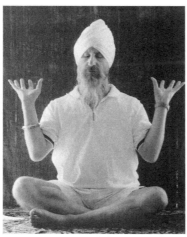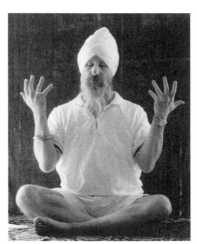

Figures 7.1 and 7.2
Meditation for Balancing and Synchronizing the Cerebral Hemispheres

7. Meditation to Balance the Jupiter and Saturn Energies: A Technique to Help Reduce Depression and Self-Destructive Behavior

Sit with a straight spine either in a chair or on the floor (see Figure 3.2, page 120). The hands are facing forward with the ends of the Jupiter (index) and Saturn (middle) fingers pointing straight up near the sides of the body at the level of the chin. The elbows are relaxed down by the sides and the hands are near the shoulders. Close the ring and little fingers down into the palm using the thumbs and keep them there against the palm during the meditation. The Jupiter (index) finger and the Saturn (middle) finger are spread open in a V shape (or closed). The eyes are closed. For 8 minutes open and close the Jupiter and Saturn fingers about once or twice per second. Make sure they spread completely open and close completely during the exercise. Simultaneously imagine the planets of Jupiter and Saturn coming together in front of you and then again going apart in synch with the finger movement—the planets should appear to go back and forth along a straight line in and out to the sides in front of you. It does not matter whether you have Jupiter or Saturn on the left or right side. Continue this imagery movement for 8 minutes along with the fingers opening and closing. (In the beginning, the imaging is difficult to do but this should not slow down the pace of the fingers, which play a more important role here). After 8 minutes, while continuing the same exercise, now begin to inhale and exhale through the nose only with the movement (inhale as the fingers are spread, exhale as the fingers close). Continue with the planets. Continue this part for 2 additional minutes. Then, for the last minute, spread the two fingers wide and hold them wide apart (now they do not open and close, they remain in the fixed V shape), keeping them very stiff (which requires considerable effort) while also keeping the mouth in an O, or ring, shape. Breathe in and out of the mouth using only the diaphragm (not the wall of the upper chest) with a rate of two to three breaths per second. After 1 minute, inhale, hold the breath in, and tense every muscle tightly (including the hands, fingers, with the "v" kept rigid, arms, back, stomach) in the body for 10 seconds. Exhale and repeat two more times for 10 seconds. Then relax.

As previously noted in Chapter 3, Yogi Bhajan said that "this meditation will help increase a person's ability to focus and concentrate and also increase the IQ of an individual over several months of practice. The mind becomes very focused and clear, the brain becomes very energized. This technique will also help eliminate depression. This technique can also enhance math skills for those who have difficulties with math. The Jupiter and Saturn energies become balanced (the brain is balanced) and this allows one to overcome any challenge, including mastery of the self. This technique also helps to eliminate self-destructive behavior and undesirable (acting out) behavior toward others. In addition, during the beginning of the technique, around the 4 to 8 minute mark, a person can feel very irritable and sometimes it can bring out deep-seated anger" (Bhajan, 1995). Note: If a person feels dizzy during the meditation, they should stop and try it again on another occasion.

8. Brain Exercise for Normalizing Frontal Lobes and Enhancing Focus, Clarity, and the Ability to Communicate (Listen and Articulate)

Sit straight and raise the hands to the shoulder level with the hands facing forward. The first three fingers (index, middle, and ring finger) are kept straight and point up (this is difficult for many in the beginning, and patients should simply do their best). The thumb tips and the tips of the little fingers continuously touch and let go at a very rapid pace (up to four to five times per second). The eyes remain closed. Continue the rapid contact and release of the thumb tips and little finger tips for three minutes maximum. After 2 minutes, the patient begins to create the effect he wants, but 3 minutes is ideal. The effects can last up to 4 hours. Once an individual develops the ability to do this technique easily for 3 minutes, he will begin to excel in his communication skills.

Techniques 9, 10, and 11 are especially useful for co-morbid patients with CD and ODD. And of course, they can be used separately. A patient with only "pure" ADHD or ADD can choose not to include techniques 9 through 11.

9. Technique for Tranquilizing an Angry Mind

This technique is usually only used when patients are experiencing significant anger. This is not a technique for latent or "cold," repressed, deep-seated anger. It is a wonderful option to be able to tranquilize a "red-hot" angry mind. There are at least a half-dozen Kundalini yoga meditation techniques for anger, and this one, in this author's opinion, is by far the simplest and most effective and can easily be implemented with young children. The results can last up to 3 days in the less-severe cases, and may require two times per day for those with severe red-hot anger.

Sit with a straight spine and close the eyes. Simply chant out loud "Jeeo, Jeeo, Jeeo, Jeeo" (pronounced likes the names for the letters *g* and *o*) continuously and rapidly for 11 minutes without stopping. Rapid chanting is about 8 to 10 repetitions per 5 seconds. During continuous chanting, the patient does not stop to take long breaths, but continues with just enough short breaths to keep the sound going continuously. Eleven minutes is all that is needed. (This technique only has real benefit if anger is a clear and immediate problem.)

10. Brain Exercise for Patience and Temperament

Sit with a straight spine. Close the eyes nine-tenths and look straight ahead at the third eye point. Interlock the middle fingers only and bring this lock in front of the heart center, 2 to 3 inches in front of the chest. The right palm faces down and the left palm faces the chest. Make sure only the middle fingers are touching and pull this lock with maximum capacity for 3 minutes while breathing slowly and deeply. This technique is usually a little painful in the middle fingers when done correctly.

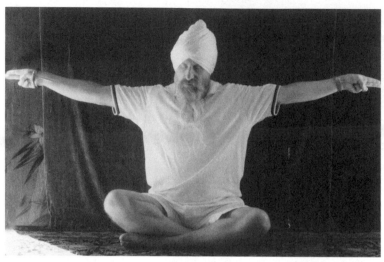

Figure 7.3
Meditation for Releasing Childhood Anger

11. Meditation for Releasing Childhood Anger

Sit straight and extend the arms stretched out straight to the sides, with no bend in the elbows (see Figure 7.3). The thumb locks down the ring and little fingers and the index and middle fingers are extended straight out to the sides, the palms facing forward. Breathe deeply by sucking the air through closed teeth and exhale through the nose for 11 minutes. To end, inhale deeply, hold the breath for 10 seconds, and stretch the spine up and the arms out straight to the sides with maximum force, then exhale, and repeat this inhale, hold, stretch two more times. This technique can be done at any time with the intended effects, but the effects are most unique when practiced in the evening (Bhajan, 2002).

Case Histories of Treatment

Case History 1: Eight-year-old Male

Gregory was age 8 the first time I saw him. He had been adopted from an Eastern European country when he was 10 months old. He was the second child, and his older sibling had also been given up for adoption. Gregory's mother was never married, was unemployed, and had a substance-abuse problem. The biological fathers of Gregory and his older sibling were both short-term boyfriends of the mother who showed no interest or any responsibility toward their offspring. Gregory's mother was living with her parents, and her father was an alcoholic and frequently physically and emotionally abusive toward her. She ultimately was given the choice of either moving out or giving up her children after each event, as she showed little responsibility toward their welfare. At the time of Gregory's adoption, his mother was 21 years of age. His mother spent most of her time with various men and meeting the needs of her substance-abuse problems. She reported that she frequently left Gregory alone for hours at a time. Gregory's adoptive parents had been unable to conceive after 10 years of trying all forms of reproductive assistance. They were both 40 years of age at the time of his adoption, and both were employed professionals in the legal field and lived a life of relative abundance. Both adoptive parents were raised as single children born into wealthy families. Neither parents had any previous experience or background with raising children. When Gregory was adopted, he had appeared malnourished, agitated, and clearly suffered from a separation-anxiety disorder. His adoptive mother spent the first 8 months at home trying to comfort him but without much success. He also suffered from food sensitivities for the first 5 years of his life until his food allergies were diagnosed by a pediatrician. When he was 2 years of age, his adoptive mother returned to work part-time. She was extremely frustrated by his inability to adapt. Gregory was first taken to a day care and then later a nanny was hired, as a request was made to remove him from the day-care center. The adoptive father worked long hours and found the difficulty of raising and managing Gregory's behavior to be "beyond his skills." When Gregory entered kindergarten, he did not get along with his schoolmates and showed early signs of ODD. It was not unusual for his mother to be called to pick him up due to his disruptive behavior and fighting with other children. When he entered second grade, his parents elected to put him into a private school where they thought he might receive a more structured environment and closer instruction and attention. Gregory showed all the classic signs of both CD and ODD by the age of 7. He had been prescribed virtually all of the stimulant medications with little positive effect on his behavior, but the medications led to sleeping difficulties and an unbalanced affinity for foods high in sugar and other carbohydrates. He failed to respond to school counselors and showed no interest in complying with the suggestions of his private therapists. When his parents finally realized he was showing sensitivity to both wheat products and dairy, they tried to eliminate both from his diet and this seemed to help to some degree, much to his chagrin. When he was first brought to me at age 8 he came with a can of soda in hand (soda is reported to have one of the highest levels of both sugar and caffeine).

On the first occasion of seeing him, he chose not to cooperate or to participate with any of the techniques. When he was 12, he agreed to return to see me and we started treatment with three 2-hour meetings per week. On the very first visit, he complied with the entire 11-part ADHD co-morbid protocol and remained in his chair for the entire 2 hours, complying with the instruction with extraordinary abilities. When we finished the protocol, I asked him how he was feeling and he said, "I feel better than I have ever felt in my life!" This may have been the first occasion that he was able to achieve anything that gave him a decent and positive sense of himself. He was beaming. His parents were not skilled at positive reinforcement and had tried every means of discipline. When his mother picked him up, she noticed he was smiling and quite calm and she asked if he would like to come back. He said "Yes, I had a good time, and I really like how I feel." I saw him three times a week for the next 4 months. After about 2 months, he started to practice part of the protocol at home on occasion. He reported that he would not do technique 11 on his own, but did occasionally enjoy techniques 5 through 7. After 4 months of seeing him on a three-times per week basis, he then saw me only weekly for two additional months and then only once a month for 2 more months. For the remainder of the year, he continued home schooling and his reading and math skills improved. He even started to read books of his own choice and developed an affinity for drawing and painting by computer. He began to mature and realized he would be much happier in the world if he was able to manage his behavior and progress again in the public school system. The last I heard from his parents, he was achieving well in his first year of high school and looked forward to going to college. He had even expressed wanting to go to medical school and possibly becoming a child psychiatrist.

Case History 2: 11-year-old Male

Ricky was 11 when he was brought to me by his mother. He was the youngest child of three from her first of two marriages. She divorced Ricky's father when Ricky was two years of age, and divorced the second husband when Ricky was eight. His biological father lived in another state in the Northwest and saw him only during holidays, and otherwise played little or no role in his life other than that of consistent financial support. His father had remarried and started a second family. Ricky was having problems in school, both in terms of his academic performance and with his behavior in and outside of the classroom. He had one older sister and brother from the same father, and one younger half-brother from his mother's second marriage. His sister was 7 years older and his brother was 4 years older. His half-brother was four years of age and Ricky had commented to me that he "felt like his brother was the one who received all of his mother's attention." Ricky had a history of problems in school since he was age 6. At age 7, he had been prescribed both methylphenidate and later dextroamphetamine. When he presented, he was on atomoxetine for his ADHD and bupropion for depression. His psychiatrist had diagnosed him with ADHD "combined," depression, an anxiety disorder, and ODD. He showed defiance toward his mother and toward his school teachers and eventually was put into a special class for behaviorally disruptive children. He developed depression at the age of 8, when his mother divorced for the second time. His mother had hoped that he would improve once the household had a chance to stabilize after her second divorce. Ricky's mother and stepfather frequently got into disputes when the stepfather was home on leave from the military. Ricky's mother had reported that her second husband showed signs of being an alcoholic and she suspected infidelity. He was occasionally verbally and emotionally abusive to her in front of the children. Ricky's mother was a school teacher and financially independent after the second divorce.

By the age of 11, no significant signs of improvement were showing in Ricky's life, either academically or behaviorally. He was preoccupied with video games, and he could spend endless hours playing on his computer in his room. Ricky's mother talked to him almost solely about his schoolwork and about not bothering his younger brother. She had taken him to a counselor on many occasions in an attempt to help resolve his emotional problems. Eventually, he told his mother in one therapy session that he was really unhappy, angry, depressed, and hopeless about his life. He said he felt like the "odd ball" in the family and that neither his father or his mother loved him. He said that everyone else in the family had a good life and he could not understand why his was such a failure. After several more months of psychotherapy, his mother heard from a school counselor about how her daughter had been helped with OCD and that maybe Kundalini yoga was something that Ricky would enjoy as a therapy because it was "very physical."

Initially, I saw Ricky once a week for 2-hour sessions for one month, and then eventually, given some signs of improvement, I saw him three times a week. Ricky enjoyed the therapy because he knew how much better he felt during treatment and also later at home. He felt much calmer and less angry and anxious. He told me, "Finally I am good at something in my life." His mother noted how his attitude had slowly changed toward his younger brother, and she progressively received less calls from the school. Eventually the school counselor also noted how he seemed to have turned around. After 3 months of therapy at three times per week, we went to twice a week for 1 month, and finally once a week for the final month. His grades and behavior were both improving. After 2 months in treatment, he was taken off bupropion, and his atomoxetine was reduced by half. Between months 4 and 5 in treatment, his atomoxetine was completely eliminated. Toward the end of treatment, his mother was so impressed she decided to take a local Kundalini yoga class to deal with her own stress. Eventually, she and Ricky would on occasion do meditation techniques together, and frequently at Ricky's request. The last report I had about Ricky was that he was getting B's on his report card in school and was no longer in a class for behaviorally disruptive children.

In 1988, I the opportunity for 2 weeks to teach Kundalini yoga to a group of 15 children, ages 6 to 12, at the San Diego Center for Children, a residential treatment center for children with emotional and behavioral problems. These children participated in a 1-hour class from 7:30 A.M. to 8:30 A.M. All of the children were diagnosed with ADHD, severe emotional disabilities, and a range of behavioral disorders. All were medicated with at least two to three medications. While funding did not permit a long-term trial, all the children that participated enjoyed their yoga practice. At that time, I had not yet developed the protocol for ADHD and co-morbid disorders. However, the children did enjoy a floor-based yoga practice. In my humble opinion, I believe that children in this age range with these classic symptoms and disorders would gladly comply with a variety of Kundalini yoga–based protocols that would help lead to significant recovery. The 11-Part ADHD and Co-morbid Disorders Protocol described earlier would be ideal for children, adolescents, and adults with ADHD, depression, anxiety disorders, CD, ODD, and ASPD.

EIGHT

Treating the Abused and Battered Psyche

Trauma victimization in the U.S. primarily results from sexual abuse, physical abuse, neglect in the case of children, and the passive witnessing of horrific events. The report of the President's New Freedom Commission on Mental Health identifies trauma as one of the four main areas for the nation to address (NFCMH, 2003). According to the director of the Center for Mental Health Services, the primary federal agency addressing mental health, "Trauma is pervasive, it is damaging, and it is an extremely serious threat to our public health" (Power, 2005). A recent report by the Surgeon General on mental health cites child abuse and neglect as one of the primary risk factors for mental disorders (Satcher, 1999). The National Child Traumatic Stress Network reported that "25% of children surveyed in one major study had experienced a traumatic event by the age of 16. Another study found that 64% of New York City school children had experienced at least one significant traumatic event before 9/11. An estimated 4 million children and youth have experienced a serious physical assault, and 9 million have witnessed serious violence. Estimates of the number of children abused, neglected, or exposed to domestic violence exceed 3 million cases annually" (Pynoos & Fairbank, 2004).

Surveys of adults for child sexual abuse in large nonclinical populations in 19 countries including the United States have found rates in line with comparable North American studies, with ranges from 7% to 36% for women and 3% to 29% for men (Finkelhor, 1994). These prevalence figures vary widely as a function of the selection and response rate, the definition used, and the method (e.g., self-report versus structured interview) by which an abuse history is obtained (Putnam, 2003). In addition, children suffer more victimizations than adults, including more conventional crimes, family violence, and abduction (Finkelhor & Dziuba-Leatherman, 1994a). One national survey of 2,000 children aged 10 to 16 years asked about victimization in the previous year only. Twenty-five percent experienced a completed victimization, 1 in 8 had experienced an injury, one in a 100 required medical attention, nonfamily physical assaults dominated, contact sexual abuse occurred with 3.2% of girls and 0.6% of boys, along with a substantial number of attempted kidnappings and violence directed toward children's genitals (Finkelhor & Dziuba-Leatherman, 1994b). However, close to 90% of sexual abuse cases are never reported to the authorities (Hanson, Resnick, Saunders, Kilpatrick, & Best, 1999). A more recent national survey of 2,030 children 10 to 17 years old and of children 2 to 9 assessed through caregiver reports showed 71% of the sample reporting at least one victimization in the last year, with an average of 2.63 victimizations per child (Finkelhor, Hamby, Ormrod, & Turner, 2005). In this study, "More than one-half of the children and youth had experienced a physical assault in the study year, more than 1 in 4 a property offense, more than 1 in 8 a form of child maltreatment, 1 in 12 a sexual victimization, and more than 1 in 3 had been a witness to violence or experienced another form of indirect victimization (Finkelhor, Ormrod, Turner, & Hamby, 2005). In addition, a variety of adult psychiatric conditions have been clinically associated with child sexual abuse, that include MDD, borderline personality disorder, somatization disorder, substance-abuse disorders, PTSD, dissociative identity disorder, bulimia nervosa, dysfunctional behaviors, and neurobiological dysregulation (Putnam, 2003). Also, "as a group, individuals with histories of child sexual abuse, irrespective of their psychiatric diagnosis, manifest significant problems with affect regulation, impulse control, somatization, sense of self, cognitive distortions, and problems with socialization" (Putnam, 2003).

The above figures with child sexual abuse and victimization begin to reveal the horrendous impact that trauma can have on our youth and how these events can either cripple or destroy a life. These figures for the most part do not include statistics in the case of war, genocide, or foreign occupation. To address those effects is beyond the scope of this book.

Perhaps the most common medical result of experiencing a major traumatic event is the development of PTSD which may affect some 2% to 3% of the general population at any one time (Davidson, Tharwani, & Connor, 2002; Ohayon & Shapiro, 2000). The National Comorbidity Survey of 5,877 Americans found that 7.8% of adults had suffered from PTSD at some time in their lives. The type of traumatic event effects rates of incidence of PTSD (Kessler, Sonnega, Bromet, Hughes, & Nelson, 1995). Physical assaults amongst women, for example, led to a lifetime prevalence of 29% and war combat for men led to a lifetime prevalence of 39%. The *Diagnostic and Statistical Manual for Mental Disorders-IV* cites a lifetime prevalence for PTSD ranging from 1% to 14% with the variability due to methods of diagnosis and the population studied (APA, 1994). PTSD has characteristic symptoms that last for more than 1 month that follow exposure to an extreme stressor that threatens death or serious injury to oneself or another person, or even learning about an unexpected or violent death, serious harm, or threat of death or injury experienced by someone close (APA, 1994). In addition to the exposure, the person's response involved intense fear, helplessness, or horror and is reexperienced in one or more of the following ways: recurrent and intrusive distressing recollections of the event through images, thoughts, perceptions, or dreams; a reliving the experience; intense distress at cues that remind the individual of the event; and a physiological reactivity on exposure to cues of the event. There is also a persistent avoidance of cues associated with the event that can include efforts to avoid anything to do with the event, some inability to recall aspects of the trauma, loss of interest in significant activities, feelings of detachment or estrangement from others, a numbing or dissociative experience, a limited range of affect, and a poor outlook on the future, persistent symptoms of arousal that can effect sleep, being irritable or angry, a hyper-vigilance and elevated startle response, or difficulty to focus attention—all of which can lead to significant distress or impairment in social and occupational or other areas of functioning (APA, 1994). The difference between PTSD and acute stress disorder is that the latter lasts for one month or less.

Severe cases of PTSD may last indefinitely. Combat veterans from the Pacific arena in World War II interviewed in the 1990s had high prevalence rates for PTSD. Among the prisoner-of-war survivors, 70% fulfilled the criteria for a current diagnosis and 78% for a lifetime diagnosis of PTSD, compared to 18% and 29%, respectively, of the other combat veterans (Sutker, Allain, & Winstead, 1993). One recent assessment of troops deployed to Iraq or Afghanistan was an anonymous survey of troops 3 to 6 months after they had returned from the war with consistent numbers, which showed somewhere between 12% and 20% prevalence of PTSD (Hoge, Castro, Messer, McGurk, Cotting, et al., 2004).

A 2002 editorial in *Nature* stated, "As you read this, 35 million humans in various parts of the world are fleeing from war. Their daily lives are severely affected by the psychological consequences of traumatic stress. Today's military actions no longer resemble those of wars long ago, in which one country's army fought the governmental forces of another. In today's wars, more than 80% of casualties are civilians" (Elbert & Schauer, 2002).

A recent Cochrane Collaboration review on psychological treatment of PTSD compared 29 randomized controlled studies for reduction of clinician-assessed PTSD symptoms that used trauma-focused cognitive behavioral therapy/exposure therapy (TFCBT), stress management (SM), other psychological therapies (excluding eye movement desensitization and reprocessing [EMDR]), and group cognitive behavioral therapy (group-CBT) (Bisson & Andrew, 2005). TFCBT did significantly better than waitlist/usual care. There was no significant difference between TFCBT and SM. TFCBT did significantly better than other therapies. Stress management did significantly better than waitlist/usual care and than other therapies. There was no significant difference between other therapies and waitlist/usual care control. Group TFCBT was significantly better than waitlist/usual care. The author concluded, "There was evidence that individual TFCBT, stress management and group TFCBT are effective in the treatment of PTSD. Other nontrauma focused psychological treatments did not reduce PTSD symptoms as significantly. There was some evidence that individual TFCBT is superior to stress management in the treatment of PTSD at between 2 and 5 months following treatment, and also that TFCBT was also more effective than other therapies. There was insufficient evidence to determine whether psychological treatment is harmful. There was some evidence of greater drop-out in active treatment groups" (Bisson & Andrew, 2005).

The pharmacological treatment of PTSD patients is complex due to the necessity of considering "a great diversity of target symptoms: (1) intrusive symptoms; (2) tendency to interpret incoming stimuli as recurrences of the trauma; (3) generalized hyper-arousal; (4) conditioned hyper-arousal to stimuli reminiscent of the trauma; (5) depressed mood, numbing, and demotivation; (6) avoidance behavior; (7) dissociative symptomatology; and (8) impulsive aggression against self and others" (Van der Kolk, 2001). Also, "only very few agents have been systematically studied. Most studies have been on male combat veterans who suffered from chronic PTSD which they first developed as adults" (Van der Kolk, 2001). One such study showed a marked difference in responsiveness to fluoxetine between a combat veteran population and a sample of non-veterans with PTSD. That study raised serious concerns that the studies of the effects of medication in combat veterans may not be generalizable to non-veteran populations, since non-veterans responded much better than veteran patients. Changes were most marked in the arousal and numbing symptom subcategories. Fluoxetine was an effective antidepressant independent of its effects on PTSD (Van der Kolk, Dreyfuss, Michaels, Shera, Berkowitz, et al., 1994).

While few large placebo-controlled trials have been reported, the largest randomized placebo-controlled trial published to date on the treatment of PTSD include only non-veterans of male and female outpatients, with women constituting the majority of the sample, and subjects ranging from 18 to 69 years, with 75% younger than 45 years and with moderate-to-severe PTSD (Davidson, Rothbaum, et al., 2001). Patients were randomized to 12 weeks of double-blind treatment with either sertraline (N = 100) in flexible daily doses in the range of 50 to 200 mg or placebo (N = 108). The Clinician-Administered PTSD Scale (CAPS-2) total severity score, the patient-rated Impact of Event Scale (IES), and the Clinical Global Impression-Severity (CGI-S) and -Improvement (CGI-I) ratings were used as assessments. Significantly steeper improvement slopes for sertraline compared with placebo were found on the CAPS-2, the IES, the CGI-I score, and the CGI-S score. An intent-to-treat end-point analysis found a 60% "responder rate" for sertraline and a 38% "responder rate for placebo." There was a clinically significant mean reduction from baseline in the range of 45% to 50% on the CAPS-2 and the IES. A 9% discontinuation rate because of adverse events was found with sertraline, compared with 5% for placebo. Adverse events that were significantly more common in subjects given sertraline compared with placebo consisted of insomnia (35% versus 22%), diarrhea (28% versus 11%), nausea (23% versus 11%), fatigue (13% versus 5%), and decreased appetite (12% versus 1%) (Davidson et al., 2001).

In general, the selective serotonin re-uptake inhibitors (SSRIs) are good first-line agents because of their broad-spectrum effectiveness over a wide range of symptoms: mood, anxiety, and impulsivity (Luxenberg, Spinazzola, Hidalgo, Hunt, & Van der Kolk, et al., 2001). SSRIs have also been shown to be effective for core symptoms of PTSD: reexperiencing, avoidance, and hyper-arousal. "However, SSRIs alone will often not be enough to contain severe symptoms. Severe states of hyper-arousal, irritability, aggression, anxiety, insomnia, psychotic-like symptoms, and dissociation may remain and will require adjunctive treatment with other classes of medications. These symptoms need to be separated as chronic or episodic" (Luxenberg et al., 2001).

However, looking again at the President's New Freedom Commission on Mental Health, the difficulties we face as a nation deserve attention here regardless of whether we are considering new conventional or nonconventional modalities of treatment. The report stated, "The services and supports our system provides are disconnected and often inadequate. It can take up to two decades before an effective treatment becomes a routine practice, and . . . our mental health workforce is ill-equipped to make use of current science, research, and practice" (NFCMH, 2003). Thus, there clearly is a need to find new and more effective modalities for treatment and prevention, especially when it comes to PTSD. A 2005 "Policy Forum" article in *Science* calls for an expansion on research "to address the enormous public health consequences of child trauma," and the "need to develop new forms of treatment" and "even the creation of a new Institute of Child Abuse and Inter-personal Violence within the NIH," due to "the emotional and economic cost of these problems" (Freyd, Putnam, Lyon, Becker-Blease, Cheit, et al., 2005).

Below I include 10 Kundalini yoga meditation techniques that help address the symptoms and conditions that can result from a range of traumas and forms of abuse. Techniques are included for specific ages, including young children, adolescents, and adults, as well as an 8-part protocol specific for PTSD. The latter would also be especially useful for war-combat veterans and victims, and is useful for those suffering from PTSD due to all other forms of trauma.

10 Kundalini Yoga Meditation Techniques for the Abused and Battered Psyche

As with all Kundalini yoga meditation practices, the first technique is the technique called "tuning in," technique 1 listed here. (Note that while it is listed first among the techniques here, technique 1 is included for all meditations and therefore isn't technically one of the 10 techniques of this particular meditation group.) This technique helps to create a "meditative state of mind" and is always used as a precursor to the other techniques. There is no upper time limit for this technique, the longer the better.

1. Technique to Induce a Meditative State: "Tuning In"

Sit with a straight spine and with the feet flat on the floor if sitting in a chair (see Figure 2.1, page 72). Put the hands together at the chest in "prayer pose"—the palms are pressed together with 10 to 15 pounds of pressure between the hands (a mild to medium pressure, nothing too intense). The area where the sides of the thumbs touch rests on the sternum with the thumbs pointing up (along the sternum), and the fingers are together and point up and out at a 60-degree angle to the ground. The eyes are closed and focused on the third eye (imagine a sun rising on the horizon, or the equivalent of the point between the eyebrows at the origin of the nose). A mantra is chanted out loud in a 1½-breath cycle. Inhale first through the nose and chant "Ong Namo" with an equal emphasis on the Ong and the Namo. Then immediately follow with a half-breath inhalation through the mouth and chant "Guru Dev Namo" with approximately equal emphasis on each word. (The O in *Ong* and *Namo* are each a long "o" sound; *Dev* sounds like *Dave*, with a long "a" sound.) The practitioner should focus on the experience of the vibrations these sounds create on the upper palate and throughout the cranium while letting the mind be carried by the sounds into a new and pleasant mental space. This should be repeated a minimum of three times. We employed it in our group about 10–12 times. This technique helps to create a "meditative state of mind" and is *always* used as a precursor to the other techniques.

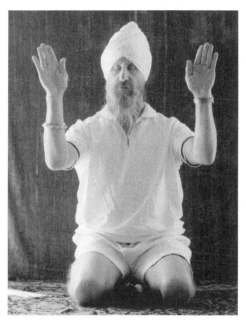

Figure 8.1
Meditation for Self-Worth and Achievement for the Very Young

2. Meditation for Self-Worth and Achievement for the Very Young
The child sits on her heels with the knees together in front and the ankles are out in back with the tops of the feet resting flat on the floor (see Figure 8.1). The arms are up with the upper arms parallel to the ground and the forearms straight up, palms open wide and facing forward. The child bows to the ground and closes her eyes and says "I am," then moves up to the original sitting position, opening her eyes, and says "somebody." This is practiced for 3 to 11 minutes.

3. Meditation for Abused and Battered Children for Developing a Balanced Psyche: The Jupiter Finger Chakra Meditation

This meditation was originally taught by Yogi Bhajan as a "children's meditation," but can also be practiced by adolescents and adults. Anyone with past trauma resulting from abuse and victimization will benefit from this practice. Even someone without past trauma can improve the balance of their personality by its use. This meditation helps to balance the chakras and meridians in the body. It will evoke many feelings that have stuck with the individual since childhood. It will help adults get rid of the "childhood syndrome," a condition where they cling to something that is already finished. This syndrome can easily ruin and limit anyone's life.

Sit with a straight spine either on the floor or in a chair. Place the left hand on the chest at the heart center with the fingers pointing toward the right. Use the index (Jupiter) finger of the right hand (keep the other fingers closed in a relaxed fist with the thumb over the other fingers) to touch, in sequence, the following points: (1) the middle of the lower lip, (2) the tip (end) of the nose, (3) the outer skin area or edge/corner of the eye socket (the region of the skull bone near the outside of the eye), and (4) a point about three-fourths of an inch above the indent of the nose, which is just below the forehead (a point that would be the mid-point between the eyebrows). Chant the mantra "Sa Ta Na Ma" out loud in sequence with the touching of the respective points. Chant "Sa" as one touches the lower lip, "Ta" as one touches the tip of the nose, "Na" as one touches the outer edge of the eye socket, and "Ma" as one touches the forehead point. But since there are two eyes and thus two outer edges of the eye socket, the patient alternates sides each time he goes up in the sequence. Start by touching the right side first. Each round of touching the points and chanting the mantra through takes about 4 to 5 seconds. Keep the eyes closed when doing this meditation. The maximum time is 33 minutes and can be practiced for the full amount of time the first time. Younger people may have to start with 11 minutes or even less. When ending the technique, inhale deeply and hold the breath, then while holding the breath feel the "inner child" by self-hypnosis. Exhale, inhale, and hypnotize oneself, picturing oneself as a child in one's own heart, where the left hand has been resting.

Concentrate, exhale, inhale, repeat the picture of oneself. Bless that child, be that child, and let the breath go.

4. A Sitting Posture to Help Reduce Aggressive Tendencies, to Be Used for "Time-Outs"

A common problem with younger children who have been abused is behavior that requires some restrictions. This technique can be used to help them learn to manage their behavior while reflecting and recovering from their actions. This technique is a more effective way of having a child sit for a "time-out."

The child should sit with the knees in front of the body and the feet behind, but she must sit in between the heels instead of on the heels. This is called sitting in "celibate pose." The eyes are kept open and focused on the tip of the nose while the patient inhales slowly through the mouth with a curled tongue (sticking out slightly and held in a "U" shape), and then slowly exhales through the nose while closing the mouth. If the tongue cannot be curled, which is a genetic ability, it should be mimicked as best as possible. Begin with 3 minutes and build to 11 minutes.

5. Meditation for the Abused and Battered Psyche: A Technique for Children, Adolescents, and Adults

Sit either on the floor with the legs crossed or on a firm chair (see Figure 8.2). The arms are extended out to the sides and up at a 60-degree angle from the ground. Curl the fingers so that the finger tips touch the region of the palm that is closest to where the fingers emerge from the hand—the pads where calluses frequently develop. Keep the thumb out and pointed straight up. Now roll the hands (and arms) in a 12-inch-diameter circle; the right hand goes in a counterclockwise direction and the left hand goes in a clockwise direction. Keep making the circles and the spine will move from top to bottom during the rotation of the arms. The eyes are closed and focused on the tip of the chin (of course the person cannot see it since their eyes are closed, but that is the direction and focus of the gaze). There is no mantra or breathing pattern, although all breathing is through the nose. This technique is to be practiced for 3 to 11 minutes.

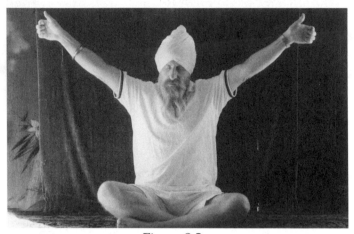

Figure 8.2
Meditation for the Abused and Battered Psyche:
A Technique for Children, Adolescents, and Adults

6. Meditation for the Abused and Battered Psyche: Advanced Technique for Adolescents and Adults

Sit either on the floor with the legs crossed or on a chair. Both arms are extended straight out in front and parallel to the ground. The left palm faces up and the right palm faces down. The eyes are open and focused on the tip of the nose, the end that cannot be seen. The tongue is pressed against the soft lower palate. The breathing pattern is only through the nose and is practiced by inhaling in four equal parts, and exhaling in one full breath. This meditation is to be practiced for 11 minutes.

7. Meditation Technique for Dyslexia

In yogic medicine, dyslexia and other learning disabilities were known to develop occasionally as a result of abuse. This meditation was thought to be effective in the treatment of dyslexia, which is understood by yogis to be a problem of processing information in general, not simply letters or words or mathematical symbols. The retarded processing of emotions is also included in this more general view of dyslexia. This technique was published previously (Shannahoff-Khalsa, 2004).

Sit in an easy pose (see Figure 8.3). The eyes are open and focused on the tip of the nose. The arms are in front of the body and extended slightly out toward the sides with the palms up, the hands at the level of the solar plexus. The finger tips touch the thumb tip in the following order with a light but definite touch. First touch the little finger tip (the Mercury finger) to the thumb tip and mentally chant "Sa." Then touch the index finger tip (the Jupiter finger) to the thumb tip and mentally chant "Ta." Touch the ring finger tip (the Sun finger) to the thumb tip and mentally chant "Na." Again touch the Jupiter finger tip to the thumb tip and mentally chant "Ma." Touch the middle finger tip (the Saturn finger) to the thumb tip and mentally chant "Wha." Again touch the Mercury finger tip to the thumb tip and mentally chant "Hay." Open the hands completely (palms are almost flat and no fingers touch) and mentally chant "Guru." The tongue tip is held constantly touching the upper palate in the top center where the palate is hard and smooth during the entire exercise; the tongue does not move. The breath has a 6-part broken-breath inhale and 1-part exhale, all through the nose only. The six parts of the broken breath of the inhale correspond to the six mental sounds of "Sa," "Ta," "Na," "Ma," "Wha," and "Hay," and the exhale corresponds to the mental sound "Guru." You mentally hear these sounds with each corresponding segment of the breath. The rate of thumb-finger tapping can increase to one complete round of going through the whole series of thumb tip to finger tips in 2 seconds. It takes some time to reach this rate, which is achieved once the practice becomes second nature, that is, when it happens automatically without thinking about the sequence. The time for this extremely powerful technique can be anywhere between 11

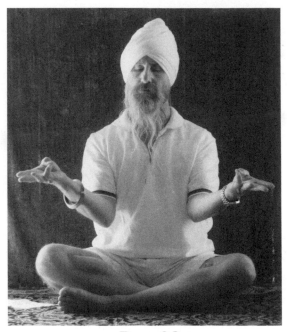

Figure 8.3
Meditation Technique for Dyslexia

minutes and 31 minutes, maximum. It is okay to start with less than 11 minutes, and most people may have to do this in the beginning. Slowly build the time up to 31 minutes. Eventually, try to complete 40 to 120 days at 31 minutes per sitting and marvel at the extraordinary effects. Individuals vary in dyslexic severity and thus each may vary in the time required to attain all benefits. At 120 days of perfected practice, virtually all of one's processing skills are said to be very much healed, with the brain attaining a near-perfect balance. End the meditation by closing the eyes, inhaling deeply, and stretching the hands up in the air above the head. Shake the arms and hands and fingers vigorously for about 30 to 60 seconds.

This technique would also be excellent for patients with ADD/ADHD; it would also be helpful for those with a battered and abused psyche to employ either or both of the two following techniques from Chapter 7 prior to this technique for dyslexia: Meditation to Balance and Synchronize the Cerebral Hemispheres (page 208) and Meditation to Balance the Jupiter and Saturn Energies: A Technique to Help Reduce Depression and Self-Destructive Behavior (page 209). The learning curve for this dyslexia technique is relatively long, but well worth the effort. This technique is very stimulating and very powerful. The yogic definition of dyslexia also includes the inability to process information or sensory feedback. Thus, we are all "dyslexic" to some degree, and what this technique can do for the average person is make his brain function at a much higher level of efficiency. This efficiency will only increase with practice over time. This technique can organize all of the major and minor regions of brain function. Once a person practices this technique for an extended time, he will begin to learn how "dyslexic" he has been.

8. Meditation for Eliminating Deep, Long-Lasting Inner Anger

Sit with a straight and erect spine, with the lower back pushed forward as if you are sitting "at attention" (see Figure 8.4). Both hands are made into fists and the starting posture is with the forearms parallel to the ground at the elbow level. The left fist moves with force toward the center of the chest area near the heart center and the right fist moves with force toward the center of the chest also, but under the left fist. They stop abruptly in front of the chest without touching the chest or touching each other. The movement is more like a hard hitting motion using full strength. Note, the hands do not hit, but move toward each other, except the left is on top. The elbows are out to the sides and the arms move in and out with the elbows remaining at the level of the fists. Chant the mantra "Har" with each hard hitting motion. Chant "Har" loudly and with force from the navel point region and repeat the action rapidly at a rate of about once every 2 seconds. The eyes remain closed and the time for this segment of the meditation is 6.5 minutes. To end this part of the meditation, inhale through the nose and make the hands and arms tight near the chest like an iron rod, making the body stiff, then exhale powerfully through the mouth, like an explosion, and repeat the inhale, tensing, and powerful exhale two more times. Place both hands over the heart center but now touching the chest with the left hand closest to the chest and the right hand touching the back of the left hand. Close the eyes and go into a state of "nonexistence"; feel and imagine "nonexistence," a state of no thoughts, and continue this for an additional 8 minutes. Then relax.

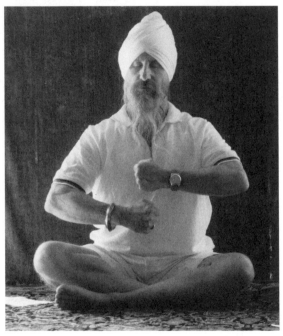

Figure 8.4
Meditation for Eliminating Deep, Long-Lasting Inner Anger

This meditation can take a patient from anger to ecstasy, and is helpful for all those who have been abused in their past. This meditation replaces the power of anger with the state of the "neutral self," a state from which all goodness comes to that person. When a person is without inner anger, he lives from a state of wisdom. One effect of inner anger is that it weakens one's intellectual caliber, and then when the intellect tells that person something useful he does not have the carrying capacity to receive and process the information, which thus leads to failure, and failure leads to more anger.

9. Meditation for Impulsive Behavior in Youth and Others

This is the same meditation for impulsive behavior that is used in Chapter 4, technique 7. Sit with a straight spine and place the left arm in front of the body with the left hand facing down and straight out in front of the heart center. The left arm and hand are parallel to the ground. The right arm is extended straight out parallel to the left arm and in front of the body, right palm facing up (see Figure 4.2, page 155). The eyes are closed. Chant the mantra "Whahay Guru Whahay Guru Whahay Guru Whahay Jeeo," with at least one entire round of the mantra per breath cycle. The sound "Wha" is like "wa" in *water*; "hay" has a long "a"; and "Jeeo" sounds like the two letters "g" and "o" run together. Practice for 18 minutes maximum, then place both hands on the chest at the heart center. The left hand is touching the chest and the palm of the right hand is on the back of the left hand. Continue chanting the mantra but in a whisper for 2 more minutes, then remain silent for 1 minute with the hands on the chest. To end, inhale deeply and hold the breath, tightening the muscles of the arms, hands (pressing against the chest), and spine. Then exhale out powerfully through the mouth like a cannon, and repeat the inhale, tightening, and exhale sequence two more times.

This meditation will also balance the "earth" and "ether" elements of the psyche. This is a useful meditation for young children who sometimes go miserably astray in life. It will increase their ability to remain stable and secure and help develop their temperament, tolerance, and restraint.

10. Meditation for Treating Grief: Especially Useful for PTSD Patients

Most abused and battered individuals suffer from grief including those with PTSD. Yogis claim that grief, anger, and anxiety play a major role in the onset of a wide range of diseases. This technique would be most beneficial when practiced with the first three techniques listed in the OCD protocol (pages 71–73). For reference, turn to Figures 3.3 and 3.4, page 124.

There are three separate parts to this technique to maximize overall benefits; however, Part 1 can be done alone. The suggested music for each part is optional, though the benefits of the music will only add to the therapeutic value.

Part 1: Siddh Shiva. "Whenever you have grief, do this exercise. It gets rid of centuries-old grief" (Bhajan, 1990). In position A (Figure 3.3), sit with a straight spine in a cross-legged position. The eyes are wide open (do not meditate). The elbows are bent by the sides, and the upper arms are kept by the sides. The forearms are parallel to the ground just above each leg, with the palms open and facing up and placed about 6 inches above the knees.

In position B (see Figure 3.4), raise the arms up so the hands quickly bounce up to the shoulders. As you do this, the tongue sticks out as far as possible (this is important because it affects the subconscious mind and helps get rid of the grief). Then return to position A. The tongue goes back into the mouth, the mouth closes, and the arms go back down to the position above the legs. Do this powerfully with the breath. Inhale through the nose as you go into position A and exhale through the mouth as you go into position B. Breathe heavily and practice this movement at a rate of two times per second. Listen to the song "Se Saraswati" by Nirinjan Kaur and Guru Prem Singh (available at the Ancient Healing Ways web site, www.a-healing.com). Do this technique for 7 minutes total. To end, inhale and hold the breath in and press the tongue against the upper palate as hard as you can for 20 seconds. Exhale. Repeat this tongue process two more times (three times total), then relax for 3 minutes.

Part 2. A second technique here is optional (taught as a companion technique by Yogi Bhajan on May 17, 1990). This exercise helps to create an inner balance that then helps to further induce healing.

Stretch the arms up over the head, elbows straight, palms very flat and stiff, facing forward with the fingers together and the thumbs extended stiffly to the sides of the hands. Begin moving the left arm in a clockwise circle overhead and over the left side of the body. Move the right arm in a counterclockwise direction overhead and over the right side of the body. The movements of the two arms do not seem to be related in any fashion. One arm gets into a certain rhythm of a circular movement while the other arm does the same. (Note: You can reverse directions if you wish.) The song "Heal Me" by Nirinjan Kaur is played (available at the Ancient Healing Ways web site, www.a-healing.com). Do this for 11 minutes and then rest for 5 minutes. Bhajan said, "The idea of the movement is that the armpits get stimulated, so make the movement of the arms just an extension of the movement of the armpits and the sides of the rib cage. Usually we condemn ourselves and we have to feel guilty to be happy. This completely breaks through that" (1990).

Part 3. The third part of this exercise is to combine the breath of life (prana) and to help balance the ida and pingala, the major left and right meridians of the body, respectively. Begin by inhaling through the left nostril by blocking the right nostril with the right thumb, then exhale only through the right nostril by blocking the left nostril with the right index finger, continuing with this pattern for 3 minutes (do not reverse nostrils). Then, firmly grasp the knees by placing the palms flat down on top of them. Begin swaying your body forward approximately one foot and then backward approximately one foot in a rhythmic fashion. The grip of the hands should be so firm that it keeps you from tilting over when you go backward. Keep your spine "tight" while doing the exercise. Play the song "Humee Hum Tumee Tum" by Livtar Singh (available at the Ancient Healing Ways web site, www.a-healing.com). Do this technique for 3 minutes. To end, inhale deeply and tighten the whole body, then shake the body as much as possible. Do this five times total, holding the breath approximately 20 seconds the first time and 15 seconds the other four times. "It is said that this posture increases the circulation in the area of the breasts for females so they will not develop breast cancer. It will develop your automatic concentration, so you can concentrate whenever you want. It will also help expel the dead cells out of the physical body" (Bhajan, 1990).

11. Gan Puttee Kriya

This technique is included in the 8-Part Protocol for Posttraumatic Stress Disorder described below; however, it can also be practiced independently for 11 to 31 minutes. See instructions below. If it is practiced independently, the end procedure is as follows: remain in the sitting posture and inhale and hold the breath for 20 to 30 seconds while shaking and moving every part of the body. Exhale and repeat this two more times to circulate the energy and to break the pattern of tapping, which affects the brain. Finally, after the shaking, sit in absolute calmness and focus the eyes on the tip of the nose with slow deep breathing for one more minute. This technique was also included in the protocol for acute stress disorders in Chapter 2 (see page 97) and for bipolar disorders in Chapter 3 (see page 130).

The 8-Part Meditation Protocol for Posttraumatic Stress Disorder*

This protocol is especially useful for war-combat victims and veterans.

1. Technique to Induce a Meditative State: "Tuning In"

For this technique, follow the instructions on page 226 under "10 Kundalini Yoga Meditation Techniques for the Abused and Bettered Psyche."

2. Gan Puttee Kriya

Sit with a straight spine, either on the floor or in a chair. The back of your hands are resting on your knees with the palms facing upwards. The eyes are nine-tenths closed (one-tenth open, but looking straight ahead into the darkness, not the light below), focused at the "third eye" point. Chant from your heart in a natural, relaxed manner, or chant in a steady, relaxed monotone. Chant out loud the sound "Sa" (the *a* sounds like "ah"), and touch your thumb tips and index-finger tips together quickly and simultaneously with about 2 pounds of pressure. Then chant "Ta" and touch the thumb tips to the middle-finger tips. Chant "Na" and touch the thumb tips to the ring-finger tips. Chant "Ma" and touch the thumb tips to the little-finger tips. Chant "Ra" and touch your thumb tips and index-finger tips. Chant "Ma" and touch the thumb tips to the middle-finger tips. Chant "Da" and touch the thumb tips to the ring-finger tips. Chant "Sa" and touch the thumb tips to the little-finger tips. Chant "Sa" and touch your thumb tips and index-finger tips. Chant "Say" (sounds like the word *say* with a long "a") and touch the thumb tips to the middle-finger tips. Chant "So" and touch the thumb tips to the ring-finger tips. Chant "Hung" and touch the thumb tips to the little-finger tips.

Chant at a rate of one sound per second. The thumb tip and finger tips touch with a very light, 2 to 3 pounds of pressure with each connection. This helps to consolidate the circuit created by each thumb-finger link. Start with 11 minutes and slowly work up to 31 minutes of practice. To finish, remain in the sitting posture and inhale, holding the breath for 20 to 30 seconds while you shake and move every part of your body. Exhale and repeat this two more times to circulate the energy and to break the pattern of tapping, which effects the brain. Then immediately proceed without rest to technique 3, "When You Do Not Know What to Do."

The sounds used in this meditation are each unique, and they have a powerful effect on the mind, both the conscious and subconscious mind. The sound "Sa" gives the mind the ability to expand to the infinite. "Ta" gives the mind the ability to experience

239

the totality of life. "Na" gives the mind the ability to conquer death. "Ma" gives the mind the ability to resurrect. "Ra" gives the mind the ability to expand in radiance (this sound purifies and energizes). "Da" gives the mind the ability to establish security on the earth plane, providing a ground for action. "Say" gives the totality of experience. "So" is the personal sense of identity, and "Hung" is the infinite as a vibrating and real force. Together, *So Hung* means "I am Thou." The unique qualities of this 12-syllable mantra help cleanse and restructure the subconscious mind and help heal the conscious mind to ultimately experience the superconsious mind. Thus, all the blocks that result from an extreme traumatic event are eliminated over time with the practice of Gan Puttee Kriya. When doing the whole protocol, 11 minutes for this technique is adequate, however, 31 minutes is even better.

3. When You Do Not Know What to Do

Sit straight, rest the back of one hand in the palm of the other with the thumbs crossing each other in one palm (see Figure 2.5, page 103). If the right hand rests in the palm of the left hand, the left thumb rests in the right palm and the right thumb then crosses over the back of the left thumb. Either this hand orientation is acceptable or the reverse, with the left hand resting in the palm of the right hand and then the right thumb is in the left palm covered by the left thumb. The hands are placed at heart-center level, about 2 inches in front of the chest, but the hands do not touch the chest, and the elbows are resting against the ribs. The eyes are open but focused on the tip of the nose (which you cannot actually see). The breathing pattern has four parts that repeat in sequence, first inhale and exhale slowly through the nose only, then inhale through the mouth with the lips puckered as if to kiss or make a whistle. After the inhalation, relax the lips and exhale through the mouth slowly, then inhale through the nose and exhale through the mouth. The last breath pattern is inhaling through the puckered lips and exhaling through the nose. Breathe slowly and deeply. Continue this cycle for 8 minutes and then take a short 2- to 3-minute rest.

4. Meditation to Balance the Jupiter and Saturn Energies:
A Technique Useful for Treating Depression, Focusing the Mind,
and Eliminating Self-Destructive Behavior

Sit with a straight spine either in a chair or on the floor (see Figure 3.2, page 120). The hands are facing forward with the ends of the Jupiter (index) and Saturn (middle) fingers pointing straight up near the sides of the body at the level of the chin. The elbows are relaxed down by the sides and the hands are near the shoulders. Close the ring and little fingers down into the palm using the thumbs and keep them there against the palm during the meditation. The Jupiter (index) finger and the Saturn (middle) finger are spread open in a V shape (or closed). The eyes are closed. For 8 minutes open and close the Jupiter and Saturn fingers about once or twice per second. Make sure they spread completely open and close completely during the exercise. Simultaneously imagine the planets of Jupiter and Saturn coming together in front of you and then again going apart in synch with the finger movement—the planets should appear to go back and forth along a straight line in and out to the sides in front of you. It does not matter whether you have Jupiter or Saturn on the left or right side. Continue this imagery movement for 8 minutes along with the fingers opening and closing. (In the beginning, the imaging is difficult to do but this should not slow down the pace of the fingers, which play a more important role here.) After 8 minutes, while continuing the same exercise, begin to inhale and exhale through the nose only with the movement (inhale as the fingers are spread, exhale as the fingers close). Continue with the planets. Continue this part for 2 additional minutes. Then, for the last minute, spread the two fingers wide and hold them wide apart (now they do not open and close, they remain in the fixed V shape), keeping them very stiff (which requires considerable effort) while also keeping the mouth in an O, or ring, shape. Breathe in and out of the mouth using only the diaphragm (not the wall of the upper chest) with a rate of one to three breaths per second. After 1 minute, inhale, hold the breath in, and tense every muscle tightly (including the hands, fingers, with the "v" kept rigid, arms, back, stomach) in the body for 10 seconds. Exhale and repeat two more times for 10 seconds. Then relax.

The effects of the meditation help the mind to become very focused and clear and the brain becomes very energized (few other 11-minute techniques compare). This technique is said to help eliminate depression. The meditation is used to coordinate and balance the Jupiter and Saturn energies, and to reduce the possibility of self-destructive and aggressive behavior. In addition, when the Jupiter and Saturn energies (functional brain areas related to the index and middle fingers, respectively) are integrated, individuals are said to be able to overcome difficult challenges more easily.

5. Ganesha Meditation for Focus and Clarity

This short 3-minute technique is also included in the protocols for acute stress disorder and MDD in Chapters 2 and 3, respectively. This technique is said to create a clear mental focus and to bring clarity to the consciousness.

Sit with a straight spine, the eyes closed (see Figure 2.4, page 100). The left thumb and little finger are sticking out from the hand. The other fingers are curled into a fist with fingertips on the moon mound (the root of the thumb area that extends down to the wrist). The left hand and elbow are parallel to the floor, with the pad of the tip of the left thumb pressing on the curved notch of the nose between the eyes. The little finger is sticking out. With right hand and elbow parallel to the floor, grasp the left little finger with the right hand and close the right hand into a fist around it, so that both hands now extend straight out from your head. Push the notch with the tip of the left thumb to the extent that you feel some soreness as you breathe long and deep. After continued practice, this soreness reduces. Do this for 3 minutes and no longer. To finish, keeping the posture with eyes closed, inhale. Push a little more and pull the naval point in by tightening the abdominal and back muscles for about 10 seconds. Then exhale, and repeat this one more time for 10 seconds. Immediately proceed to the next technique.

6. *Meditation for Deep Relaxation*

This technique was first taught by Yogi Bhajan on July 2, 1998, for improving health. Bhajan claimed that "There is no more powerful relaxation than this. When you are very nervous, and you have too many thoughts, and you are being ground up by everything, do this for 3 minutes. You will be shocked—things will disappear. There is nothing more relaxing."

Sit and maintain a straight spine on the floor, or if in a chair, keep both feet flat on the ground without crossing the legs. Open the mouth to make an O shape. Stick the tongue out of the right side of the mouth to form a Q shape with the tongue and mouth. Keep the tongue stretched out. If the patient has trouble holding the tongue out in this position, they can hold it slightly between the teeth. (Note, the tongue should not be straight out, but extended out to the right side of the mouth only). Breathe slowly and deeply through the mouth, keeping the tongue extended out and stretched the entire time. The eyes are kept closed. Any beautiful music can be played or no music at all. The practice time here is only 3 minutes. To end, keeping the spine straight and eyes closed, inhale and hold the breath for 13 seconds, then squeeze the breath out with a powerful exhale through the mouth. Repeat this but hold the breath the second time for only 11 seconds. Again squeeze the breath out with a powerful exhale through the mouth, and one last time inhale and hold for 7 seconds. Squeeze the breath out with a powerful exhale through the mouth. Bhajan commented: "Karma will be over. It is called 'pre-experience.' Your 'Q' should be perfect."

The first part of the protocol is now complete. These techniques help take the patient through the shock, anger, fear, and guilt that is common for many PTSD patients. Now immediately begin the second part with the next meditation.

7. A Tantric Meditation Technique to Create a Normal and Supernormal State of Consciousness

This technique was also published previously (Shannahoff-Khalsa, 2003). This is said to be a very powerful healing meditation that helps to organize and normalize the various regions of the brain. It is called a *tantric meditation* because of the hand posture, although it is not a "White Tantric yoga" meditation technique. This is a very sacred technique because of its power to produce rapid changes in brain states.

Sit with a straight spine (see Figure 8.5). The eyes are closed and focused at the third eye point, the point where the nose meets the forehead. The hands are interlocked with the right thumb dominant to the left thumb, all the fingers are interlaced, and the left little finger is on the bottom. (This finger-to-finger relationship is to be used even if one naturally has a left thumb that is dominant to the right, when the fingers are interlaced, with a right little finger on the bottom.) The right middle (or Saturn) finger is brought into the space between the hands, and points toward the region of the wrists. The hands are then closed and the right Saturn finger becomes enclosed in a cave-like structure. The hands are held at the heart-center level about nine inches in front of the chest with the elbows resting at the sides. Sit and relax in this posture for 3 to 5 minutes with the breath regulating itself. Then keeping everything the same, begin to consciously regulate the breath, where the inhale, holding of the breath, and exhale are of equal lengths of time (there is no holding the breath out). The breath cycle can approach 1 minute where the inhale, holding in, and exhale are each 20 seconds in duration. However, 5 seconds for the three phases is a good starting time. Have a conscious relationship with the experience and sensations of the hand posture and the sensations in the head simultaneously. This technique can frequently produce unique physical sensations in the head. Practice this for a total of 11 minutes. A break of 5 minutes is recommended here before going on to the final meditation, and depends on the health of the patient.

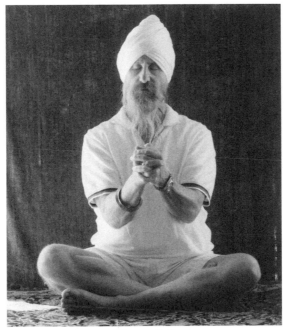

Figure 8.5
A Tantric Meditation Technique to Create a Normal
and Supernormal State of Consciousness

8. Meditation to Be Done When You Want to Command Your Own Consciousness to a Higher Consciousness*

Sit in an easy crossed-legged pose and maintain a straight spine, or sit in a chair and keep both feet flat on the ground without crossing the legs (see Figure 8.6). The hands are relaxed in the lap. Grasp the left thumb with the right hand and wrap the fingers of the left hand around the back of the right hand. The eyes are nine-tenths closed and focused on the tip of the nose (the end not visible to the practitioner's eye). This eye posture is called ajna bond and translates to "mind lock." The effect of this eye posture is to help stabilize the activity of the frontal lobes. The following mantra is chanted three

* This technique was originally taught by Yogi Bhajan on September 21, 1978, and first published in Shannahoff-Khalsa, 2005.

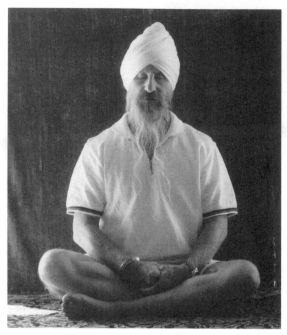

Figure 8.6
Meditation to be done When You Want to Command
Your Own Consciousness to Higher Consciousness

times in one breath: "Hari Nam Tat Sat Tat Sat Hari." Three times in one breath may be difficult for some beginners but with practice and good lungs it can easily be achieved. Chant more rapidly if necessary to complete the three cycles. The word Hari is pronounced like "Har" in the name Harvey and the "i" sounds like "ee." The word Nam sounds like "Nam" in Viet Nam, with a short "a" sound. The "a" in Tat and Sat sounds like "ah." This mantra is said to awaken the infinite creative power within. The time for practice is 11 minutes. For a few minutes immediately after the 11 minutes, chant "Sat Nam Sat Nam Sat Nam Sat Nam Sat Nam Sat Nam Whahay Guru" in an eight-beat rhythm (one beat for each "Sat Nam," one beat for "Whahay," and one beat for "Guru"). The sounds of "Sat" and "Nam" are the same as in the first mantra, and the word *Whahay* is "wha" and feels like the word water in the mouth without the "ter." "Hay" sounds like the word that is the correlate of straw with a long "a."

Case Histories of Treatment

Case History 1: A Female with PTSD, Anorexia Nervosa, MDD, and Anger to the Bone

Jackie was a single female (age 26) living on Social Security disability when I met her. She was raised in a dysfunctional family. Her father and mother were both alcoholics; the father physically and emotionally beat the mother and both her and her older sister. The mother did her best to ignore the abuse and when Jackie was 18 her mother died of cervical cancer. Jackie was then left living with the father for a short period of time, but then felt that if she wanted to survive she would have to move out. During the time when the family was "intact," Jackie said what was really most difficult for her was that her older sister would also abuse and beat her. At age 14, Jackie was raped. Jackie had anorexia nervosa and bulimia. Her self-concept was grossly stifled, as if she was aware of her surroundings but locked into the past, and presented more as a child than as an adult female. At the time I met her, she was renting a room in the house of an older couple, who knew of my work and sent Jackie to me and assisted in her financial needs. When I spoke with her and asked her what seemed to be the most overpowering result from her years of trauma, she said, "I am angry, just angry and very depressed and frequently I feel like I do not exist. I feel numb." I said you do not look angry, and she said, "I know, but I am, I can hardly move." This comment made a deep impression on me, and I knew what she was talking about—the anger was just below the surface, and went clear to the bone. It was "cold anger," the type that comes when someone feels violated either from one severe event or years of trauma.

Jackie was a typical case of years of chronic abuse. She suffered from acute (rape) and frequent and chronic abuses that left her feeling absolutely powerless and disenfranchised in life. She had reported two occasions when she had attempted suicide, both by medication overdoses. She had a typical array of psychiatric disorders that included MDD, anorexia and bulimia nervosa, and PTSD. The question was how best to treat her. I could have given her two-dozen techniques that would have helped, but I decided to teach her technique 8 in this chapter, called Meditation for Eliminating Deep, Long-Lasting Inner Anger, as the core technique for her practice. I taught her to tune in, spine flexes, shoulder shrugs (see Chapter 2, techniques 2 and 3), Gan Puttee Kriya for 31 minutes, and technique 8. She complied well on the first visit, and saw me almost every week for the next 2 months. After about another three months of near-daily practice she decided to return to school in a community college and eventually to seek a career in counseling.

Case History 2: A Female with OCD, PTSD, MDD, Eating Disorders, TMJ, ADHD, and Self-mutilation

Anna was 26 years of age, married to her second husband, and without children. She presented with depression ("her worst enemy," suicidal thoughts), OCD, an eating disorder in the form of bingeing and purging with a history of restricted diets, temporal mandibular joint (TMJ) syndrome, PTSD with significant numbing and dissociation, ADHD, severe anxiety, and intermittent self-mutilation in the form of cutting or cigarette burns. She was referred to me by a psychiatrist in the Los Angeles area who thought my work on OCD might benefit her patient. Anna's OCD symptoms had not improved with trials of clomipramine, nortriptyline, and a series of SSRIs. In addition, she had poor therapeutic responses to other medications and frequently intolerable side effects. When I first saw her, she was on nortriptyline 10 mg, Ativan 2 mg (for sleep), Straterra 25 mg, and Seroquel 12.5 mg. Earlier she had been prescribed a range of medications that in part included Abilify and Risperdal in an effort to treat her numbing and dissociation, Wellbutrin for depression, and methylphenidate 5 mg BID for ADHD. Her psychiatric care had involved a revolving and apparently ineffective regimen of medications. Her psychotherapy with a female clinician had helped her to understand somewhat the complications of her life and feelings of being a victim and basically an "undeserving person," but did little to help ameliorate her wide range of psychiatric symptoms.

Anna had a 10-year history of sexual abuse from her grandfather while living with her mother. Her father and mother were divorced when Anna was 3 years of age. At that point, Anna and her mother moved in with Anna's mother's parents who lived on a farm in Tennessee. The sexual abuse (touching, penetration, oral sex) continued until Anna reached puberty. Her grandfather had threatened her and told her that if she ever told what he did that she and her mother would be "forced to move out and live on the street." When Anna was in her senior year of high school she married her boyfriend, who had joined the military. This made it possible for her to move out from the house and to another state to escape the household stress of living with her grandfather, even though the sexual abuse had ended, but the secrets remained. Anna's marriage lasted 3 years and in the interim she entered college, but found the stress of school too much to endure, since some of her obsessions were perfection-based with rereading and rewriting, and her attention skills were also severely affected. When stressed, her TMJ problems were also exacerbated and her self-hatred, anger, and "inability to achieve anything significant" led to her bouts of depression and intermittent self-mutilation and bingeing and purging routines.

The first time I saw Anna, she had been in weekly therapy with both her psychiatrist and her psychotherapist for approximately 8 months. During previous years, she had also been in therapy and attempted treatment through medication with several other psychiatrists. Both of her therapists had agreed she may gain some relief at least for her OCD by learning the Kundalini yoga protocol for OCD. I saw her twice a month for 2 months and she achieved a substantial reduction in her OCD symptoms. "It is 30% to 40% of what it was when I first saw you," she told me. In addition, her self-mutilation and bingeing and purging habits had reduced to the lowest levels she had remembered in 5 years. But due to the half-day round-trip required to see me, she chose to end contact and told me she would continue her practice on her own. When I was seeing her, she used my video for the OCD protocol on occasion and would practice without it usually for the immediate week after seeing me. However, she could not manage to establish a regular at-home practice with any lasting continuity and her practice never went beyond 2 weeks. Several months later, she again reentered therapy with me but only on a monthly basis. In that interim, all of her symptoms had worsened since she had completely given up her practice. She thought if she were to see me again it might help her to establish a more regular practice.

During this period, her psychiatrist had attempted on a near-weekly basis to titrate her medication doses or to change medications in an effort to help eliminate the side effects that were making her feel nauseous, gave her headaches, and generally made her feel uncomfortable in her body, with near-constant fatigue and listlessness. She also reported sleeping difficulties and occasional nightmares. It was not clear how much of this was medication induced or purely symptomatic of her various disorders. I taught her techniques for mental focus and depression (Ganesha Meditation [page 242], Fighting Brain Fatigue [page 117], the Jupiter-Saturn Meditation [page 241]), ADHD (technique 6 in Chapter 7, Meditation to Balance and Synchronize the Cerebral Hemispheres [page 208]), and PTSD (Gan Puttee Kriya [pag 239]). At that time, I had not yet developed the Kundalini yoga 8-Part Meditation Protocol for PTSD. I suggested that she alternate practice days between the OCD protocol and several of those that I taught her for her depression, ADHD, and PTSD. She complied again, but usually only for a week or 2 at most in the interim between monthly appointments. Her general complaint was that her usual malaise and fatigue were too frustrating and she could not get herself to do the yoga.

With the guidance of her psychiatrist, Anna was instructed which medications to lessen or end and what schedule to follow, with two visits per week with her psychiatrist. She had also continued her weekly psychotherapy. Once off the medications she was feeling physically much better and her energy levels had returned to pre-medication days, but her psychiatric symptoms remained unchanged. She then started seeing me at bi-weekly intervals for 3 months. Anna continued her at-home practice and had far fewer severe episodes or crises. She also started to go to regular Kundalini yoga classes twice a week in the Los Angeles area, and this helped to inspire her to commit to a near-daily practice on other days. After 6 months, she returned to school and managed to enter nursing school. She eventually received a degree as a registered nurse and became employed in a large community hospital. She continued to go to Kundalini yoga classes and to practice at home. She told me her OCD symptoms were at most subclinical, only intermittent, and rarely affected her, and that when they did she could easily tolerate the few minor obsessions. She also reported much less fear and anxiety and had stopped all of her bingeing, purging, and self-mutilation. She told me that she had seen a dentist specializing in TMJ and she started to wear a mouth guard during sleep, which helped to eliminate the jaw pain, headaches, and the grinding of her teeth.

Case History 3: A Female with OCD, PTSD, Anorexia and Bulima Nervosa, Depression, and Psychosis

Lisa was born in Switzerland in 1976. Her father sought my assistance in January 2002 for her OCD. Lisa was diagnosed with OCD, PTSD, anorexia and bulimia nervosa, self-mutilation, depression, and a psychosis. She has a younger brother with severe to extreme OCD. The following is a very lengthy and detailed case history in Lisa's own words that depicts the history and extent of her disorders and her efforts and success with treatment. This description was completed in February, 2005.

"According to my father, as a little girl I probably was more anxious than other children. He noted that at the age of 3 I had this anxious look in my eyes, constantly observing the environment with a need to protect my brother. At 11, I developed the compulsive behavior of turning the light switch definitively off. I could only stop this compulsive ritual when I had a good feeling, which might have been a sign for me that nothing negative would happen. During my childhood, I always felt that my father had no interest in me, my brother, or my mother. My father was diagnosed with manic-depressive disorder and has been taking lithium for about 25 years. At 12, I had my first problems with neurodermitis. At 13, I had an enormous anxiety for my mother where I started to torment her with my compulsive questions about her state of health. I feared so much that my mother would get ill and die. That's why I had to observe her all the time. When she sneezed, I felt this very uncomfortable anxiety inside of me and I had to ask her immediately, "Is anything wrong with you?" She told me this behavior ruined many holidays. Years later I was diagnosed with OCD. For me this fear for others was tormenting. I had to observe others around me and look for a sign of illness. The biggest fear I had was that my mother would not eat enough and that she would lose weight. At 15, I had my first sign of a disturbed eating behavior. I had the fixed idea that I didn't want to put on weight anymore (my weight was 52 kg [115 lbs] at a height of 1.76m [5' 7"]). I started to throw food out of my window to avoid articles of food with fat and a lot of calories in them, and tried to do a lot of sports. But this behavior only lasted for a year.

"At 15, I had a ritual with my slippers before going to bed and every night I had to look once or twice under my bed to make sure that there were no monsters or murderers underneath. I also developed a touching ritual with the traffic-shield in front of my house and a stepping ritual over a garden wall before returning home. However, only the compulsions with my mother and brother and my eating behavior made me suffer. At 16, I finally realized that something strange was going on inside my head that was tormenting me and that I didn't understand. I remember that I switched away from uncomfortable and tormenting feelings and compulsive thoughts by using my compulsive sentences. This often left me depressed because I couldn't enjoy conversations with friends, watch TV, or relax on my bed anymore. During these years in school my hands, face, and neck were covered with neurodermitis and it hurt, and I often scratched, and I did not want to be seen with this ugly skin. This led to low self-assurance.

"After high school, I started university studies for the science of medicine. But I had to give this up after 5 weeks in the fall of 1996 because of health problems. I was depressed and I wasn't able to learn, read, think, or comprehend anymore. My thoughts didn't flow. I wasn't able to experience emotions like joy, happiness, sadness, or anger anymore. I always felt the same dullness. Besides school stress, a girl friend had a borderline personality disorder and my closeness to her led to a burdensome relationship. After one incident, she wrote me that she did not want to see me anymore and that she wouldn't lose a single tear at my funeral if I died now. During my first psychiatric crisis, which when compared to later ones was only mild, I took only St. John's Wort tea, and then went to my brother's psychiatrist, who told me I did not need treatment. By the spring of 1997, my condition slowly improved and I started my first relationship with a boy that I enjoyed, and this was my first real love. But sometimes I was concerned that this could be perhaps a hypo-manic state, as my father and brother were both diagnosed with depression and mania. In the summer of 1997, I had problems with my eating behavior again and I began to feel dizzy and unable to think clearly because of the lack of food. In the autumn of 1997, I got terribly hurt by my boyfriend. During sex, when I wanted to completely give myself to him, he shouted out the name of the man he was in love with. I think this experience caused the extreme hatred toward my body that I've had since then, and is the main reason why I hated myself so much and wanted so desperately to die over the next 5 years. After this terrible experience, I again was unable to experience my feelings. Listening to my favorite music, for example, no longer gave me any feelings. I couldn't notice the difference between being in nature or inside the house. I was very exhausted after going for a walk.

"Finally, I went to see a psychiatrist at the University Hospital in Bern. He prescribed thioridazine and lorazepam, which didn't help. Later he suggested that I go to a private psychiatric clinic in Münchenbuchsee. I agreed because I did not want to stress my family anymore. I was extremely scared that my mother, father, and brother would get ill because of the stress of my illness. I was in this clinic from the beginning of October 1997 through March 1998. It was an extremely terrible time for me, not only because of my symptoms, but also because of how my therapists treated me. I had the impression that they didn't believe I was suffering, but only paid attention to my actions or looks. I often felt enormously overwhelmed by their expectations of me, which proved to me that they didn't understand my terrible state of mind. In this clinic, I was diagnosed with a psychosis and major depression. I was initially prescribed trimipramine and risperidone. Later resperidone was substituted with flupenthixol. Later Rhotrimine was added. In January these medications were substituted by lithium and citalopram. I had to take part in sports, feeding animals, body and music therapy, and handicrafts, which was too much for me and not helpful. I also went with my mother to an acupuncturist outside the clinic. He gave me acupuncture and magnesium, which also wasn't helpful.

"The first days in this clinic, I was enormously afraid of the other patients and that I would become as ill as I thought they were. I remember two states of mind while I was there. One was that my feelings had died. The other was a fear that something very horrible would happen, for example, I would go out of my room naked without noticing it, or really lose control, or everybody would laugh at me. My biggest fear was that I was going totally crazy and losing my mind, that I would have to suffer in this state for the rest of my life, and nobody would be able to save me. I developed my first permanent compulsive sentence to protect me against all my terrible fears: "*Dass nüt passiert*" (that nothing bad is going to happen). Later I created the second part of this compulsive sentence: "*la los—egau*" (let go—nothing matters). The latter part came from the advice of my music therapist in the clinic. She was the only person in the clinic who I felt understood me and took me seriously. And she probably saved my life at that time.

"I had to silently say '*la los—egau*' to myself almost every second to help protect me from my fears and to give me advice on how to act, behave, and do things, as I lost my identity more and more, including almost all my memories, my knowledge of myself, my relationship to life, to my education, to my friends, and also to myself, all became extremely foreign and enormously distant to me. From this time on, my compulsive sentences were continuously circulating in my mind. This compulsion became more severe in the following years, and the number of sentences also increased.

"While in the Klinik Wyss, and perhaps as a result of the trauma with my ex-boyfriend, I felt like parts of my ego got chipped away, and I had an enormous longing for death. I did not understand what was going on. I think this is one reason for my very strong need to tell myself compulsive sentences. I needed something to hold onto, as I wouldn't have been able to live in the emptiness otherwise.

"I also started to have eating attacks, and I gained 10 kg. I ate, bought, and sometimes even stole food with a lot of fat and sugar that I would not have eaten before during my two anorexic phases. On one hand, I did this for comfort, since I really couldn't stand my situation anymore. On the other, I several times celebrated with a big eating attack, my 'last meal,' since I was going to commit suicide the next day. While in the clinic, before my eating attacks started, I first experienced my body as extremely fat.

"After 5.5 months, my parents took me home from the clinic. I agreed with my mother, who said that the stay there hadn't helped me at all. I probably was calmer after leaving, but also much more numb, and the stay made my health worse. From the end of March to the end of June 1998, I was only on lithium, which my mother made me try. In the middle of June, I started therapy at a day clinic at the Universitäte Psychiatrische Dienste because I wasn't able to make decisions or to think clearly. I spent the days in the clinic and the evenings and nights at home. I went there for 2.5 years. The average stay in this clinic is about 3 to 5 months maximum. In this clinic, I had different therapies such as cooking with other patients for the group, sports, painting, and other creative therapies, and group discussion. For me, most of the therapies were only a way to make time pass more quickly. I felt overwhelmed in group conversation because I could not under-stand what the people were saying and I was not able to take part in it. One therapist said that this clinic wasn't adapted for my disorder. For example, I felt very excluded, when other patients were talking about their feelings the therapists very often forgot that I wasn't able to notice my feelings. But nobody knew a better place for me. While there, I was so dissociated from myself and the things around me, I was only able to say a few words and I wasn't able to understand the effects of making a point while playing badminton, even though I was automatically still able to play.

"In July 1998, my therapist at this clinic prescribed Deroxat/Paxil in addition to lithium. This increased my activity, but did not improve my perception. After several months at the day clinic, I started to see the head physician twice a week. At the end of November 1998, he prescribed zuclopenthixol in addition to Deroxat/Paxil. Some months later he increased both Deroxat and Paxil to a very high dose, which made my physical condition worse. I had to repeat quotes from my therapists—why I really mustn't kill myself. A tiny part of me wanted to live. I had to tell myself again and again quotes from my therapists saying that I wasn't guilty for causing my illness in order to overcome the fear and belief that I had caused it. There was a lot of advice from my therapist telling me how to be and what to do, as I really had lost myself and didn't know what to do anymore. I depended almost completely on others. For example, I had to tell myself 'So wie's isch' (as it is) before entering the clinic in the morning. What made me really panic (only on an intellectual level, without being able to feel it), was when the advice I got from others was contradictory. This led to a painful fight inside my mind. I wasn't able to choose the advice that I thought was best for me, so everybody had to advise me more or less the same to avoid total confusion.

"In late 1998, I started receiving a disability pension. At the end of 1999, my psychiatrist replaced Deroxat/Paxil with Temesta/Ativan, Clopixol and lithium. He told my parents that the severe depression was over now (for example, I could cry again from time to time, but without being able to experience emotions inside my body). He said that now I suffered from a neurotic disorder caused by difficult family circumstances, and that I suffered from a dissociative disorder, and also from a borderline personality disorder (BPD). He said I had BPD because I suffered from a separation, where a very small part of me wanted to live, but a very strong and destructive part wanted to suffer and die. He added that my enormous self-hatred and black-or-white thinking were also signs of BPD. For example, it only took one negative thought about a person I liked and idealized to instantly change my opinion from love to hate. I often had the impression that something inside me had broken and that I was losing the ground under my feet. My enormous self-hatred was so extreme that one day I had the impression that even water was far too good for me.

"After about 1 year in the day clinic, I was a little more present and active, but mostly in a very self-destructive way. I began to harm myself, the first time only with a needle, then by cutting with knives, but mostly with fragments of glass. I cut my arms, legs, belly, and several times. I also burned myself (hand and foot) with cigarettes. Once, after a terrible eating attack, I hated myself even more than before and I could no longer bear my extremely fat body. So I also stuck a needle four times deeply in my unbearably fat thigh. I wanted to know if I could touch my bone with a needle.

"There were two partly contradictory reasons for my self-mutilation. This was a way I could punish myself, since I really had a very strong belief that I was an extremely bad creature that has to be eliminated with a method that is as painful as possible, and at the same time, my self-destructive part was also very proud. When others noticed my bandages and wounds, this was evidence of how bad I was, and thus fulfilled the expectations that I thought others had of me. I couldn't imagine that anyone could love such a monster. On the other hand, self-mutilation also became like a friend. It was something that belonged only to me. If I really couldn't stand my state anymore, or if I didn't feel that my therapist understood me, I knew that there was the self-mutilation that I could rely on to make my condition more bearable. For example, instead of listening to my therapist's explanations, which I couldn't understand, I planned my next act of self-mutilation. I also thought that my wounds would convince people how terribly I suffered. However, I often hid my wounds, being afraid of being blamed by somebody for my deed. Rather often, while being angry with somebody (without being able to notice my feeling of anger), or feeling badly treated by somebody, I directed the anger against myself by self-mutilating, since I wasn't able to take the anger out on that person, or to deal with my anger. My need to cut myself became compulsive. Just like the feelings I had to kill myself, or to use compulsive sentences. My therapist was strictly against my self-destructive behavior. He told me to end therapy and leave the clinic if I were to continue. This prohibition had (as far as I remember) almost no effect on my self-destructive behavior.

"In the beginning of 2000, I developed a strong noise sensitivity, perhaps due to stress, so I had to protect myself with ear plugs all day. Sometimes I almost completely lost contact with the world around me and with myself. I suffered with quite extreme dissociative states. Sometimes I felt like I was melting into the chair and the boundaries between me and the chair were disappearing, or I was dissolving and couldn't detect the difference between my legs, feet, hands, and the air, or in a room with people I knew, they would start to feel foreign, or I might think that my hand didn't belong to me anmore. I couldn't control these frightening experiences at all.

"I lost more than 10 kg during those 2.5 years in the day clinic. I always ate only a small salad at our common midday meal, while most of the other patients ate the whole meal. I wanted to keep my weight at 59 kg (130 lbs), and being 59.5 kg (or 131 lbs) was a tragedy for me, since I thought the other people around me would notice my increase in weight and despise me because of it. If I gained weight I had to eat even less. My weight told me if I was worth being loved at least a little bit or if I was here to be eliminated. I often felt very fat (though I wasn't fat at all). I looked compulsively in a mirror to make sure I hadn't gotten fat.

"After 1 year in that clinic, I started bingeing again in the evening and at night. While I had control during the day, I ate all the food that was forbidden during the night. Afterward, I always hated myself even more. I tried several times to vomit afterward by putting my finger into my throat, but I never managed to do it. One day, I suddenly had the idea to chew the food and instead of swallowing it, spit it in the toilet, or in napkins that I later through away.

"In June 2000, my psychiatrist at the day clinic prescribed clomipramine in addition to zuclopenthixol, lorazepam, and lithium, because my compulsive sentences became very strong and I also developed the need to read them again and again on little notes. For example, while being in a store with my mother, I had to read these sentences on my notes to insure that I did not have a wrong perception and that I had no hallucinations and that I could trust my own perception. For example, I wasn't sure at all anymore if the people around me were really there or if I was just imagining them. Or if there might be a big hole in the ground that I wasn't noticing.

"In July 2000, my therapist stopped lithium and substituted zuclopennthixol with penfluridol, which was supposed to help prevent my self-mutilation and my almost permanent suicidal thoughts. Around this time, my brother had his first psychotic breakdown and the situation at home became too burdensome for me. So I slept 2 weeks in the Kriseninterventionszentrum, a center for dealing with crisis attacks. One night in this center, I cried and shouted hysterically because I thought that the woman in my room had to suffer because of me. This ended with me pressing a burning cigarette several times on my hand in front of the doctor. At this point, my therapist prescribed haloperidol in addition to the other medications.

"Over the next 2 months, I slept at my great-aunt's home and in real emergencies at the Kriseninterventionszentrum, when my fear became so strong that I was convinced for a short time that our new therapist was a psychopath who wanted to kill us and was only pretending that he wanted to help us. I would also stay in the center at night when my need for committing suicide was too strong and when everything around me seemed to say 'kill yourself!'

"In November 2000, my therapist increased the clomipramine to 300 mg per day, and this almost stopped the compulsive sentences and looking at notes.

"Then for 1 month I moved into the Chalet Margharita in Kersatz, a domicile for people with (severe) psychiatric disorders, while still at the day clinic. Since I wasn't able to plan my future, my therapist in the day clinic suggested that I go to a therapeutic farm called Chly Linde in Hinterfultigen together with four or five other female patients my age. My therapists thought it was time for a change, since after 2.5 years, in his opinion and in mine, there was no significant improvement. However, they did help prevent me from committing suicide.

"In February 2001, after 3 weeks at Chly Linde, I attempted suicide by swallowing 16 pills of lorazepam that I was hiding. During these weeks, my condition had gotten more and more unbearable. I felt that the demands of the work were too much. Also, I had the strong impression of being so different from the other patients. I was only able to speak a few words a day and wasn't able to experience myself as a young woman. I also feared that the others hated me because of it. In addition to my suicidal thoughts, I had very strong bingeing attacks again. I had to eat constantly and I had to interrupt my work to run to the refrigerator to eat anything several times a day. I was so desperate that I even ate dog food and stole food from the deep freezer. While on this farm, I saw my therapist at the day clinic twice a week 30 minutes away in Bern. On these trips I bought and ate so much forbidden food that it probably would have taken a normal person several days to eat it. Before attempting suicide, I also had the strong feeling that I would kill the two horses on the farm. They were very important in the life of the therapist who owned them. I also had the fear that I would kill people around me while they were sleeping. I did not feel like I was being understood by my therapist at the day clinic or by my new therapists at the farm. They wanted me to take responsibility and to make decisions, like getting healthy, which I felt was totally impossible for me in my state, and this made me feel even worse and more desperate.

"After my suicide attempt, I went to a closed psychiatric ward at the University Hospital in Berne. In my mind this place was where hopeless cases were sent that could not be managed in a private psychiatric clinic. There I had to sleep several nights alone in a closed room with belts on my wrists, belly, and ankles for protection against committing suicide. The psychiatrist on this closed ward stopped the clomipramine and prescribed clozapine, sertraline, and lorazepam. He said that I was suffering from a severe psychosis. My therapist at the day clinic that I had seen for more than 2.5 years came to visit me in this hospital and told me that our therapy was finished because of my suicide attempt, which was forbidden by our contract. Learning this was very hard for me, and I was glad that I was only able to realize it very superficially, because I was too dissociated to realize more. At the hospital my therapies included handicrafts, cooking, sports, and group discussions that I could not follow or contribute to. I also had physiotherapy, since I had dislocated my right shoulder earlier while in the day clinic. I continued my bingeing and sometimes stole food from other patients; I also continued smoking. During this time I was either obsessed with my thoughts of killing myself or about eating, and my tormenting need to tell myself compulsive sentences and little notes returned, probably because my therapist had stopped the clomipramine.

"In the beginning of April 2001, I went into an anorexic phase to lose weight. For about 2 months I only ate half a piece of bread with a little jam for breakfast, small portions of salad and vegetables for lunch, and half a piece of bread with yogurt for dinner. I did a lot of gymnastics on my bed and every day I spent 2.5 hours on the stationary cycle in the ward. I lost over 10 kg again within 2 or 3 months and weighed 61 kg (or 134 lbs). I think because of my dissociative disorder, I was not able to notice being hungry or able to experience the sweat running down my body after my daily cycling program. I also had to get on the scale, sometimes 40 times a day, to check my weight to stop my enormous fear of having put on weight again. I also had to look in the mirror again and again. I repeatedly touched my ribs and bones on my face and hips to see if I could feel the bones and that they were not covered by fat. I compulsively told myself again and again what I was allowed to eat. My thoughts were almost only about food and being fat. In the beginning of May, I was prescribed mirtazapine for depression in addition to my other medications. The doctor also tried to substitute lorazepam with diazepam, and this did not help. At this point, I stopped menstruating.

"Later, I was diagnosed by the head psychiatrist on the ward with a schizoaffective disorder, and this was confirmed by the professor of the Waldau clinic. He told my parents and me that there had been a quarrel between the psychologists and the psychiatrists on the ward, and that the psychologists didn't agree with their diagnosis. The psychologists diagnosed a severe anxiety disorder. They also stopped mirtazapine, as it was not helping. In addition to the other medications, they prescribed amisulpride, and my parents said I started to walk like a robot. At this time my neurodermitis came back and it was treated with cortisone-pomade. In the middle of July, the therapists stopped clozapine.

"I started to spit out food again. I compulsively bought large amounts of food to later chew and spit in the toilet. I was very ashamed of this because someone might be able to hear the sound of me chewing on the toilet, but I wasn't able to stop. Sometimes this behavior came very suddenly, from one moment to the next, induced by a question like 'Are you hungry?' I never talked with the therapists about my eating disorder in this clinic. I was only able to tell them that I really couldn't stand my suffering any longer. Other subjects were much too complicated for me to discuss or to understand, as I had almost completely lost contact with myself. At the end of July, my parents took me home from the clinic. The doctor told them this would not be easy for them.

"From August 2001 until the end of January 2003, I went to my father's psychiatrist, who he had seen for 30 years. She injected me three or four times with a neuroleptic that did not improve my condition. At the end of August 2001, she also substituted amisulpride with quetiapine (350 mg per day) and added sertraline (200 mg per day). When I was in the Waldau Clinic, I had been prescribed 2.5 mg of reboxetine, which she increased to 12 mg per day. But I suffered terribly and had the firm impression that my condition was getting worse and more unbearable every day. I was only able to communicate a few stereotypical sentences like 'I don't understand anything anymore,' and 'I really can't stand my situation anymore.' I started having bingeing attacks again and my parents had to lock the door of the kitchen. These attacks were combined with spitting out food. Again the only thing I wanted in addition to my enormous will to commit suicide was to lose weight. I wanted to reduce my weight from the horrible 71 kg to 59 kg by taking less than 500 kcal per day. In the middle of September 2001, my therapist prescribed in addition to the other medications 20 mg of Deroxat and 3 mg of bromazepan per day. I still had to tell my compulsive sentences. These thoughts made me panic and I desperately tried to contradict them and prove them wrong by looking for arguments against them. But they never disappeared and they always had the last word.

"Next I met Peggy Claude-Pierre, who had the Montreux Clinic in Canada for treating severe eating disorders and self-mutilation. She was in Switzerland with her husband, and my father arranged a meeting at our home. For the very small part in me that wanted to go on living, a stay at her clinic was apparently the only remaining possibility. She tried to communicate with me for about 2 hours, while her husband talked with my father. At the end she said I could not go to her clinic in Canada, since they only help people that could guarantee not to hurt themselves physically or try to commit suicide, or attack others. I could not guarantee, not even a little bit. But she promised to stay in contact with my father and encouraged him to practice her therapy with me.

"When she left, I had horrible and very fast thoughts about how I could kill myself at once, and also how I could kill my family, and I now thought I might be a psychopath and a wholesale murderer. From this day on my father had to lock me in the attic while my parents and my brother lived on the ground floor because I wanted to commit suicide by jumping from a bridge in Bern. I was also really convinced that without being locked up, I would kill my family or people on the street. I behaved totally crazy at that time. I threw cups and other things around in my room, made loud sounds like an animal, hit my head against the wall, laughed like I was crazy and shouted, and made movements like a psychopath. I mostly behaved like this in my room. I was only able to leave my room with my mother or my father. When outside, I was only able to say very little and I was so numb and so dissociated that I did not notice people standing near me, or even the cold of the winter.

"At the end of December 2001, my parents started to reduce the quetiapine without telling the therapist, who was strictly against it. I also was not told and didn't notice the reduction, as my parents replaced the missing pills with magnesium pills that looked the same. This took 2 weeks. Around this time the therapist discontinued reboxetine and paroxetine. Also at this time my therapist prescribed clomipramine, starting with 25 mg then slowly increasing it to 225 mg by the middle of April. This came from a request of my father who was reading everything he could find on psychiatric disorders, and he thought I had a very severe case of OCD. In the beginning of January 2002, bromazepan was discontinued, and I was prescribed lithium for my self-destructive impulses. I had the firm idea to put out my eyes. Lithium was slowly increased to two tablets a day with every second day 2.5 tablets. Ever since then I have been taking lithium at this dose. In the middle of January 2002, my therapist officially started to reduce quetiapine.

"In January 2002, my father found David's Kundalini yoga protocol for OCD in a book and he started to do parts of the protocol. In the beginning, my father tried to do the OCD breath (OCDB) with me, but he had to force me by shouting at me and sometimes hitting me, which I didn't feel because I was too dissociated. My resistance against this protocol, like everything else, was enormous. Evening after evening there were hard fights between my father and the part of me that so desperately wanted to die. My enormous fears led to my resistance against starting Kundalini yoga. I was convinced that I would be terribly punished or that my mother would die if I did these techniques. Finally, thanks to my father's almost endless patience, I began to do the OCDB with his help (without tuning in with "Ong Namo"). My father used a watch and told me at each five-second interval what I had to do—breathe in, stop, breathe out, stop. First I did every phase for about 5 seconds for 10 minutes in the morning, 10 minutes at midday, and then 10 minutes in the evening, with several breaks during each 10-minute effort. Some days later I did the OCDB for 31 minutes with 5 seconds per phase with several breaks during it. After about half a month I managed to do 5 seconds inhale, 15 seconds hold, 5 seconds exhale, 15 seconds hold out. Since I was so dissociated at that time, I was not able to experience my enormous fear or anything about my body while doing the OCDB and also during the rest of the day. I think that's the reason for my ability to hold the breath in and especially out for 15 seconds at that time: I just didn't feel anything at all while doing the OCDB. But I had to continuously use my compulsive sentences while doing the OCDB. Often I had to enumerate to myself during the 31 minutes of the OCDB what I was allowed to eat and to compare with what I had already eaten at my last meal to prove that I hadn't eaten too much.

"Near the end of January or the beginning of February 2002, I had two important experiences. One evening, I was able to remember some of my concepts in my head ('fixed false beliefs'), which I told my father with a normal and clear voice, and this was extraordinary for me at that time. I was able to tell him that I always had the strong belief that my mother loved my younger brother more than me and that he didn't love me. During this conversation, my father told me for the first time (as far as I can remember) that he did love me, which was very important for me to know. He also told me and my brother that he loved my mother (despite the fact that I always thought that the marriage of my parents was rather loveless) and that we were a family. Thanks to my father I realized that evening that we can think wrong things and that a lot of my firm convictions and thoughts during that time didn't correspond to reality.

"After the conversation that evening, I wasn't able to feel my pulse anymore. I also closed my nose with my hand while holding my mouth closed and had no reaction at all to this action. Nothing inside of me seemed to fight against a death through suffocation. I was totally convinced that I would die. I told my father this. Instead of panicking, he went out of my room, locked me inside and left me alone. This was terrible for me. I laid down in my bed, wrote a farewell letter to my family, and waited for death. The next morning I was still alive. This was important, because I interpreted to mean that 'God doesn't want me to die now.' This experience also showed me that the universe gives me the right to live, or otherwise I wouldn't have woken up again. It was like I had put my life into the hands of something bigger and let it decide whether I should go on living or dying now. I also realized after my father left me alone in my misery that he couldn't make me healthy, and that I would have to do it alone with the help of others.

"I think this experience was a turning point for me, away from the very firm will to kill myself to a loving behavior toward myself. Perhaps this was where my long way back to life started again.

"The day after this experience, while on a walk with my mother, I was able to hop for a few seconds. This was very surprising, because I was able to notice the physical impulse inside of me of the hopping movement. Probably I returned briefly to an awareness of my body again. During this walk I was also able to feel my ponytail again, which was moving with my steps.

"At that time I also began to trust in people around me a little bit, especially in my parents and also in my great-aunt. I told them about my terrible suffering, and I also asked questions to help understand the still very powerful self-destructive part inside of me who was a liar. This part was telling me for example that my great-aunt hated me. I found out by asking her that this was not true.

"While I still felt like I was unbearably fat in some areas, I finally learned from my father that seeing oneself as fatter than they really are, is a symptom of an eating disorder and that this did not correspond to reality.

"In the middle of February, my father hired two female students to help me with the OCDB and the technique for managing fears. So for the next 2 or 3 months I did the OCDB with their help twice a day (still without "tuning in"), followed each time by the fear technique, which I did three times in a row. In the beginning I was only able to say a few words to the students. The psychology student later told me that when we first met, it seemed like I was not present at all, and not even in the room.

"From the beginning of February 2002 until the middle of April 2002, with my parent's support, I managed to increase my weight from 58 kg to 65 kg. In my opinion, this was a great achievement. In spite of the terrible fearful thoughts about gaining weight, after four months, without the aid of a therapist, I was able to eat normal meals. By June 2002, I was able to stop spitting food in the toilet or throwing it away. I was also able to stop compulsively telling myself what I 'was allowed' to eat during a meal or the whole day. I think this amazing progress was the result of doing Kundalini Yoga, especially the OCDB, which I know from David and my own experience is able to help eating disorders.

"Today (at a weight of about 68 kg), I'm able again to eat without that terrible big fear I used to experience during meals. I'm also able to communicate with the people I eat with and I can also smell and taste the food, something I could not do for about 5 or 6 years. I also don't suffer from eating attacks or spitting food anymore. Only very seldomly do I see myself in the mirror as fatter than I really am.

"By the end of February 2002, I was able to go without my father's company to my therapist. She noticed that I talked more compared to the month before. At that time, I began to experience something in my body. I felt an enormous pressure and pain in the region of my heart chakra that may have been related to my enormous fear. Until this time, I wasn't able to notice the physical symptoms of this terrible fear as I had dissociated from these symptoms like all the other feelings.

"In the beginning of March 2002, I told my father that my compulsive thoughts were a little bit less important and more distant than when they had tortured me most.

"In mid April 2002, my psychiatrist told me that I could try to reduce the clomipramine, as my need to tell myself compulsive sentences was weaker. By mid July I reduced it from 225 mg per day to 75 mg per day.

"In mid May 2002, I read a book about sexually abused women and realized I had a lot of the symptoms that they develop. I had enormous self-hatred, feelings of being terribly dirty inside, the very firm conviction of being absolutely bad, dissociative symptoms, self-mutilation, extreme disgust and fear of the male sexual organ, and other symptoms. Suddenly I could remember again small parts of the horrible experience with my ex-boxfriend that I had completely blocked out. The rediscovery and the memories concerning the experience with my ex-boyfriend made my state worse for at least 2 or 3 weeks. I began to understand the effects that this experience had on me, some of which are still with me today. I know that my ex-boyfriend did not violate me, but in my opinion he nevertheless misused me. Today I think this experience was part of the reason, but not the only reason, for my severe psychiatric condition.

"In early June 2002, I traveled alone by train to a see a spiritual-energetic healer in Dornach about an hour away from Bern. I still go to see her with other people about twice a year. She told me that during our first meeting, she quickly realized that she could only treat me from a distance of about 1 meter, because of my fears.

"At the end of June 2002, I started a dance therapy class in Bern that I still attend today. Besides dance therapy and painting, my therapist would occasionally also lead me in imaginary journeys. I entered into dance therapy with the hope of getting more in touch with my feelings and body.

"At the end of July 2002, I managed to do the OCDB for the first time alone while looking at a watch. About the same time, my psychiatrist recommended an increase in clomipramine because my self-destructive part was a little stronger again, and I had the experience of fear at my heart-center again that led to more compulsive sentences. Perhaps it was because I got closer to life and to my body that I felt the fear in my chest more and more. That's why my therapist and I agreed to increase the clomipramine. I was glad we did, as I could experience the positive effects of this medication. My compulsive sentences and fear at my heart-center got really weaker and even disappeared for a short time, and it got more quiet in my head. Unfortunately, my OCD symptoms reappeared again after about a week. That's why I increased clomipramine more and more up to my highest dose of 525 mg per day at the end of March 2003. My therapist gave me the permission to reduce or increase it as long as I had informed her what I was doing with the medication. (I later learned from

David when I told him about my dose that 700 mg per day can be deadly and 525 mg per day was nearly twice the maximum dose that is ever prescribed in the U.S.A.)

"In the beginning of December 2002, I finally followed my father's advice and extended my Kundalini yoga program, which I was doing almost everyday. I started to include Ong Namo, spine flexes, and shoulder shrugs. A little later I included the fourth and fifth meditation techniques and the mantra for anger. The only technique of the protocol that I did not include was the sixth technique to avoid dislocating my right shoulder again. It took me almost a year to get around to doing the entire OCD protocol.

"In mid January 2003, my therapist suggested that I go to a behavior therapist to learn how to deal with my compulsions in addition to the techniques of the OCD protocol. I do not think she believed in the effects of the OCD protocol, although she noticed the progress I was making. I think she wanted me to go to a new therapist because she noticed that I really depended too much on her and that I had too close a relationship with her. Of course this change of therapist was very hard on me, as I again had the impression that nobody wanted me.

"In mid February 2003, I started with a new therapist at Muri near Bern who is a psychologist, psychotherapist, and a general practitioner. Still today I usually go once a week to him for therapy. I frequently disagree with him because he is not as familiar with spiritual issues as my other therapists. But he is a good therapist for me because he is very down to earth and helps me with every-day-life issues. He diagnosed me with dissociative disorder, OCD, borderline, and eating disorders. He primarily focuses on treating my dissociative disorder since he thinks this is now my major problem.

"In mid March 2003, my dance therapist recommended a Sufi teacher in Bern and reading books on Sufism. This was the first time somebody told me that I was not only psychically ill, but that I was also going through a spiritual transformation. A little bit later, I got very similar insights from David. I'm really glad that he is able to combine spiritual wisdom and knowledge about psychiatric disorders. He is the only therapist I have that is able to do this.

"Since the end of March 2003 I have gone several times a year to meetings of different spiritual teachers in Bern, or on occasion to Zurich, or Lucerne. And in mid April 2003, I started going almost weekly to a Sufi meditation group.

"At the end of March 2003, my therapist was afraid that the very high dose of clomipramine (525 mg per day) could begin to seriously harm me. I also had side effects—dryness of the mouth, sometimes trembling hands and less frequently trembling legs, fatigue, profuse perspiration. So my therapist slowly began to reduce it and to substitute it with BuSpar. He also prescribed zinc and vitamin B6. I'm quite sure that I wouldn't have been able to reduce clomipramine without the pressure of my therapist and the advice of David. In the middle of April 2003, I was on 375 mg of clomipramine, 15mg of BuSpar, and lithium. I was able to reduce clomipramine to 150 mg per day at the end of September 2003. At that point, my therapist helped me to slowly reduce Buspar to zero by February 2004.

"At the end of March 2003, I was able to write my first short e-mail to David. Prior to that time, only my father had been sporadically writing to him for about 1 year. From this point on I started writing David e-mails, sometimes weekly, to ask him questions about my fears and about my Kundalini yoga practice. David's advice and fast answers to my often quite long e-mails are very important and helpful.

"At the beginning of our e-mail correspondence, David suggested that I mentally use the "Ek Ong Kar Sat Gurprasad Sat Gurprasad Ek Ong Kar" mantra instead of telling myself compulsive sentences. This was very hard for me because at that time I still had to tell myself compulsive sentences and my mind always told me that doing the "Ek Ong Kar" mantra was wrong. But when I managed to use it, I realized how much a relief this was and how healing it can be for me. He also told me to use the mantra "Wha

Hay Guru" during the OCDB instead of telling myself compulsive sentences.

"In May 2003, I learned from David that it was important to keep the four phases of the OCDB at the same length, and then I realized that until that point I hadn't practiced the OCDB correctly, because I was doing it with 5-second inhales, 15-second holding in, 5-second exhales, and 15-second holding out. In the beginning of September 2003, I started to do the OCDB with 10 seconds per phase.

"In mid June 2003, I started a job for about 1 or 2 hours per day without salary. My therapist recommended that I start work again part-time. For 3 weeks I picked strawberries in a field about 20 minutes away by train.

"In the beginning of July 2003, when the strawberry season was over, I started a new job about 2 hours a day in a garden near Bern for about 2.5 months. I went to work on a bicycle and this was the first time in about 5 years that I was able to cycle alone. Doing these two jobs was very difficult for me, since I often experienced the unbearable fear at my heart chakra and had to constantly tell myself compulsive sentences, which during those times I managed only for very short periods to substitute with the "Ek Ong Kar" mantra.

"In early July 2003, I had my first phone conversation with David. Since then I have talked with him five times on the phone. Every time I found these 1.5- to 2.5-hour conversations very helpful. During the evening after the first conversation there were almost no compulsive sentences in my mind, which was extraordinary for me. In this conversation he also taught me how to equalize all five senses and how to use the Pratyhar meditation (Shannahoff-Khalsa, 2003) for achieving a state of mental silence and stability that could be used in place of compulsive sentences or mantras. I had written to him that I really longed for silence in my head. From the middle of July until today I have been doing the Pratyhar meditation frequently. I like doing it. One day I was thinking about food all the time again and I experienced the desire and urge to binge. After doing the Pratyhar meditation these problems were completely gone! Doing this technique also helps me to hold my mental space much more stable and to live and be rooted more and more in this state of silence not only while doing these techniques, but also during everyday life.

"During our first phone conversation, David told me that in the beginning I had a rather severe or extreme case of OCD and that I also suffered from PTSD, which I had probably developed from the sexual experience with my ex-boyfriend, and that this probably accounts for my ability to dissociate. To heal my PTSD symptoms, David taught me Gan Puttee Kriya and I have been doing it somewhat regularly since late July 2003.

"In one of our first phone conversations, David asked me what plans I had for my future. For me, this was a very unexpected and unusual question, because since the first time I went to the clinic in 1997, it was very clear to me that I would have no future because I would probably kill myself. It may have been in this conversation when David also suggested that I become a Kundalini yoga teacher and specialize in treating OCD and PTSD. This idea gave me a totally new perspective. For the first time in about 6 years I had the thought that I might have a future. Today I sometimes think that I would like to become a teacher. I always wanted to help people, and if I learned this profession I could better understand psychiatric patients because of my own suffering.

"In August 2003, I wrote David that I had the perception of an identity within me that was observing my thoughts. David told me that this wasn't an illness or craziness, as I had feared, but that I was blessed to have the awareness of my true eternal identity, my eternal spiritual self that one can frequently experience through meditation. This is another example of why David's guidance is so important to me. I think most Western-trained therapists don't know enough about spiritual or altered states and therefore often confound these experiences with psychiatric disorders that can lead to improper treatment. In 1997, when I had a similar experience, my brother's former psychiatrist told me that it was very dangerous to observe one's own thoughts and that I should stop trying to do that. I can imagine that most psychiatrists would have diagnosed these experiences as symptoms of a psychiatric disorder. And without having developed my spirituality, I would never have found the way out of psychiatric clinics.

"I began to learn from David that when I had uncomfortable feelings caused by my compulsive thoughts to allow my fears and everything else (sensations, memories, etc.) to come and go without reacting to them, while holding the stable space and state of mind produced that I learned while practicing the Pratyhar meditation. I can't always do it, but I am able to do it more and more these days.

"While I still sometimes suffer from the compulsion to ask my mother about her health, it happens less frequently today and is certainly less intense. I think it's so hard for me to stop because it's probably my oldest compulsion, the one I've used most, and because I don't try hard enough on this one.

"In mid 2003, another old compulsion returned. I had to interrupt my Kundalini yoga practice to look at my compulsive sentences that were written on many little notes lying on the floor or to look in one of my books. Sometimes I stopped the OCDB up to four or five times to look at my compulsive sentences. At that time I wasn't able to just allow my compulsive questions that resulted from my fears without looking for sentences and answers to calm myself. It's clear that these interruptions diminished the benefits of the technique.

"In mid 2003, at David's suggestion, I started to fall asleep to the sounds of the fear tape; he said this is another way to work on my mind since the subconscious mind is always awake and absorbing.

"In August 2003, I told David that most of the time I'm not aware of the effects of the yoga techniques because I can't experience and feel them or anything else during the day. I was not used to feeling or experiencing anything that I do. But I also told him that I was slowly getting better and slowly getting in contact with my body again.

"One of the first effects of Kundalini yoga I was able to notice consciously (near the end of March 2003) was that sometimes during or after the OCDB my unbearable feeling of fear that manifested at my heart center and the intense need to tell myself compulsive sentences really got weaker. Later, when doing the OCDB, I suddenly realized that I was now inside my head again and not out of my head anymore, where I probably had been for about 6 years without being able to notice. I was also able to feel the movements of my belly again while breathing.

"In mid September 2003, David sent me a Kundalini yoga exercise set called Nabhi Kriya to help me feel my body better again and to increase my energy. Prior to this exercise set, I had to sleep every afternoon for about 1 or 2 hours. He also told me this set would make me more earthy, stable, and centered. Today I do Nabhi Kriya about twice a week and I am finally able to do at least parts of this exercise set without compulsive sentences.

"In October 2003, my therapist recommended that I start part-time work. I had been working about three times a week for about 2 hours (seldom up to 4 hours) in a small local grocery. In the beginning I frequently had to tell myself compulsive sentences and also write down new compulsive questions (when nobody was looking). I was so dissociated that I wasn't able to experience that I was working in a store and that I was very distant from customers or other workers. Also, I could only say a few words because I felt so out of touch with the world and daily life that I wouldn't have known what to talk about with normal people. In the early days there, my main attention was on my compulsive sentences. However, today I almost never tell myself compulsive sentences while working in the store. I'm much more present and in touch with everyday life. Now I notice what season it is and when decorations in the store change and I even make suggestions for them. Now my mind is less narrow and dark and I am able to talk about my life and listen with interest to what others tell me about theirs.

"In November 2003, I was able to do the OCDB frequently with 10 seconds per phase and to do it using a mantra ("Wha Hay Guru") instead of compulsive sentences. However, at that point I had the impression that doing the OCDB was more difficult because I was a little bit more in my body and consequently holding the breath out was more difficult. I had to stop two, three, or four times mostly in the beginning while doing the breath hold-out phase to get more air. I had to stop because I really had the impression that I couldn't stand it anymore and that I might suffocate. I also started to avoid the hold out phase by directly breathing in again without holding the breath out. David told me several times to stop this behavior and not to interrupt the OCDB. He also said that the hold out phase was the most important phase of the OCDB as it helped me to learn to overcome my fears. At that time, and sometimes today, doing the OCDB is really very trying for me, but I know that I have to do it to get completely healed.

"Also in the beginning of November 2003, David sent me two new Kundalini yoga techniques—the meditation technique for dyslexia and another short one for fear. Many times, David told me that I could give my intellectual mind a rest and to just experience and enjoy the effects of the techniques. He said it was more important for me to experience the process than to understand it intellectually. Today I'm able to notice a big difference if I am either deeply rooted in the state of mind that I learned while doing the Pratyhar meditation, or if I am only experiencing the activity of my intellectual mind. Only in the latter do I ever use compulsive sentences, though very rarely now.

"In mid November 2003, I finally realized how unpresent I was and how separate I was from life. I realized that I needed to come back to an earthly life and to see, notice, and experience life with my own eyes! I knew I had to learn again to be aware of everything that belongs to me, my feelings, thoughts, actions, and the environment. I think this realization was very important for me, since for more than 5 years all I really wanted was to extinguish myself totally and to notice, sense, and experience nothing.

"In mid January 2004, I started to have the experience of the empty, silent, and stable space that is produced while doing the Prathyhar meditation and while doing the OCDB, especially near the end. I noticed that the state produced during the OCDB gave me a new stability where I had no need to do compulsive sentences or to switch away. That's when I really began to experience the very agreeable effects of the OCDB.

"From the beginning of March 2004 until the end of July 2004, I was able to reduce clomipramine further from 112.5 mg to 37.5 mg In April 2004, I went on my first holiday in 7 years. I went to a 4-day Sufi retreat near Zurich. In September 2004, I was able to go abroad again for the first time in 7 years.

"In October 2004, I had two unpleasant dissociative experiences triggered by stress and nervousness. I had the impression of leaving my body through the top of my head and being on the ceiling, although I was not able to view my body from outside. I also experienced again that the boundaries of things in a room were melting and everything merged. I felt like all the people in the room and even my own face were suddenly very foreign to me. Although I didn't like these experiences, I realized that contrary to all my prior dissociative feelings, I was able to experience these two events more consciously. Before I was only able to note that something was terribly wrong with me and that I couldn't stand that state and I really didn't know what to do in those situations. I also discovered that by breathing deeply or by knocking parts of my body against the floor (without hurting myself) that I could come back into my body again.

"David later told me that I should learn to enjoy these experiences if they happen and that people work for years to learn to achieve such states, although they develop a conscious control with such events and use them as a valuable experience. He also taught me to chant the mantra "Ong Namo Guru Dev Namo" and other mantras during any dissociative event to give a greater sense of comfort and protection. Contrary to the past, I'm much more conscious during an event and I also panic less and use the mantras to help protect and guide me during a dissociative experience.

"In late November 2004, I had a severe lumbago that triggered a 10-day renewed interest in committing suicide. However, during these days I realized that my old and rather firm conviction that after death everything will be totally over, was a complete illusion. The wisdom that you can't extinguish your suffering by committing suicide is very important for me today, although it is now only a rare event.

"In mid January 2005, I started living alone in an apartment paid by disability insurance. During the first 1 or 2 weeks a lot of fears and old memories were coming up and I had some disagreeable dissociative experiences where everything around me appeared very foreign to me. The Tomatis therapist and the Kundalini yoga techniques helped me to overcome these fears. And my condition got better and more stable again, although it is not as good yet as it used to be, before I moved. But going home almost every day to eat a warm meal and having my mother do my laundry and parental support is very helpful.

"In February 2005, I had surgery on my right shoulder to prevent it from dislocating. After some recovery I started doing Kundalini yoga about 6 days a week for 1.5 to 2.5 hours in the morning. This practice included the OCD protocol, except for shoulder shrugs and technique 6, which are both too much for my shoulder, and I rarely do the technique for anger or the victory breath. About twice a week I do Nabhi Kriya to help my back, be more centered, and for my energy levels. And sometimes I practice Gan Puttee Kriya or the Pratyhar meditation before going to bed. I realized that doing the OCDB is much easier for me after doing most of the other techniques in the OCD protocol, rather than just tuning in and doing it. Before moving into my apartment, I was able to do the OCDB at 13 seconds per phase, or 14 seconds per phase, and sometimes up to 15 seconds per phase, but only for the first 8 minutes. And I was able to practice it without stopping, though I would still leave out the hold-out phase about 10 times during the 31-minute practice. In my apartment, I do the OCDB now mostly with 13 seconds per phase and occasionally with 12 seconds, and after input from David I now try not to leave out the hold-out phase, but still do about three times throughout the practice.

"Today (February 2005), I'm not healed yet. I'm not able yet to feel my body in a 'normal' way, or to experience my feelings like I did before my illness. But now I can sometimes experience joy and excitement. I am not able to associate with all of the things that I have dissociated myself from. I still experience states of psychiatric disorders, but less often, less intense, and for much shorter times. Despite that, life has a much better quality again. I'm much less compulsive, and I am living more in the present. I no longer self-mutilate. I now believe that I will recover completely and that this is possible even for someone who started out in an extremely bad condition as I did.

"I'm convinced and know deep inside that Kundalini yoga and David's assistance has helped saved my life. Step by step, I am healing more every day. I can't imagine how else my very ill mind would have been cured from my endless compulsive sentences; the OCDB helped me to purge my thoughts and trained me how not to do anything on an intellectual level other than breathe."

Lisa was completely off clomipramine by May 2005. The only medication she has been on from that date until the date of this transcript (December 28, 2005) has been lithium (2 tablets per day, every second day 2.5 tablets). From March 28, 2003, when she made her first personal contact with me, until February 2005, when she provided her last input for this case history (other than the last medications entry), I have had about 40 e-mail exchanges and five phone calls with her.

PART THREE

Therapy for Individuals, Couples, and Groups

NINE

Integrating Kundalini Yoga Meditation Techniques into Therapy

This chapter is primarily directed toward psychiatrists, psychologists, social workers, and other clinicians who work directly with patients as individuals and/or in groups. The first rule of thumb for a therapist seeking to achieve a successful therapeutic outcome is simple: the more direct personal experience that therapist has with a specific technique or protocol, the more likely he will be able to inspire the patient to comply with therapy. In part, this is true because the therapist plays a role as a coach and as a salesperson. It is incumbent on the therapist to point out the hurdles in therapy and to inspire the patient to overcome each hurdle. The height of the hurdle and number of hurdles is both dependent on the disorder and the patient's severity and condition. In addition, the patient may have several disorders, and will want to have some guidance and insight into what the therapy will entail, and how quickly he can expect a resolution to his condition. Direct experience by the therapist with each technique or protocol leads to the best source of motivation for the patient. If the therapist can say with conviction, "These are very powerful techniques and they can lead to near-immediate relief, I have tried them, and I am amazed by their incredible efficacy," clearly he will be able to inspire the patient much more successfully than by saying, "I have heard they are very good and do wonders; why don't you try them?" Therefore, the first hurdle is to get the patient to experience the technique or protocol. The second and usually last hurdle is compliance and perfection over time.

The second general rule of thumb in therapy is that the choice of most patients is to do as little as possible to achieve relief. Regardless of what you teach them, the majority of patients, perhaps 60%, will titrate their practice to the minimal dose required to lessen their symptoms to an acceptable degree of discomfort. Most patients do not see a need to achieve complete relief and are willing to live with some level of discomfort rather than to develop a strong and consistent discipline with their practice. That is to say, they are more motivated by their suffering and not by their levels of mental excellence and well-being. This is true of patients who I have seen privately and also mostly true with those participating in clinical trials. However, those attending a clinical trial tend to be somewhat more motivated because they usually have made one or more failed attempts at therapy and are more committed because they may have been suffering much longer. This has clearly been the case with OCD patients. Also, being in a group setting has several advantages, and this in part probably helps make the difference in terms of a successful outcome. First, the patient is a little less self-conscious while practicing the techniques. Secondly, it leads to an opportunity for comparison with others' progress, and a mild but subtle form of competition usually develops with those out-performing others in the group. Patients are frequently inspired by other members. Those lagging behind see that others achieving certain "mile stones" in their practice are usually doing so because their at-home practice is more frequent, and the leaders in the group are doing the whole protocol at home. In my experience, almost all patients work hard in a group and less hard when they are not in the group. Of course, there are many reasons why they might fail to work hard outside of the group—hectic home activities, demanding responsibilities and schedules, family members who are not supportive or in fact reject their choice of therapy, or perhaps they do not suffer enough.

The third rule of thumb is that the therapist should do the protocol along with the patient(s). In an individual session, the patient will feel far less self-conscious if he is not expected to do it alone. If the therapist wants to help the patient, he will not request that they practice the technique alone. In a group situation, the patients still prefer to see the therapist participating rather than simply telling them what to do. However, regardless of whether therapy is conducted in a group or with a single patient, the therapist must pay enough attention to the patient(s) to ensure that the patient is practicing the techniques correctly. Once it is clear that the patient understands the techniques and practices them correctly, less immediate attention is required. In general, larger groups usually have a more powerful and pleasant group energy. This energy helps to inspire and carry the individuals who tend to lag behind.

The therapist who is set up to see patients in individual therapy and in groups is obviously going to be able to offer the best opportunities for patients. Some patients will prefer one-on-one therapy, and some will prefer group therapy. Some may choose to start out in one-on-one therapy, and then enter a group once they feel like they have discussed their own personal situation and issues adequately. Then they realize it is only a matter of keeping up with the techniques over time. Obviously, practicing with a group is more cost effective, and for some more pleasant.

Compliance in therapy is a challenge regardless of whether the therapy is meditation, medication, psychotherapy, or cognitive behavioral therapy. Each disorder also presents with its own challenges, however, that topic is beyond the scope of this chapter. When medication is the modality of treatment, and there are side effects without a complete remission, the therapist frequently considers dosing frequency, medication choices, and other techniques to increase adherence for an improved long-term outcome. There are analogous considerations with meditation, however, the questions arise for somewhat different reasons. With meditation there are no side effects (with some exceptions, such as practicing Shabd Kriya for several weeks), and frequently, a healthy dose will yield a complete but short-lived relief. The problem of course is that meditation takes time and effort even if the rewards are profound. Perhaps the two most common questions from patients are the following: (1) Do I have to do the whole protocol to get well? and (2) Do I have to do the therapy every day? Of course, in most circumstances, the answer is no and no. What the patient is telling you is that he/she really does not want to do anything that he/she does not have to do (an attempt to titrate work and suffering—rule of thumb number 2). So while the therapist is not negotiating over the recommended daily dose, he can work out a reasonable level for starting out so that the patient does not fail. However, the first responsibility is to set the "hooks of experience" with the patient. The patient must know how effective the techniques are, even if the effects are only temporary.

Perhaps 20% to 30% of patients are highly self-motivated. This can be for at least two reasons. They may have suffered for years or even decades and all their life they have been looking for a cure, and now that they believe they may have found one, they are exceptionally grateful and want to take every opportunity to improve their lives and overcome their suffering and lead a normal and healthy life. Secondly, they may know that the consequences they face if they do not overcome their problems are otherwise horrendous and unacceptable. They may know that they will go to jail if they are an addict and do not overcome their addiction. Or, if they are bipolar and also have a personality disorder, they may realize that unless they really work hard to overcome their instability, they will live at best in a halfway house. For some patients the choice is black and white, but for most, they are again looking for a settlement. Thus, they seek to titrate their miseries to an acceptable level.

When starting out with a patient, it is best to explain his choices and provide him with a range of opportunities so that he feels like he has complete freedom with how he can approach treatment. When I see a client for the first time, I almost always take at least 2 hours to teach him everything he needs to know, set the "hooks of experience," and to explain the options for further treatment. Most have a hunch they will not go home and do the therapy on their own in a reliable way. But at least they know it will give them temporary relief if they do practice it, and this lifts a huge burden off their shoulders. They have hope. They now know they have a solution and if their suffering gets bad enough, they can do something if they have too. But they also know it is now a test of their willpower to keep up. Most patients need to see their therapist once a week or attend a group at least once a week. Patients in residential programs need to practice a protocol at least once a day if not more often. Much depends on the nature and severity of the disorder(s). Lisa's case history in Chapter 8 with OCD, PTSD, eating disorders, psychosis, self-mutilation, and depression is not so rare in terms of the combination of disorders, but it is rare that an individual will comply so well with Kundalini yoga meditation without the in-person guidance of a trained therapist. However, Lisa's father helped her, and he hired others to help her in the simplest way, even though they had no training in therapy. On the other hand, she was partly motivated due to the course of her numerous previous failed attempts with other therapies. In addition, she did obtain relief with meditation, and knew she probably had no other choices in her life.

It is important not to set up a patient to fail. Rare is the patient who will take a protocol home and practice diligently day after day. Scheduling a patient on a weekly basis and telling him that this is his best option in the beginning makes sense and gives him the assurance of care. In addition, it is frequently helpful to start patients off with only parts of the protocol and for very short times. The initial recommended "dose" is best kept within reason and is again based on the circumstances. If an OCD patient thinks that she will have to do the OCDB perfectly in the beginning, she will be left without hope, and if the addict or bipolar patient believes that they will have to be able to do their respective protocols to completion within a few days to achieve recovery, they will give up before they start. Patients must be conditioned by the benefits over time and with a reasonable expectation of how much they can perform. There is obviously a wide variance here for how much experience patients require initially and what their future hurdles entail. This gives some insight into frequency and dose. Patients vary in severity, willpower, and basic health. Protocols vary in difficulty. And patients' home circumstances and what a therapist can provide in terms of options for recovery will vary.

With medication as therapy, we often think about "other techniques to increase adherence." With Kundalini yoga, the very best "technique" to use to increase adherence is the direct benefits of the techniques themselves. Experience of a complete but temporary relief is the best method to increase adherence over time. Kundalini yoga is a system based on experience, not on beliefs. A regular schedule for treatment is the best strategy, whether it is regular individual sessions or regular weekly or daily groups. These groups can be run by the therapist or they can be run by a qualified Kundalini yoga teacher who has experience with that specific protocol and patients with a specific disorder. Clearly, the patients prefer and benefit most by engaging in treatment with a therapist who has the ability and past experience to understand their disorder, their current state of mind, and who can also perform the protocol exactly as they are expected to do it. They want to know that it is really possible to do the protocol. If it is the OCDB, can the therapist also breathe at one breath per minute with the four 15-second intervals for 31 minutes? Is it really possible or is this simply an ancient reported tale? Again, witnessing the therapist perform that technique gives assurance. Does this mean a therapist should not teach the patient the protocol if they cannot do the entire protocol perfectly and for the maximum specified time? The answer is no. However, we are trying to optimize the therapeutic encounter for the patient. Here again, the therapist plays the role of a coach. In addition, the therapist's own experience in learning to perform the protocol gives him insight into the hurdles, difficulties, and challenges that the patient will encounter. He can then better provide an answer to specific questions. The most common answer to questions is simply, "Keep up, keep going." This is believable and realistic, because the therapist has already set the "hooks of experience" and has demonstrated that it can be done, at least that the Kundalini yoga teacher can do it.

Adherence to therapy is primarily set by the talents of the therapist, but also by the environment and what the patient needs to avoid prior to their practice. If the patient comes to therapy just after a big meal, they will feel too lethargic and less capable of performing. This would be similar to any athletic event. Eating prior to performance is always a detriment. Demands for blood are usually set by the requirements of the muscles, the digestive system, and the brain. While a patient does not need to feel relaxed prior to Kundalini yoga therapy, eating or too much physical exercise prior to therapy lead to performance difficulties. Too much caffeine is also a detriment, and in the experience of all Kundalini yoga practitioners and patients over time, eating foods with added processed sugar also leads to problems. This does not imply that low blood sugar is beneficial, in fact it is a handicap. Fruit juice without added sugar can be helpful if the patient is feeling fatigued. Many practitioners and patients also learn that a cold shower, or ending a shower with cold water before practice can lead to renewed energy and calm as well as the will and motivation to practice.

Once therapists have taught the patient in a previous session how to practice the technique or protocol, they may recognize that starting new sessions with a technique or protocol leads to increased clarity for the patient, so that the concerns the patient had when he arrived may have changed, and insights into himself, his practice, and his problems will be more clear and reasonable. A clear and stable mind is a great asset to the patient toward progress. When I do therapy with individual patients, I first ask whether they have any immediate concerns, and frequently the answer is no, then we proceed to practice. We end with a discussion about the results and how they have been progressing, and then discuss other problems that they may face.

The next question is what other forms of therapy can the patient employ while learning and practicing a specific Kundalini yoga protocol. More than 50% of the patients I see are already on at least one medication. It is possible and acceptable and medically feasible to work with medicated patients. There is no a priori reason not to accept a medicated patient. Sometimes patients are of course both benefiting and suffering from their medications. For example, a patient with psychosis may no longer suffer from delusions or hallucinations, but he or she may be experiencing slurred speech, reduced energy, "brain fog," and any number of side effects. Medications can also handicap a patient's practice. However, only licensed physicians should make the decision to reduce or change medications. In my opinion, if a patient shows interest in Kundalini yoga as a treatment modality, in general, she should be encouraged to attempt treatment initially without medication if she is capable of living independently and is not delusional or dangerous to herself or others. Again, many of these issues go beyond the scope of this book. Rare is the patient who does not need some counseling and guidance in addition to Kundalini yoga. Also, for example, with OCD patients, they are more likely to be able to do other forms of therapy more efficiently after practicing the Kundalini yoga OCD protocol. However, most OCD patients find that everyday life provides ample opportunity to engage their fears and that all they really need to do is keep practicing the protocol and resisting as best they can as the day goes on.

One very important point has to be made to some patients. It is very dangerous to practice Kundalini yoga and take marihuana, cocaine, or any other illegal substances at the same time. Also, people who smoke cigarettes will have greater difficulty employing some of these techniques because they have reduced lung capacity, and the excessive toxins will affect brain function.

Group Procedures

The amount of time necessary for each disorder and protocol will vary. The OCD group-therapy sessions for the clinical trials addressed in Appendix Three were scheduled for every Wednesday evening from 6:30 P.M. to 8:30 P.M. We almost never started on time but set a 10-minute grace period and held to it. We also frequently finished a little late because members enjoyed sharing their experiences from the meditations and conversing about other worldly events. They developed a wonderful feeling of comradery. Too much time resting or discussing in between techniques diminishes the overall effects, so we only took a few minutes at most between techniques as required for rest, and we did not encourage discussion during the practice of the protocol. The maximum time required for the OCD protocol, if all of the eight primary techniques are practiced for the full amount of time, is 64 minutes back-to-back without rest. This includes practicing techniques 4 and 5 for 11 minutes each and the OCDB for the full 31 minutes. It took the group in the second clinical trial about 4.5 months to begin doing the OCDB in class for 31 minutes, although this was not at one breath per minute. Patients in the first uncontrolled trial took a little less time. Each protocol and population will vary with the abilities to achieve specific milestones in practice.

The OCD group practiced while sitting in chairs around a big conference table in the second study and in a small circle in the first study. When practicing in a group, the "group effects" are increased by having a circular orientation if possible. This also provides a more personal atmosphere for everyone. There is no requirement to sit on the floor with most protocols. Maintaining a straight spine is much easier while sitting in a chair for the beginning patient. The chairs should not be too soft, where they tend to sink backwards, or too hard leading to discomfort over prolonged sitting times. During the practice of the techniques, patients should avoid resting their backs against the chairs. The lower spine should be pushed forward slightly. This effort helps keep the spine slightly bowed, with the abdomen very slightly extended forward. This posture helps patients remain alert.

When the patients practice, they should be in a quiet and peaceful environment where they are not disturbed. Battery-operated digital timers are helpful for either the therapist or patient so that he is not forced to look at a clock during the practice of the techniques. Any distraction while practicing a technique, like looking to see how much time remains, reduces the benefits. Certain positions for the eyes, when described, are meant to be held constant to achieve the maximum benefit. The patient should always be encouraged to practice each and every technique without stopping or shifting a position. The ability to endure will vary for each patient and technique.

Again, this chapter is only included to help the therapist with some of the most basic questions when he considers employing Kundalini yoga as either a sole therapy or as an adjunct to other therapies. Various issues may arise during treatment, and first hand experience with techniques and experience over time with various patient populations is usually an adequate source of information for answering these questions, along with some common sense. There are too many possible scenarios that can arise given the various disorders covered in this book and various ranges of severity and circumstances that may accompany patients to try and cover them in greater depth here. However, there is no a priori reason not to attempt therapy with any population discussed in this book once the therapist has some working knowledge of these techniques and protocols. The therapist may also find it helpful to set up groups with Kundalini yoga teachers who have some experience with psychiatric patients and a thorough working knowledge of the specific protocols to be employed. A joint effort by a therapist and Kundalini yoga teacher may be the most reasonable approach for some therapists.

TEN

Using "Venus Kriya" Meditation Techniques for Couples Therapy

The term *Venus kriya* refers to an array of unique meditation techniques taught by Yogi Bhajan that are to be practiced together by a man and a woman or any committed couple. The intent with these techniques is to help heal and bring greater depth, dimension, and growth to a committed relationship. These techniques are very useful for helping to awaken the spiritual dimension in a relationship, and they are also very useful for helping to work out the problems of trust, fidelity, and communication. In ancient times, they were used as a form of marital therapy and also as a means to simply enhance a healthy relationship. The word *Venus* refers to the goddess of love, and the Sanskrit word *kriya* translates to a "completed action." This chapter presents a number of techniques that are Venus kriyas as well as two other meditation techniques to be used by couples. These last two are not technically Venus kriyas, although they serve the same purpose. One essential difference between the Venus kriyas and these two techniques is the length of time for practice, as the Venus kriyas are limited to three minutes in duration but the other two are not, and may be practiced for periods up to 31 minutes. The time limit for Venus kriyas is due to their powerful effects, and teachers are taught not to practice more than one an hour. The protocol described here is for their specific use. Also, Venus kriyas *look* similar to the meditation techniques practiced in what is called "White Tantric yoga," but they are not the same. Venus kriyas are powerful techniques and thus are considered sacred and should only be practiced with the intent to elevate and heal a relationship. They were not taught for the purposes of sexually exploiting a partner, or for exploiting the partner in any way. However, this does not mean that they cannot be used as therapeutic tools for enhancing the loving practices of a committed relationship. The purpose for including these techniques in this book is first for their value for enhancing committed relationships and as a therapy for the prevention of marital problems, as well as their potential use in marital therapy for troubled relationships.

Procedures for Using Venus Kriyas

The first step in the Venus kriya protocol is the same as that in any other Kundalini yoga meditation protocol taught in this book, or in any other book or manual on Kundalini yoga as taught by Yogi Bhajan. That step is to use the mantra "Ong Namo Guru Dev Namo" for tuning in (see technique 1 below). However, the only variation here with tuning in is that couples start by facing each other. This is the first mandatory step, and the other is not to go beyond the time limits prescribed, either with a Venus kriya or another meditation for couples. While it is not mandatory, it is highly recommended that the environment be peaceful, pleasant, and serene. Additionally, it is recommended that a couple set the stage by using another Kundalini yoga meditation technique or even a complete Kundalini exercise set prior to the use of a Venus kriya. This will ultimately enhance the practice and benefits of a Venus kriya. The other techniques in this chapter for couples would be ideal for this purpose, or, for example, the technique called Gan Puttee Kriya described in Chapter 8.

1. Technique to Induce a Meditative State: "Tuning In"

Sit with a straight spine and with the feet flat on the floor if sitting in a chair (see Figure 2.1, page 72). Put the hands together at the chest in "prayer pose"—the palms are pressed together with 10 to 15 pounds of pressure between the hands (a mild to medium pressure, nothing too intense). The area where the sides of the thumbs touch rests on the sternum with the thumbs pointing up (along the sternum), and the fingers are together and point up and out at a 60-degree angle to the ground. The eyes are closed and focused on the third eye (imagine a sun rising on the horizon, or the equivalent of the point between the eyebrows at the origin of the nose). A mantra is chanted out loud in a 1½-breath cycle. Inhale first through the nose and chant "Ong Namo" with an equal emphasis on the Ong and the Namo. Then immediately follow with a half-breath inhalation through the mouth and chant "Guru Dev Namo" with approximately equal emphasis on each word. (The O in *Ong* and *Namo* are each a long "o" sound; *Dev* sounds like *Dave*, with a long "a" sound.) The practitioner should focus on the experience of the vibrations these sounds create on the upper palate and throughout the cranium while letting the mind be carried by the sounds into a new and pleasant mental space. This should be repeated a minimum of three times. This technique helps to create a meditative state of mind and is *always* used as a precursor to other Kundalini yoga techniques.

The second requirement before the practice of any Venus kriya is the chanting of the following mantra: "Aad Guray Nameh Jugaad Guray Nameh Sat Guray Nameh Siri Guru Devay Nameh" in a monotone. The same hand and eye postures are used here that are used in technique 1. Again, three times or more are suggested. This mantra helps to provide the experience of a protected meditative space and further clear any negativity from the mind.

At this point, either one of the meditation techniques for couples listed below can be practiced or any other suitable meditation technique. A complete Kundalini yoga exercise set can also be practiced to enhance the couple's overall sense of well-being. It is also acceptable to simply practice one Venus kriya. However, prior to the practice of a Venus kriya, it is suggested that the couple look into each other's eyes and reflect momentarily on the soulful nature of their partner with acceptance and humility for that person's graceful, divine nature.

When a Venus kriya is completed, the partners should each close their eyes (if the technique was practiced with eyes open) and stretch their arms up over their heads, breathing slowly and deeply several times, making every effort to stretch the spine upward as much as possible. Each partner then twists his or her body from side to side while inhaling, twisting to the left and exhaling, then twisting to the right with eyes closed. Bow toward each other, saying thank-you with a most sincere and loving appreciation for each other. Then partners can take turns massaging each other and relaxing, or simply relax together and enjoy the effects.

Venus Kriya 1: "Pushing Palms"

There are two versions of this technique, and the difference is the mantra employed. Partners sit facing each other in a cross-legged position with a straight spine. The right knee touches the left knee of the partner. Sitting in chairs is acceptable, but the knees must still touch. The eyes are open, looking directly into the partner's eyes. The hands are up at shoulder level with the palms facing forward, and the left palm of each partner touches the right palm of the other. Start with the palms at an equal distance between each other (the line just over where the knees meet). Then push the right palms forward, the left palms moving back toward the shoulder. With this movement the woman chants the word "Gobinday." The left palms push forward and the right palms come back toward the shoulder. During this movement the man chants "Mukanday" (sounds like "mookanday"). The next movement is again with the right hands moving forward and left hands moving back, and the woman chants "Udaray" (sounds like "oohdaray").

Again the left hand is then pushed forward while the man chants "Aparay" (the "A" sounds like "ah"). These alternating pushing movements continue as the woman chants "Harying" (sounds like "hareeing") and the man chants "Karying" (sounds like "kareeing"). The woman then chants "Nirnamay" (sounds like "nearnamay") and the man chants "Akamay" (sounds like "aahkamay"). Then the entire mantra is repeated, again with the woman only chanting "Gobinday" and the man only chanting "Mukanday," and so on. Note, the woman chants when the right hands go forward and the man chants when the left hands go forward. Couples do not chant together, but alternate the use of the eight sounds. Only the woman chants "Gobinday, Udaray, Harying, Nirnamay," and only the man chants "Mukanday, Aparay, Karying, and Akamay." The respective meaning of the eight sounds are the following: "sustainer," "liberator," "enlightener," "infinite," "destroyer," "creator," "nameless," "desireless." The rate of chanting and moving the arms in the pushing movement is about one sound per movement per second. The total time limit for practice is 3 minutes. When finished, make sure to follow the procedures described above.

This 8-part mantra is the first version of "Pushing Palms." The second version is as follows. Using the mantra ("Sa Ta Na Ma"), the woman chants "Sa" (the "a" sounds like the "a" sound in "father" throughout the mantra) as the right hands are pushed forward and the man chants "Ta" as the left hands are pushed forward. The woman chants "Na" as the right hands are pushed forward and the man chants "Ma" as the left hands are pushed forward. This 4-part mantra is repeated in the same sequence for a maximum time of three minutes. All other aspects of the practice are the same as the first version with the 8-part mantra. Note also that this is chanting out loud; it is not a silent chant. The sound "Sa" gives the mind the ability to expand to the infinite; the sound "Ta" gives the mind the ability to experience the totality of life; the sound "Na" gives the mind the ability to conquer death; and the sound "Ma" gives the mind the ability to resurrect, and also means "rebirth." In short, the mantra can translate to mean "infinity, life, death, and rebirth." This is a very powerful mantra for cleansing and restructuring the subconscious mind and helping to set a mental framework in the conscious mind to experience higher states of consciousness (Shannahoff-Khalsa & Bhajan, 1988; Shannahoff-Khalsa & Bhajan, 1991). Both mantras help to awaken the individual from his or her finite identity and to live in higher states of consciousness. The first version has been my favorite Venus kriya. There is some virtue to learning and practicing all of the different Venus kriyas, however, a couple can choose just one to practice consistently over time. If couples choose the latter, I recommend this kriya and version one for its general overall benefits.

Venus Kriya 2: "Washing Windows"

Partners face each other and each partner sits on his or her heels with the ankles together underneath and the thighs touching. The knees of each partner touch those of the other. Place the left palm against the right palm of the partner and move the hands independently as if washing windows with each hand. The eyes are open and looking into the partner's eyes. The breath employs the pranayam technique called "breath of fire" or *kapalabhati*—a very rapid and shallow breath through the nose only with a respiration rate of two to three breaths per second. The navel point moves in and out like a bellows pump; the breath is shallow and only abdominal in nature and is not a thoracic movement. The effort is on forcing the breath out through the nose as the navel is contracted quickly and pulled slightly back toward the spine, and the inhalation occurs through a relaxation of the abdominal muscles. It is best if this breath technique is learned prior to attempting this Venus kriya. The upper time limit is 3 minutes.

Venus Kriya 3: "3-Part Kriya"

Sit on the heels facing the partner. Stare into each other's eyes without blinking and radiate love toward each other. See yourself in the other person's eyes and continue for 1 minute. When this minute is up, stand and face each other and join hands and look into each other's eyes again, projecting love. Then squat down together into "crow pose" (keep the feet flat on the floor and squat down as far as possible, bringing the buttocks as close to the floor as possible), keeping the spine straight and head forward, still looking into the eyes of the partner. Then again stand up, keeping the feet flat and holding hands. Keep the eyes open and looking into the eyes of the partner the entire time. Inhale while raising up, hold the breath in while standing erect, then exhale and squat. When down, hold the breath out. Then inhale up and so on, repeating the entire breath and movement cycle five times. When finished, sit on your heels once more facing your partner. While keeping the eyes open and looking into each other's eyes, inhale, hold in, exhale, and hold out five more times. All of the breathing is done in synchrony with the partner. When finished, relax.

Venus Kriya 4: "Venus Rock Pose"

Sit on the heels in rock pose (heels under buttocks, knees together, the top of the feet flat on the floor; you do not support yourself with the toes). This time the knees do not touch the partner's knees. The hands are resting on your own thighs just above the knees. Look into each other's eyes without blinking and project love and divine light. Continue with normal breathing while applying *mulbhand* (pulling up on the rectum and sex organs and in toward the navel point) for 90 seconds. Then do breath of fire (*kapalabhati*) for 90 seconds. When finished, apply *mahabhand*, or the "great lock" (pulling in on the chin slightly toward the spine to straighten the cervical vertebrae and pulling up on the diaphragm and the abdominal muscles) and *mulbhand* (pulling up and in toward the navel). After the exhale, apply *mahabhand* two more times and then relax.

Venus Kriya 5: "Touching Finger Tips"

It is said that this kriya will also help to improve the eyesight. You can feel the life force flow between partners through the finger tips. Sit on the heels in rock pose facing each other. Partners knees touch in this kriya. The hands face forward and the finger tips touch the respective fingers of the partner. The eyes are open, projecting divine love. Consciously experience the flow of energy through the finger tips while projecting love. Hold the position for 3 minutes, then inhale, hold 10 seconds, and exhale. Again inhale, hold 10 seconds, exhale, then relax.

Venus Kriya 6: "To Get Rid of Grudges"

Sit back to back with your partner and bring your knees up against your chest with your arms wrapped around the knees. Meditate on your heart and hear the sounds of your heart while simultaneously meditating on the sun, bringing the light and warmth of the sun into your heart to burn out all bitterness you have felt throughout the years. Continue for 3 minutes.

Venus Kriya 7: "Heart Lotus"

Sit in an easy cross-legged posture facing your partner. Form your hands into a lotus: all the fingers and thumbs point upward and are separated while the ridge along the little fingers to the base of the hands and along the sides of the thumbs touch, the elbows resting down toward the sides. The man puts his little fingers under the woman's little fingers, and these are the only fingers of the partners that touch, making a heart lotus. Look into the soul and heart of the partner through the eyes. Continue for 90 seconds. Then place one hand over the other at your own heart center and close your eyes. Meditate on your own heart, going deep within to the center of your own being for 90 seconds. When the time is up, inhale deeply and exhale deeply three times, then relax.

Venus Kriya 8: "Easy 60-Degree Lean"

Sit on the floor with the legs stretched out in front of you and lean back at 60 degrees using the arms (elbows locked) to support you.

The soles of the feet touch those of the partner, and the eyes are open and focusing into each other's eyes. Do breath of fire (*kapalabhati*) for 3 minutes. Then inhale and exhale three times and relax.

Venus Kriya 9: "Legs Stretched Out/Breath of Fire"

Sit on the floor with the legs stretched out in front of you and grasp the respective hands of the partner, with the right hand holding the left hand. The soles of the feet touch those of the partner, and the eyes are open and focusing into each other's eyes. Do breath of fire (*kapalabhati*) for 3 minutes. Then inhale and exhale three times and relax.

Venus Kriya 10: "Seeing Yourself in Your Partner"

Sit in rock pose with the heels under the buttocks and the tops of the feet flat on the ground. The knees touch the partner's, and your hands are in your own laps in Venus lock: the fingers are interlaced, and the male has the right thumb dominating over the left thumb, which dominates over the right index finger, which dominates over the left index finger, and so on until the left little finger is on the bottom; the woman's fingers are reversed, with the left thumb dominating over the right thumb, and so on until the right little finger is on the bottom. The eyes are open and looking into the partner's eyes. Concentrate on seeing yourself in your partner. Project love and continue for 3 minutes, then relax.

Venus Kriya 11: "Venus Back Roles"

Sit in an easy cross-legged posture, back to back, with the backs touching. The hands are interlaced and placed in the lap. Partners breathe in synchrony while one partner bends forward and brings the head toward the ground. The other partner leans back against the back of the partner who is leaning forward. Then the partner leaning forward inhales and sits up, leaning against the other partner as that partner then straightens up and leans forward, bringing the head toward the ground. The backs remain touching as if the vertebrae are locked. The partner leaning forward exhales and so does the one leaning backward. Then they both inhale to sit up and exhale in synchrony. The time for this is 3 minutes, followed by relaxation.

Venus Kriya 12: "Double Back Bend"

Sit on the heels in rock pose with the knees of the partners touching. Clasp the hands of the partner, both partners leaning backward as far as possible, hands hang backwards and the eyes are closed. The breathing technique is optional: (1) no breath control, (2) slow, deep abdominal breathing, and (3) breath of fire (*kapalabhati*). Continue for 3 minutes and relax.

Meditations for Couples (Non-Venus Kriya Meditations)

1. Long "Ek Ong Kar"

Version 1. Sit in an easy cross-legged posture facing each other with the knees of the partners touching. The hands are in "bear grip" (open fists with fingers together and hooked onto the hands of the partner). Both partners have the left palm facing up and right palm facing down. The eyes start out open, looking into the eyes of the partner. Chant out loud the mantra "Ek Ong Kar Sat Nam Siri Whahay Guru" in the following manner, with neck locked (pull the chin in slightly toward the chest to straighten the cervical vertebrae) (Shannahoff-Khalsa & Bhajan, 1991): First, inhale deeply through the nose and chant "Ek" with a sharp cracking sound, pulling in at the navel region. It is very short. Continue to use the same breath to vibrate "Ong" (accentuating the nasalized "ng" as the sound stretches out) for equal time with "Kar" (accentuating the rolled "rrrr" as the sound stretches out). Be sure to chant powerfully and vibrate "Ong" at the back of the neck. Then again, inhale deeply and fully through the nose only and chant "Sat," but very short (like "Ek"), and feel the cracking sound while pulling in at the navel point. Using almost all of the same breath, chant a long "Nam," with an emphasis on "m" over time. Before completely running out of breath, finish with "Siri" (pronounced "Sree," not "Sri," "Shri," or "Seri"). Then again inhale, but only a half breath through the mouth, and chant "Wha" (like the sound "wa" in *water*), "Hay" (long "a"), "Guru" (pronounced "Gurruuu," rolling the *r* and accentuating the "ru" after "Gu") but not extending it too far. Continue this chanting in synchrony with each other for 11 minutes. When finished, close the eyes and maintain the image of your partner at the third eye region, the point where the eyebrows meet.

Version 2. Sit back to back with the hands in ghyan mudra (the thumb tip and index finger tip touch on each hand with the palms facing up, the backs of the hands relaxed on the knees). Again the first part is for 11 minutes but the eyes are closed. The second part remains the same, visualizing the partner at the third eye region. This mantra is very powerful and it is said to work on all eight chakras to help heal and repair and open them correctly and to help lead to a state of enlightenment and liberation (Shannahoff-Khalsa & Bhajan, 1991).

2. Kirtan Kriya to Clear the Clouds

Sit in an easy pose back to back with the partner. The backs of the hands rest against the tops of the knees. The eyes are closed and focused on the third eye point (the point where the eyebrows meet and where the nose originates in the forehead). The mantra to be used is called "Panch Shabd," and is "Sa Ta Na Ma" (Shannahoff-Khalsa & Bhajan, 1988). It is composed of the five primal sounds that are proportional in their combined vibration to the totality of creation. "Sa" means infinity, "Ta" means life, "Na" means death, and "Ma" means resurrection. The fifth sound is the "ah" sound common to all four. "Ah" is the creative sound of the universe.

As you chant, the thumb tips touch each fingertip in rhythm with the mantra (applying two to three pounds of pressure each time) in order to channel the energy through the nerve endings in the fingers that are connected to the brain centers relating to intuition, patience, vitality, and communication, respectively (Shannahoff-Khalsa & Bhajan, 1988). On the sound of "Sa," touch the thumb tip to the first finger tip (index); with "Ta," the thumb tip touches the second finger tip (middle); with "Na," the third finger tip (ring finger); and with "Ma," the fourth finger tip (little finger). Each round of the mantra takes 3 to 4 seconds. Chant the mantra in three ways: out loud, in the voice of the human being; whispering, in the voice of the lover; and in the silence of your own consciousness, the voice of God (as described below). From the depth of your silent meditation, come back to the whisper and then to the full voice. Throughout the meditation, each syllable of the mantra should be projected mentally like a light from the top of the head, down to the center of the head, and then straight out the third eye. Chant the mantra out loud for 5 minutes, whisper for 5 minutes, and then silently meditate on it in this way for 10 minutes. Then again chant in a whisper for 5 minutes and then 5 minutes out loud. The finger tapping is maintained through all stages. Now inhale, holding the breath and stretch the arms up over the head, shaking the fingers wildly. Hold the position and exhale. Inhale again, shake the fingers, and exhale for three consecutive breaths. Make sure to keep the proportion of 5 minutes out loud, 5 minutes loud whisper, 10 minutes silent, 5 minutes loud whisper, and 5 minutes out loud when doing this technique. Never vary the ratio and always complete the exercise with stretching the arms up and shaking the fingers for one minute. Using this technique, you can experience your own infinity and balance the total energy of your nervous system (Shannahoff-Khalsa & Bhajan, 1988). When finished, completely relax. Now, proceed with a Venus Kriya.

A New Dimension for Psychiatry: Kundalini Yoga Meditation as a Novel Approach for Prevention and Treatment

When we consider the current high incidence rates reported in earlier chapters for the variants of anxiety, depression, addictions and impulsivity, sleep disorders, ADHD and co-morbidities, and the effects of battering and abuse, along with the other prevalent psychiatric disorders that are not addressed in this book, we are duly reminded that if prevention is possible, clearly it would be the wiser, more important, and more cost-effective mental health-care strategy. However, let's not neglect the marker of youth and violence as a definitive sign of a need for change.

The Commission for the Prevention of Youth Violence states that the U.S. has the highest youth homicide and suicide rates of the 26 wealthiest nations, and this report concluded that "youth violence is an epidemic, comparable to the impact of war" (Benoit, Bagley, et al., 2000). Among the many "cold facts" listed in the commission's report, the following selected facts give insight into the scope of this U.S. epidemic. In 1933, 75% of deaths among youth aged 15 to 19 were from natural causes; in 1993, 80% were the result of homicide and unintentional injury (Mann, Borowsky, Stolz, Latts, Cart, et al., 1998). Among youth aged 10 to 14, homicide and suicide are the third and fourth leading causes of death, respectively; and for those 15 to 19 years of age, they are second and third (Cohen & Potter, 1999; Spivak, Christoffel, Gray, Hayes, Jenkins, et al., 1999). About 1 in 8 people murdered each year are under the age of 18 (Rennison, 2000). Almost 16 million adolescents, including 70% to 95% of children in our inner cities, have witnessed some form of violent assault, including robbery, stabbing, shooting, murder, or domestic abuse (Mann et al., 1998; Ayne, Pynoos, & Cardenos, 2001). And tragically, 8% to 10% of high school students carry guns to school every day (Ayne et al., 2001). The final sentence in the commission's executive report stated "More school suspensions and more prisons are not the answer. The answer, rooted in public health, is prevention" (Benoit, Bagley, Spivak, Addington, Hill, et al., 2000).

To add further clarity and dimension to the U.S. health care crisis, the 2003 presidential address to the American Association for the Advancement of Science stated: "A growing problem of major proportions has been staring us in the face for many decades. Until solved, this long-neglected problem presents a gigantic obstacle to the application of the discoveries flowing from biomedical research into deliverable standards of medical practice that could benefit all of society, both in the United States and globally. This problem is the imminent collapse of the American health system. Unless steps are taken soon to undertake a comprehensive restoration of our system, the profound advances in biomedical research so rapidly accruing today may never be effectively transformed into meaningful advances in health care for society" (Bloom, 2003). In that same speech we are told, "Scientists must now unite to insist that the system be prepared for the discoveries of the future and that we fulfill as quickly as possible the major needs of today's global health problems" (Bloom, 2003). In addition, Bloom presented an overarching analysis and argued that a consensus for change for the health care system at large "must consider restoring the incentive to be a physician or nurse; restoring medical care and treatment affordable by the consumer, the provider, and the payer; standardizing the best practices for diagnosis, treatment, and outcome assessment so that systems of care provision can be compared; reducing the occurrence of practice errors by implementation of a modern system of communication; accelerating the recovery from the diverse published literature of information on clinical issues and their interactions; and implementing preventive medicine with a renewed emphasis on public good health in which the consumers of health services accept responsibility for their own health maintenance" (2003). He further argued that "we must create a translational health system in which research discoveries flow to clinical trials to best-practice standards" and that "we must restore a system that can welcome the new insights and exploit them" (2003). Again we hear the necessity for prevention and accepting responsibility for one's own health and affordable treatment.

To further understand the extent of the mental health-care crisis, we have only to look at how many people in the U.S. and worldwide are currently not utilizing health services. According to the World Health Organization, worldwide the median treatment gaps are as follows, "schizophrenia and other non-affective psychosis, 32.2%; depression, 56.3%; dysthymia, 56.0%; bipolar disorder, 50.2%; panic disorder, 55.9%; GAD, 57.5%; OCD, 57.3%; and alcohol abuse and dependence has the widest treatment gap, 78.1%" (Kohn, Saxena, Levav, & Saraceno, 2004). The figures for the U.S., respectively, are 35.7%, 46.1%, 57.9%, 39.1%, 41.2%, (GAD not reported), 54.9%, and 78.0% (Kohn et al., 2004). The report concluded "The treatment gap for mental disorders is universally large, though variable across countries" (Kohn et al., 2004). These authors further claim that this reported gap is underestimated due to the unavailability of community-based data from developing countries. However, these figures indicate that the U.S. fairs no better than the world at large.

One intention of this book is to argue that not only do we need new advances in psychiatry for treatment and prevention, but that Kundalini yoga meditation techniques provide a novel, powerful, and unique opportunity, and potentially a whole new dimension for psychiatry. In ancient times, when Kundalini yoga was a common practice for the householder, people went to their physician to avoid sickness. If they got sick, frequently they would find a new physician. Times have changed. Today, if we can afford it, we go to a specialist to be treated for a disease, and sometimes the fortunate go to their family practice physician for routine exams to screen for disease. And if necessary, patients are given the advice to quit smoking, reduce alcohol, increase aerobic exercise, eat a healthy diet, and reduce weight. Today this sound advice is considered to be "prevention." However, it is clearly inadequate.

The bottleneck that restricts personal change is based on one's own mental patterns, opportunities, and level of awareness. While we are habit forming creatures by nature, the habits that we tend to develop are very difficult to change, and all too often not favorable toward health. In addition, whether we call it ignorance or short-sightedness, we are frequently ruled by our emotions, desires, and misconceived notions of reality—rather than a clear, objective, and realistic view of the world—and the impact of our actions. This is one way that Kundalini yoga can be a useful and important adjunct toward change and growth. Yogis discovered numerous techniques for altering and restructuring mental patterns and elevating one's awareness. Every technique in this book is an example for how mental patterns can be affected, and frequently, when necessary, by the use of a disorder-specific technique. The obvious implication here is that thousands of years ago, society was far more mentally and spiritually advanced than society today. When Yogi Bhajan first started teaching Kundalini yoga in the West, he called meditation a "huge technology of the mind." What he taught openly had been kept secret for thousands of years, and for the most part, many today who believe they have a working knowledge of yoga, unfortunately misconceive of it as only an ancient system of postures with but a handful of meditation techniques. This has been part of the problem in communicating the real content of this ancient science, which includes about 5,000 different meditation techniques. People simply have no awareness of the vastness of this system. Even science fiction writers have never conjured up a science so vast. Today, now that this work and knowledge is coming more to the forefront of medical science, many may challenge its credibility, and understandably so. In my view, it will be hundreds of years before we understand the brain mechanisms activated by these advanced techniques, but only a few decades before a large number of techniques and protocols are tested for their purported efficacy, and thus help carry us into a better, brighter, and healthier future.

One vital point has to be made abundantly clear. The experience of these techniques can easily lead to a clear and stable state of mind, and one that borders on a state of bliss and ecstasy. The power and impact of these techniques are not only useful for treating psychiatric disorders and quickly helping to ameliorate the most acute and intense suffering, but they can also play a vital role in providing an alternative to drugs and alcohol for our youth. Perhaps there is no greater deterrent to the inebriated states of mind produced by drugs and alcohol, than the natural "high" and expanded bliss-like state that can easily be experienced using Kundalini yoga. Indeed, in the late sixties and early seventies, and still today, many youthful and older individuals have found the effects of Kundalini yoga to be a wonderful and positive experience that quickly leads to a new path of wellness, delight, inner peace, clarity, optimism, with a healthier sense of direction and purpose.

In addition, there are many potential uses that need to be investigated that can help turn our health care crisis around and lead to a more hopeful, healthy, creative, productive, and peaceful future. Kundalini yoga meditation techniques can be employed to enhance education at all levels, rehabilitation and maintenance in prisons, enhanced creativity, performance, and productivity with reduced stress throughout all aspects of the economy, and even enhance skills and readiness within the military. A "technology of the mind" can help to alter our future, bringing us security, peace, and unlimited opportunities for renewal.

PART FOUR

APPENDICES

APPENDIX ONE

Kundalini Yoga Meditation Techniques and Protocols

Chapter 2
Treating the Anxiety Disorders

The 11-Part Kundalini Yoga Meditation Protocol
for Treating OCD

1. Technique to Induce a Meditative State: "Tuning In" (p. 72)
2. Spine-Flexing Technique for Vitality (p. 72)
3. Shoulder-Shrug Technique for Vitality (p. 73)
4. Technique for Reducing Anxiety, Stress, and Mental Tension (for the treatment of insanity; p. 73)
5. Technique for Reducing Anxiety, Stress, and Mental Tension (for rejuvenating the heart center and alleviating emotional stress; p. 74)
6. Technique for Reducing Anxiety, Stress, and Mental Tension (1–2 minute meditation for emotional stress; p. 75)
7. Technique for Managing Fears (3-minute meditation; p. 76)
8. Technique for Treating Obsessive Compulsive Disorders (p. 77)
9. Technique for Meeting Mental Challenges: The "Vic-tor-y Breath" (p. 78)

Chapter 4
Treating the Addictive, Impulse Control, and Eating Disorders

A 7-Part Meditation Protocol Specific for the Treatment of Addictive, Impulse Control, and Eating Disorders

Chapter 7
Treating Attention Deficit Hyperactivity and Co-morbid Disorders

11-Part Kundalini Yoga Protocol for Attention Deficit Hyperactivity Disorder and Co-morbid Disorders

1. Technique to Induce a Meditative State: "Tuning In" (p. 204)
2. Spine-Flexing Technique for Vitality (p. 205)
3. Spine Twists for Reducing Tension (p. 206)
4. Ganesha Meditation for Focus and Clarity (3-minute meditation to help understand, focus, and create a clear consciousness; p. 206)
5. Meditation for Learning Disabilities, ADD, and ADHD (p. 207)
6. Meditation to Balance and Synchronize the Cerebral Hemispheres (p. 208)
7. Meditation to Balance the Jupiter and Saturn Energies: A Technique to Help Reduce Depression and Self-Destructive Behavior (p. 209)
8. Brain Exercise for Normalizing Frontal Lobes and Enhancing Focus, Clarity, and the Ability to Communicate (Listen and Articulate; p. 210)
9. Technique for Tranquilizing an Angry Mind (p. 211)
10. Brain Exercise for Patience and Temperament (p. 211)
11. Meditation for Releasing Childhood Anger (p. 212)

Chapter 8
Treating the Abused and Battered Psyche

10 Kundalini Yoga Meditation Techniques for the Abused and Battered Psyche

1. Technique to Induce a Meditative State: "Tuning In" (p. 226)

2. Meditation for Self-Worth and Achievement for the Very Young (p. 227)
3. Meditation for Abused and Battered Children for Developing a Balanced Psyche: The Jupiter Finger Chakra Meditation (p. 227)
4. A Sitting Posture to Help Reduce Aggressive Tendencies to Be Used for "Time-Outs" (p. 229)
5. Meditation for the Abused and Battered Psyche: A Technique for Children, Adolescents, and Adults (p. 229)
6. Meditation for the Abused and Battered Psyche: Advanced Technique for Adolescents and Adults (p. 230)
7. Meditation Technique for Dyslexia (an abuse-related learning disorder; p. 231)
8. Meditation for Eliminating Deep, Long-Lasting Inner Anger (p. 233)
9. Meditation for Impulsive Behavior in Youth and Others (p. 235)
10. Meditation for Treating Grief: Especially Useful for PTSD Patients (p. 235)
11. Gan Puttee Kriya (a technique to help treat psychic scarring and ASD; p. 238)

8-Part Meditation Protocol for Posttraumatic Stress Disorder

1. Technique to Induce a Meditative State: "Tuning In" (p. 238)
2. Gan Puttee Kriya (p. 239)
3. When You Do Not Know What to Do (to help eliminate anxiety from the most restless mind; p. 240)
4. Meditation to Balance the Jupiter and Saturn Energies: A Technique Useful for Treating Depression, Focusing the Mind, and Eliminating Self-Destructive Behavior (p. 241)
5. Ganesha Meditation for Focus and Clarity (3-minute meditation to help understand, focus, and create a clear consciousness; p. 242)
6. Meditation for Deep Relaxation (Q-tongue technique; p. 243)

7. A Tantric Meditation Technique to Create a Normal and Supernormal State of Consciousness (p. 244)
8. Meditation to Be Done When You Want to Command Your Own Consciousness to a Higher Consciousness (p. 245)

Chapter 10

Using Venus Kriya Meditation Techniques for Couples Therapy

Meditations for Couples (Non-Venus Kriya Meditations)

Further Studies on UFNB

n 1989, one study of UFNB on cognitive performance showed a mixed pattern of hemispheric activation with males appearing to have an ipsilateral increase in performance, but "unilateral breathing influences female performance contralaterally, but only on the spatial task" (Block, Arnott, Quigley, & Lynch, 1989). These results were obtained after only 5 minutes of UFNB. In contrast to the results of past studies, they state, "These differences within and between sexes may exist because unilateral nostril breathing differently activates the two hemispheres and thereby facilitates performance, or because attempts of the brain to control the NC unilaterally interfere with performance." However, in 1994, an attempt to replicate the Block et al. study (1989) exactly as conducted found no nostril-to-condition related performance for either males or females with a 5-minute exercise period using identical psychological tasks (Sanders, Lattimore, Smith, & Dierker, 1994). The Klein et al. study (1986) found similar nostril dominance and hemisphere (contralateral) relations between the two sexes during rest. It is not likely that ANS circuitry differs between sexes. In addition, another study found that UFNB through the dominant nostril also led to greater cognitive performance in the contralateral hemisphere (Schiff & Rump, 1995).

However, this study did not investigate the UFNB effects in the nondominant congested nostril. In sum, it may be concluded that the results of these studies are in part dependent on the true lateralized nature of the cognitive tests employed, the breathing times and efforts, and keeping the nostril blocked during the final testing period.

An EEG study (Velikonja, Weiss, & Corning, 1993) also failed to find a nostril-hemisphere effect. However, that study only captured four 1-minute samples of EEG by having subjects lie in the lateral recumbent position while occluding the contralateral nostril. They only analyzed high alpha (10 Hz to 12 Hz) and low beta (12 Hz to 18 Hz) EEG frequency bands. This study also differs from that of Werntz et al. (1987) in that it did not analyze a continuous measure of EEG activity over all the entire recording period. One-minute samples of data, compared to a continuous recording of relative left/right power, can easily lead to missampling due to the Mayer Wave (0.1 Hz to 0.008 Hz) activity that produces substantial intermittent increases in power. Longer, continuous, and filtered recordings are less affected by this normal autonomic event when relative hemispheric powers are compared.

In 1991, another study (Stancak, Honig, Wackermann, Lepicovska, & Dostalek, 1991) compared UFNB to bilateral breathing and reported that the peak power of beta 2 activity in the frontal leads was lower during UFNB than in bilateral breathing. They also report that they found a homolateral relationship between nostril activity and EEG theta activity, but attribute this result to "increased upper airway resistance and to lateralized modulation of the subcortical generators of EEG theta rhythm during unilateral nostril breathing."

In 1997, a study on memory attempted to detect the hemisphere-specific effects of UFNB; however, the testing was done on a day after 10 successive days of the intervention (Naveen, Nagarathna Nagendua, & Telles, 1997). They compared right UFNB, left UFNB, alternate-nostril breathing, breath awareness, and a control group with no breathing practices. All four breathing groups showed only increases in spatial skills, where an "average increase in spatial memory scores for the trained groups was 84%." Again, hemisphere-related cognitive testing was not done during a breathing exercise, but only one day later after 10 days of practice.

When considering the peripheral effects of UFNB, perhaps the earliest Western scientific study to demonstrate a normal half-sided reaction in autonomic function was that of the relationship of the nose and lung (Sercer, 1930; Samzelius-Lejdstrom, 1939; Stoksted, 1960; Drettner, 1970). There is a unilateral nasal-pulmonary reflex mechanism that is clearly elicited when there is a forced inhalation through one nostril producing a significant increase in inflation of the homolateral lung. In 1939, Samzelius-Lejdstrom studied 182 individuals and showed that the movements of one thoracal half were much more inflated compared to the contralateral lung in 94% of the subjects. She also observed that "variations in width of one-half of the nasal cavity caused variations in the amplitude of the movements of the homolateral thoracal half." While it is not clear if she was aware of the nasal cycle, she observed how differences in nasal congestion could affect the lung. Her work did not pursue possible effects of continuous UFNB. However, she did report that in cases of tuberculosis where there is primarily a lateralized deficit, there is a simultaneous pathological phenomenon of the homolateral nasal and thoracal halves (Samzelius-Lejdstrom, 1939). The enhanced ipsilateral inflation of the lung is explained by noting that sympathetic activity in the lung increases blood flow through vasodilation of the vessels, and in most organs, including the brain, and other tissues, sympathetic activation leads to vasoconstriction. One group studied rabbits under experimental conditions and showed that if coal dust was inhaled through one nasal opening, it was deposited in much larger quantities in the homolateral lung (Wotzilka & Schramek, 1930). These studies all indicate that lateralized ultradian rhythms of alternating lung inflation are likely to parallel the NC since a neural reflex exists between the nose and lung. However, this does not discount the possibility of a CNS-mediated rhythm of alternating lung dominance through sympathetic fibers directly innervating the lungs.

Backon and colleagues (Backon, 1988; Backon & Kullok, 1989; Backon, Matamoros, & Ticho, 1989) have demonstrated the effects of UFNB on several unique autonomic dependent phenomena. As proposed earlier (Werntz et al., 1983, 1987), right-nostril dominance correlates with the "activity phase" of the BRAC, the time during which sympathetic activity in general exceeds parasympathetic activity throughout the body. Backon (1988) showed how right UFNB significantly increases blood glucose levels and how left UFNB lowers it, thus supporting this thesis. Backon and Kullock (1989) also showed how UFNB can differentially affect involuntary eye-blink rates. They found that right UFNB reduced blink rates and that left UFNB increased involuntary blink rates. Backon et al. (1989) also showed how intraocular pressure can be selectively altered by UFNB patterns. Their paper cited references that suggest that vagal tone is increased in glaucoma simplex, reflecting high intraocular pressure. They found that right UFNB leads to an average and significant decrease of 23% in intraocular pressure and that left UFNB increases intraocular pressure by an average but insignificant value of 4.5%. The mean value changes here are the mean of both left and right eye-pressure changes across subjects. This is further evidence that right UFNB increases the generalized sympathetic tone of the body, thus correlating with the "active phase" of the BRAC. Another study also found that right UFNB reduced intraocular pressure, and again left UFNB failed to increase it significantly, when using the average of both eyes to calculate changes (Mohan, Reddy, & Wei, 2001). A more recent study also showed how right UFNB significantly decreased intraocular pressure and again the effect of left UFNB was insignificant (Chen, Brown, & Schmid, 2004). They showed that with right UFNB the intraocular pressure for the right eye dropped by a significant value of 9.6% and the left eye pressure dropped by a significant 6.7%, and that left UFNB resulted in a trend toward higher pressure with a mean increase of 5.7% and 2.5% in the right and left eye respectively (Chen et al., 2004). However, another study showed that both right and left UFNB in men significantly reduces intraocular pressure in both eyes, and in women right UFNB did not affect pressure in either eye, and left UFNB had no effect on the pressure of the right eye, but did significantly decrease pressure of the left eye (Kocer, Dane, Demirel, Demirel, & Kohn, 2002). This study seems to conflict with the findings of the other three trials that all showed similar results (Backon, Matamoros, et al., 1989; Mohan et al., 2001; Chen et al., 2004).

The sympathetic and parasympathetic branches of the ANS each have separate trunks on the two sides of the body (Saper et al., 1976) and thus affect bilateral structures and organs differentially where one side or organ is dominant and the other resting, in a relative sense (Shannahoff-Khalsa, 1991a). An early review showed how some bilateral structures (e.g., kidneys) are regulated with resting and active patterns (Beickert, 1951). A more recent study showed how ultradian rhythms can exhibit in the blood flow patterns of the adrenals with either the left or right gland dominating (Benton & Yates, 1990). However, this differential ANS pattern of organ innervation can also have interesting effects on organs that are not represented as bilateral structures, for example with the heart. Levy and Martin (1979) reviewed studies on the neural innervation and control of the heart and discussed lateral differences. There is considerable right-left asymmetry in the distribution of the sympathetic fibers to the heart (Levy, Ng, & Zieske, 1966; Furnival, Linden, & Snow, 1973). In studies of the dog, Levy et al. (1966) found that stimulation of the right stellate ganglion can increase heart rate (HR) by 85 beats per minute while the effects of left-sided stimulation produce a much smaller increase, and that right-sided stimulation can increase left ventricular systolic pressure (LVSP) by 50 mm Hg, while left-sided stimulation increases LVSP $>>$ 50 mm Hg. They concluded that right-sided stellate ganglion stimulation has greater chronotropic effects, while the left produces greater inotropic effects; right stellate ganglion stimulation decreases systolic duration and left-sided increases mean arterial pressure. Thus the right sympathetic trunk via the right stellate ganglion has relatively greater effect on HR, while the left sympathetic trunk has relatively greater effect on left ventricular function. There are also right and left vagal differences; the right vagus has a greater cardiac deceleratory effect compared to the left vagus (Hondeghem, Mouton, Stassen, & De Geest, 1975), and right vagal transection causes a greater cardiac acceleration than left transection, suggesting the right vagus exerts greater restraint on the sino-atrial node than the left vagus (Hamlin & Smith, 1968). And the heart period is more prolonged when a stimulus is given to the right vagus compared to the left (Hondeghem et al., 1975).

In addition to the following results below looking at the effects of UFNB on the heart, the left versus right differences in sympathetic and vagal innervation have been exploited through the use of unilateral vagal nerve stimulation (VNS) via implanted pacemakers as a modality for treating epilepsy (V.N.S.S. Group, 1999), depression (George, Sackeim, Marangell, Husain, Nahas, et al., 2000; Rush, George, Sackein, Maranscll, Husain, et al., 2000), and obsessive compulsive disorder (Husted & Shapira, 2004). "It is concluded that although the precise mechanism of action of VNS is still unknown, the search for the mechanism has the potential to lend new insight into the neuropathology of depression" (Groves & Brown, 2005). Therefore, one might conclude that the effects of VNS may also be mediated through a mechanism similar to that of UFNB. In fact, yogis refer to the vagus as the "mind nerve" (Bhajan, personal communication). One can only conclude that selective unilateral autonomic activation would have importance for the treatment of a variety of psychiatric disorders, and perhaps other health conditions.

Yogis knew that UFNB had differential effects on HR. And HR has an ultradian periodicity in the 1–4 hour range (Orr & Hoffman, 1974; Livnat, Zehr, & Buoten, 1984), and ultradian rhythms of blood pressure are coupled to HR (Livnat et al., 1984). Some researchers conclude that the sympathetic nervous system drives the ultradian rhythms of the heart (Shimada & Marsh, 1979). In addition, now it has been shown that the ultradian rhythms of HR and blood pressure are coupled to the nasal cycle and markers of other major bodily systems (Shannahoff-Khalsa et al., 1996, 1997; Shannahoff-Khalsa & Yates, 2000). Shannahoff-Khalsa and Kennedy (1993) suggested that the ultradian rhythms of HR are also governed by the alternating rhythmic influences of the right and left branches of the ANS with increased HR resulting from right sympathetic and left parasympathetic dominance.

Shannahoff-Khalsa and Kennedy (1993) conducted three experiments that employed impedance cardiography to monitor the beat-to-beat effects on the heart using UFNB in resting subjects. Two experiments employed a respiratory rate of 6 breaths per minute and one experiment employed a rapid rate (2–3 breaths/second) with shallow respiration using a yogic technique called "breath of fire" or *kapalabhatti*. These studies showed that right UFNB increases HR compared to left UFNB, which lowers HR (at a rate of 6 breaths per minute). They also showed that stroke volume is higher with left UFNB and that left UFNB increases end diastolic volume (Shannahoff-Khalsa & Kennedy, 1993). Another study with 58 resting subjects showed that left UFNB significantly reduced HR in the subjects that were initially right-nostril dominant, but failed to in those who were initially left-nostril dominant, and also failed to show any effects of right UFNB in subjects who were either left- or right-nostril dominant initially (Mohan & Wei, 2002). In yet another study, but measured only after running to achieve a HR within about 30% maximum, instead of resting, left and right UFNB increased HR and SBP (but not DBP) in men, but in women they found that right UFNB increased and left UFNB decreased SBP and DBP (Dane, Caliskan, Kavasen, & Oztasan, 2002).

In addition, right UFNB, left UFNB, and alternate nostril breathing have been compared for their effects on metabolism measured by oxygen consumption (Telles, Nagarathna, & Nagendra, 1994). These researchers studied the effects of having

"27 respiratory cycles, repeated 4 times a day for one month" and found that right UFNB produced a 37% increase in baseline oxygen consumption, and that left UFNB produced a 24% increase and alternate nostril breathing increased baseline values by 18%. They also found that the left UFNB group showed an increase in volar galvanic skin resistance, interpreted as a reduction in sympathetic activity supplying the sweat glands. In another study they found that a one-time 45-minute practice of right UFNB increased oxygen consumption by 17%, increased systolic blood pressure by 9.4 mm Hg, and decreased digital pulse volume by 45.7% (Telles, Nagarathna, & Nagendra 1996). They did not compare against left UFNB in this study, only against normal breathing. These results and the relevant understanding of the ANS innervation of the heart perhaps help to explain the findings of an open clinical trial using alternate nostril breathing as an effective therapy for the treatment of angina pectoris (Friedell, 1948).

Kundalini Yoga Meditation for OCD: Two Successful Clinical Trials

Two published peer-reviewed scientific studies have demonstrated how Kundalini yoga meditation techniques can be used to treat what has long been recognized as the most recalcitrant, difficult-to-treat psychiatric disorder. The first was a 12-month pilot study that was designed to test an 11-part Kundalini yoga meditation protocol that had not yet been put to trial and which included a yogic breathing technique claimed to be specific to treating OCD. All of the eight patients who entered the trial had not achieved adequate success with conventional therapy (Shannahoff-Khalsa & Beckett, 1996). The second trial was a randomized controlled trial (RCT) comparing the same Kundalini yoga meditation protocol against another meditation protocol as the control group to test whether the expectation of doing "meditation" and the time and attention in a group could account for the results (Shannahoff-Khalsa, Ray, Levine, Gallen, Schwartz, et al., 1999). Patients in both studies met once a week on Wednesday evenings for two hours from 6:30 P.M. to 8:30 P.M. The RCT was funded by the National Institutes of Health, Office of Alternative Medicine. Detailed descriptions of the entire 11-part protocol were first published along with the preliminary results of the RCT in 1997 (Shannahoff-Khalsa, 1997).

Both clinical trials were conducted at the University of California in San Diego (UCSD) in collaboration with faculty in the department of psychiatry. The first study was conducted in collaboration with Liana R. Beckett, MS, MFCC, who was at that time the clinical coordinator for the OCD treatment program at UCSD's Gifford Center for Outpatient Psychiatry. The second study was conducted with Professor Saul Levine, MD, the director of the division of child and adolescent psychiatry at UCSD and the chairman of the department of psychiatry at Children's Hospital in San Diego, along with Leslie E. Ray, MS, MFCC, who ran the control group, Christopher C. Gallen, MD, PhD, and Barry J. Schwartz, PhD, who were both at the Scripps Research Institute, La Jolla, California, at that time, and John J. Sidorowich, PhD, who along with the primary author were in the Institute for Nonlinear Science at UCSD.

Study One

The first study (Shannahoff-Khalsa & Beckett, 1996) was an uncontrolled clinical trial where patients only received the Kundalini yoga protocol. There was no comparison group. The patients in this study had all previously received at least one or more forms of conventional therapy (medication, behavior therapy, or psychotherapy) from very accomplished clinicians without achieving satisfactory relief. Of the eight patients in this study four had already attempted all three conventional modalities, and some of these therapies were used conjointly. One other patient had previously attempted treatment with ERP and psychotherapy, two others had tried medication alone, and one other failed to improve using only psychotherapy. It is also well known that OCD patients are the most unlikely psychiatric patients to recover over time if they are not treated, and that they do not respond significantly to placebo. These two facts partially make up for the lack of rigor in our uncontrolled study, which did not include a comparison therapy or placebo.

In this trial, three out of five of the patients who were well stabilized on medication at the beginning were free of medication five months before the end of the 12-month study. The other two medicated patients were significantly reduced, and after a one-year follow-up, four of the five were completely free of all medication. What is outstanding is that as a group these patients dramatically improved. Studies tell us that "Patients who respond to drug treatment are often reluctant to discontinue medication secondary to the fear that their symptoms will recur" (Rasmussen et al., 1993). In addition, an earlier study observed a relapse rate of 90% within 2 to 4 months following abrupt discontinuation of Anaphranil in 18 patients considered to be in "remission" on the drug (Pato et al., 1988). In the study, Anaphranil was substituted by desipramine, an antidepressant and close relative of Anaphranil, and most of these patients relapsed within two months of beginning desipramine (Leonard et al., 1991). Similar results of a rapid relapse were found in a study of patients who discontinued fluoxetine after having a good initial response (Fontaine & Chouinard, 1989). Therefore, the results reported here on our patients who were previously well stabilized on fluoxetine for a long period prior to inclusion in our study suggest that the yogic therapy is not only a novel approach but verges on being a curative therapy. Three of our five medicated patients had discontinued fluoxetine for what would be considered very long times without relapses prior to the end of our 12-month study. One discontinued for five months prior to the end, another for seven months, and a third for eight months. The two others reduced their dosages significantly and for reasonable periods prior to the 12-month end point. One year after the study, four of our five patients were off medication for 9, 16, 18, and 19 months. All of these subjects reported continued psychological improvement. Of the five of eight to complete the study, the end result showed a mean improvement of 55.5% on the Y-BOCS, with individual improvements of 83%, 79%, 65%, 61%, and -18%. The one subject who did not improve (−18%) by the Y-BOCS did improve by another scale (24% using the Symptom Checklist 90-R ([SCL-90-

R]). The other subjects showed consistency between the Y-BOCS and the OCD scale in the SCL-90-R scores. The three patients who had an 83%, 79%, and 65% improvement also had one zero, which means no symptoms, for either their obsession or compulsion Y-BOCS score. Of the three patients who dropped out at the three-month time point, one showed a 32% improvement, another a 26% improvement, and the third a decrease of 14%. These three patients dropped out due to uncontrollable circumstances—work/school schedule conflicts, end-stage pregnancy (eight months), and idiopathic fibromyalgia, respectively.

Three of our five patients that finished at 12 months no longer met the standard psychiatric criteria for having OCD. And one subject with a 61% improvement (no meds), obsessing 15 to 40 minutes per day was marginal since the criteria state that the symptoms "take more than an hour a day, or significantly interfere" (American Psychiatric Association, 1994). Another scale (SCL-90-R) widely used to compare the severity of symptoms of nine psychiatric disorders that include OCD, anxiety, depression, paranoid ideation, somatization, interpersonal sensitivity, hostility, phobic anxiety, psychoticism, and a global severity index, showed a marked and statistically significant improvement. There was a 53.3% improvement for OCD symptoms, 62.5% improvement with anxiety, and according to the Global Severity Index (GSI) scale, which is a summary for all of the nine independent scales, there was a 53.25% improvement. The subjects also demonstrated that they perceived 39% less stress in their lives, according to the Perceived Stress Scales (PSS) test.

Study Two

The second study (Shannahoff-Khalsa, 1997; Shannahoff-Khalsa et al., 1999) was a controlled experiment that met all the rigorous standards that are imposed to assure that the result is not due to chance or placebo. This RCT compared the 11-part Kundalini yoga meditation protocol with a combination of two other popular meditation techniques. These two treatment protocols were compared in matched groups where both the subjects and therapists were unaware of which protocol, if any, would prove to yield a better result. Prior to entering the study, all patients were informed that two meditation protocols would be compared and that if one proved to yield better results, the group that started with what later proved to be the less-effective therapy would then join the group employing the more effective therapy and get 12 additional months of treatment. They understood that the experiment would be conducted over 12 months and that differences in the two therapies could be determined at any one of the three-month test periods to follow. This experimental design was employed to give everyone the confidence that everybody would eventually have an equal opportunity if one therapy proved to be more efficacious. Both groups had 10 adults and were almost identically matched at the beginning of the experiment for ages, sex, medication status, and the severity of symptoms.

The 11-part Kundalini yoga protocol is described in Chapter 2. We chose to compare it with the popular Relaxation Response (RR) meditation technique (Benson, 1975) that is almost identical to the Transcendental Meditation (TM) technique brought to the West in the 1960s by Maharishi Mahesh Yogi. The difference between the TM technique and the RR technique is that you choose your own mantra or affirmation in either English or any other language for the RR technique. This is done to ensure that your word or phrase has a personal meaning and appeal. With the TM technique a Sanskrit mantra is provided. The RR has been studied primarily at the Harvard Medical School by Herbert Benson, MD, and his group since the 1970s. Benson is now the director of Harvard's Mind-Body Institute, where they employ this technique in their stress-management and health-promotion programs. This technique has also been widely studied at other universities. We also chose the Mindfulness Meditation (MM) technique (Kabat-Zinn, 1990) (sometimes called the Vipassana

Mediation technique), to include along with the RR technique. This technique is also very popular and has been avidly promoted through clinical programs at the University of Massachusetts by Dr. John Kabat-Zinn, and the technique is now employed in a program in more than 200 hospitals across the country for stress management. It has been studied as an effective clinical treatment for generalized anxiety (Miller, Fletcher, & Kabat-Zinn, 1995), so it seemed appropriate to test it as a treatment for OCD. Both techniques were to be practiced for 30 minutes each to equal the hour approximately required for the Kundalini yoga protocol. This group is now referred to here as the RRMM group. Leslie E. Ray, the therapist for the RRMM group, had practiced both techniques personally for 12 years and taught groups and private clients using these two techniques. She was not aware of the contents of the Kundalini yoga protocol prior to or during the trial.

Each group had three adult subjects drop out prior to the first three-month tests for symptom severity. Before these dropouts, the mean severity according to the Y-BOCS for both groups was almost identical (Y-BOCS = 22.80 and 22.75). After each group lost three members, the mean severity at the 0-month baseline changed but statistics failed to reveal a significant difference in the recalculated 0-month baseline Y-BOCS scores for the two groups, even though the new calculation of the baseline (before therapy) for the Kundalini yoga group's mean score increased (showed greater severity) and the RRMM group's mean score decreased. This change left a four-point difference between the groups. This statistically insignificant difference in baseline Y-BOCS scores between the two groups nonetheless could be interpreted to indicate that the RRMM group was marginally less severe at baseline. One might expect that if a group is less severe they may more readily comply and benefit from treatment. However, the mean change in Y-BOCS scores (Kundalini yoga group = −9.43, RRMM group = −2.86) for the first three months clearly indicated that the Kundalini yoga therapy was far more efficacious, yielding a 38.4% versus a 13.9% improvement. The 13.9% improvement for the RRMM group was not statistically significant. In the second three-month period, when the patients in the RRMM group joined the Kundalini yoga group they showed a 44% improvement using the Kundalini yoga protocol. In addition to the Y-BOCS, SCL-90R (OC scale and GSI scale), and PSS, we also used the Profile of Moods State (POMS) and the Purpose-in-Life scale (PIL).

To compare the intergroup differences, we performed a two-way mixed model Analysis of Variance (ANOVA), pre-therapy versus post-therapy differences, and the group interaction for the first three months of therapy. The three-month Y-BOCS totals for the Kundalini yoga group and the RRMM group were 15.14 (STD=6.2, N=7) and 17.71 (STD=2.98, N=7), respectively. The interaction term of the ANOVA model reflects the potential differential effects of each therapy over time. This term was significant—$F(1,12)=4.89$, $p < 0.0471$—indicating that the change in the Kundalini yoga group from baseline to three months was greater than the RRMM group. In addition, the results of the SCL-90-R OCD and GSI scales, POMS, PSS, and PIL test for the first three months of therapy were compared using a Student's Independent Groups T-test (two-tailed). The respective results for those five scales are p=0.003, 0.035, 0.046, 0.207, and 0.071. The Kundalini yoga protocol proved significantly superior to the RRMM protocol on four of six scales (Y-BOCS, SCL-90-R OCD, GSI scales, and POMS), and better but not significant on the PSS and PIL tests.

A paired T-test (two-tailed) was used to compare within group differences for zero and three months for all six scales. The Y-BOCS, SCL-90-R OC scale and GSI scale, POMS, PSS, and PIL all showed significance for the Kundalini therapy, N=7 (p values of 0.013, 0.01, 0.017, 0.004, 0.034, and 0.004, respectively). Respective improvements were 38.36%, 47.68%, 49.44%, 62.41%, 30.05%, and 10.60%. No scale was significant for the RRMM Group (N=7) with respective percent changes of 13.9%, -3.87%, 0.63%, −2.51%, 8.92%, and −1.10%. Based on the Y-BOCS results, groups were merged at three months.

When comparing the 0-month baseline (N=14) mean to the 15-month mean (N=11), the improvements at 15-months were 70.62% (Y-BOCS), 61.96% (SCL-90-R OC scale), 66.16% (SCL-90-R GSI scale), 73.90% (POMS), 39.03% (PSS), and 22.97% (PIL test). For these 11 patients, the Y-BOCS "totals" included three 0 scores, one 1, two 5's, one 6, and an 11, 14, 15, and 16. Six of the twelve medicated patients to enter completed the study. Three of these six were free of medication for a minimum of six months prior to the study's end. The others reduced.

In addition, four female subjects scored 0's for the obsessions and/or compulsions by the nine-month time point. One woman with hoarding and arranging rituals with a moderate case (baseline of 19) entering at three months was able to achieve 0's for both her obsessions and compulsions by six months. Another woman (baseline of 21) scored 0's for both obsessions and compulsions at both her first three-month and six-month Kundalini yoga time points. She initiated treatment with the RRMM therapy and went from a 21 to 20 for those three months. Of these four subjects, only one subject started on medication. She initially went from 19 to 21 for her Y-BOCS scores while using the RRMM therapy for the first three months, and with the Kundalini yoga therapy she went to 12 (from 21) and four for the first and second quarter, respectively, and finally to 0's for both her 9- and 12-month scores. In the first study, among the five patients remaining in the group, we had three with the respective final Y-BOCS scores of 3, 4, and 6. Each of these patients had a 0 for either their obsession or compulsion sub-score. In the second study, we had 4 of the final 11 score in the remission or cure range. One patient scored a 0 for obsessions and a 1 for compulsions, and three other patients scored 0's for both their obsessions and compulsions.

At the beginning of the study, OCD patients see the one yogic technique specific for OCD (the "OCDB") in the Kundalini yoga protocol as very difficult if not impossible to perform. However, in study 1, 60% of the patients developed the ability to perform the OCDB at one breath per minute for the entire 31 minutes during the first 8 months of a 12-month program. In study 2, only one subject, an unmedicated female age 38, was able to consistently complete the OCDB for 31 minutes at one breath per minute. However, two males were also able by the end of the study to on occasion reach the one-breath-per-minute level for the entire 31 minutes. Those patients who made a serious commitment to achieving the one-breath-per-minute rate for 31 minutes and had enough youthful vitality were all able to accomplish this important milestone in their practice.

In sum, study 1 showed a group mean Y-BOCS improvement of 55.5% and study 2 showed a group mean improvement of 71%. In study 2, we also measured for the perceived stress in the patient's lives. There was a 48.4% mean reduction in the amount of stress that they perceived after 12 months. This is an improvement over study 1, where the mean reduction of perceived stress was 39%. Also, in study 2 we used the PIL scale to measure a factor that indicates how much personal meaning the patient perceives in their own life. We found that there was a 20% mean increase by this scale at three months, but only with the Kundalini yoga therapy. We also used a test to measure their mood ratings using the POMS. The Kundalini yoga group showed a 62% improvement in the first three months and the RRMM Group showed a 2% decrease, a dramatic difference in therapies. And again we used the SCL-90-R scales to rate OCD, somatization, interpersonal sensitivity, depression, anxiety, hostility, phobic anxiety, psychoticism, and paranoid ideation as we had in study 1. The Kundalini yoga group improved 47.5% according to the OCD scale of the SCL-90-R test and the RRMM group regressed 5.5% in the first three months. Also, using the global severity index, which measures changes for all of the nine different psychiatric scales, the Kundalini yoga group improved 49.3% and the RRMM group had an insignificant increase of only 0.4%.

It is the near-immediate and rapid relief achieved with the Kundalini yoga therapy that kept patients returning to the groups. The self-described case history of the 20-year-old female on page

59 who had OCD, BDD, and social phobias is fairly representative of the experience of people in the group. However, the rigor of a daily, or near daily, consistent discipline over time was difficult and imposing for those subjects who dropped out early in study 2, who also tended to be much younger than the others in the group. Maturity plays an important role in success.

Also, with respect to prior experience with "meditation," only 2 of 8 people in the first study and 3 of 20 in the second had any previous experience with meditation, and their experience was very limited. They had used only very simple techniques and none had a daily or even irregular meditation practice prior to either study. None of our patients had ever achieved substantial relief for their OCD symptoms prior to using the Kundalini yoga techniques. Past experience with meditation techniques is not necessary but may be helpful.

References

Abramowitz, J. S. (1997). Effectiveness of psychological and pharmacological treatments for obsessive-compulsive disorder: A quantitative review. *Journal of Consulting and Clinical Psychology, 65*(1), 44–52.

American Psychiatric Association (APA). (1994). *Diagnostic and statistical manual of mental disorders DSM-IV* (4th ed.). Washington, D.C.: Author.

Ancient Healing Ways (2006). "Chakkra Chattra Varti" audio tape. Retrieved June 7, 2006, from *www.a-healing.com*.

Applegate, B., Lahey, B. B., Hart, E. L., Biederman, J., Hynd, G. W., Barkley, R. A., et al. (1997). Validity of the age-of-onset criterion for ADHD: A report from the DSM-IV field trials. *Journal of the American Academy of Child and Adolescent Psychiatry, 36*(9), 1211–1221.

Aschoff, J., & Gerkema, M. (1985). *On the diversity and uniformity of ultradian rhythms* (Experimental Brain Research, supplement vol. 12). Berlin: Springer-Verlag.

Ashley, C. C., & Lea, T. J. (1978). A method for studying the cyclic changes in nasal resistance in the anaesthetized pig. *Journal of Physiology, 282*, 1p–2p.

Ator, N. A. (2005). Contributions of gaba receptor subtype selectivity to abuse liability and dependence potential of pharmacological treatments for anxiety and sleep disorders. *CNS Spectrums: The International Journal of Neuropsychiatric Medicine, 10*(1), 31–39.

Aubin, D. (2004). Adult ADHD costs Americans $77 billion in lost income. Retrieved from http://www.medscape.com/viewarticle/489002

Ayne, C., Pynoos, R., & Cardenas, J. I. (Eds.). (2001). Wounded adolescence: School-based psychotherapy for adolescents who sustained or witnessed violent injury. In M. Shafii & S. Shafii (Eds.), *School violence: Contributing factors, management and prevention*. Washington, DC: American Psychiatric Press.

Backon, J. (1988). Changes in blood glucose levels induced by differential forced unilateral nostril breathing, a technique which affects both brain hemisphericity and autonomic activity. *Medical Science Research, 16*, 1197–1199.

Backon, J., & Kullok, S. (1989). Effect of forced unilateral nostril breathing on blink rates: Relevance to hemispheric lateralization of dopamine. *International Journal of Neuroscience, 46*(1–2), 53–59.

Backon, J., Matamoros, N., & Ticho, U. (1989). Changes in intraocular pressure induced by differential forced unilateral nostril breathing, a technique that affects both brain hemisphericity and autonomic activity. A pilot study. *Graefes Archive for Clinical and Experimental Ophthalmology, 227*(6), 575–577.

Bamford, O. S., & Eccles, R. (1982). The central reciprocal control of nasal vasomotor oscillations. *Pflugers Archive European Journal of Physiology, 394*, 139–143.

Bates, D. W., Schmitt, W., Buchwald, D., Ware, N. C., Lee, J., Thoyer, E., et al. (1993). Prevalence of fatigue and chronic fatigue syndrome in a primary care practice. *Archives of Internal Medicine, 153*(24), 2759–2765.

Beickert, P. (1951). Halbseitenrhythmus der vegetativen innervation. *Archiv fur Ohren-, Nasen- und Kehlkopfheilkunde, Vereinigt mit Zeitschrift fur Hals-, Nasen- und Ohrenheilkunde, 157*, 404–411.

Benoit, M., Bagley, B., Spivak, H., Addington, W., Hill, J., Nielsen, N., et al. (2000). *Youth and violence—medicine, nursing, and public health: Connecting the dots to prevent violence*. Chicago, IL: American Medical Association.

Benson, H. (1975). *The relaxation response*. New York: Morrow.

Benton, L. A., & Yates, F. E. (1990). Ultradian adrenocortical and circulatory oscillations in conscious dogs. *American Journal of Physiology, 258*(3 pt. 2), R578–R590.

Bhajan, Y. (1976). *Kundalini yoga: Sadhana guidelines*. Espanola, NM: Kundalini Research Institute Publications.

Bhajan, Y. (1980). *Survival kit: Meditations and exercises for stress and pressure of the times*. Espanola, NM: Kundalini Research Institute Publications.

Bhajan, Y. (1981). *Kundalini lectures: Man to man Part 5, the real strength of the man*. Espanola, NM: Kundalini Research Institute Publications.

Bhajan, Y. (1982). *The ancient art of self-healing*. Eugene, OR: West Anandpur.

References

Bhajan, Y. (1990). Grief meditation. Lecture, Los Angeles, CA, May 17, 1990.

Bhajan, Y. (1995). Meditation to balance the Jupiter and Saturn energies: A technique useful for treating depression, focusing the mind, and eliminating destructive behavior. Lecture, Los Angeles, CA, December 12, 2005.

Bhajan, Y. (1998). *Self-knowledge: Kundalini yoga as taught by Yogi Bhajan.* Espanola, NM: Kundalini Research Institute Publications.

Bhajan, Y. (2000). *Self-experience: Kundalini yoga as taught by Yogi Bhajan.* Espanola, NM: Kundalini Research Institute Publications.

Bhajan, Y. (2002). *Reaching me in me.* Espanola, NM: Kundalini Research Institute Publications.

Bhajan, Y., & Khalsa, G. (1975). *Kundalini meditation manual for intermediate students.* Espanola, NM: Kundalini Research Institute Publications.

Bhajan, Y., & Khalsa, G. (1998). *The Mind: Its projections and multiple facets* (1st ed.). Espanola, NM: Kundalini Research Institute Publications.

Biederman, J., & Faraone, S. V. (2005). Attention-deficit hyperactivity disorder. *Lancet, 366*(9481), 237–248.

Biederman, J., Mick, E., & Faraone, S. V. (1998). Normalized functioning in youths with persistent attention-deficit/hyperactivity disorder. *Journal of Pediatrics, 133*(4), 544–551.

Bisson, J., & Andrew, M. (2005). Psychological treatment of post-traumatic stress disorder (PTSD). *Cochrane Database Systematic Reviews* (2), CD003388.

Block, R. A., Arnott, D. P., Quigley, B., & Lynch, W. C. (1989). Unilateral nostril breathing influences lateralized cognitive performance. *Brain and Cognition, 9*(2), 181–190.

Bloom, F. E. (2003). Presidential address. Science as a way of life: Perplexities of a physician-scientist. *Science, 300*(5626), 1680–1685.

Bojsen-Moller, F., & Fahrenkrug, J. (1971). Nasal swell-bodies and cyclic changes in the air passage of the rat and rabbit nose. *Journal of Anatomy, 110*, 25–37.

Bouayd-Amine, D., Cupissol, D., Nougier-Soule, J., Bres, J., Gestin-Boyer, C., Rene, C., et al. (1993). Variations ultradiennes des concentrations en interleukine-1 beta, interferon-gamma et recepteur soluble d'il-2 chez l'homme volontaire sain. *Comptes rendus des seances de la Societe de biologie et de ses filiales, 187*, 542–553.

Brown, E., Heimberg, R., & Juster, H. (1995). Social phobia subtype and avoidant personality disorder: Effect on severity of social phobia impairment and outcome of cognitive-behavioral treatment. *Behavior Therapy, 26*, 467–481.

Buchwald, D., Umali, P., Umali, J., Kith, P., Pearlman, T., & Komaroff, A. L. (1995). Chronic fatigue and the chronic fatigue syndrome: Prevalence in a Pacific northwest health care system. *Annals of Internal Medicine, 123*(2), 81–88.

CASA. (2005). *Under the counter: The diversion and abuse of controlled prescription drugs in the U.S.* New York: The National Center on Addiction and Substance Abuse at Columbia University.

Cassell, G., Demitrack, M., & Engel, C. M. H., McCully, K., Reeves, W. C., Sharpe, M., Shaver, J., Wessely, S., White, L. R., Wilson, B. (2000). National Institutes of Health chronic fatigue syndrome state-of-the-science consultation. Bethesda, MD: National Institutes of Health.

Chen, J. C., Brown, B., & Schmid, K. L. (2004). Effect of unilateral forced nostril breathing on tonic accommodation and intraocular pressure. *Clinical Autonomic Research, 14*(6), 396–400.

Cohen, L. R., & Potter, L. B. (1999). Injuries and violence: Risk factors and opportunities for prevention during adolescence. *Adolescent Medicine, 10*(1), 125–135, VI.

Cole, P., & Haight, J. (1986). Posture and the nasal cycle. *American Otology, Rhinology, and Laryngology, 95,* 233–237.

Coleman, R. M., Roffwarg, H. P., Kennedy, S. J., Guilleminault, C., Cinque, J., Cohn, M. A., et al. (1982). Sleep-wake disorders based on a polysomnographic diagnosis: A national cooperative study. *Journal of the American Medical Association, 247*(7), 997–1003.

Costa e Silva, J. A. (1999). A forward in report of an international consensus conference, Versailles, October 13–15, 1996. *Sleep, 22* (Suppl. #3), S416.

Cottraux, J., Bouvard, M. A., & Milliery, M. (2005). Combining pharmacotherapy with cognitive-behavioral interventions for obsessive-compulsive disorder. *Cognitive Behavioral Therapy, 34*(3), 185–192.

Cottraux, J., Mollard, E., Bouvard, M., & Marks, I. (1993). Exposure therapy, fluvoxamine, or combination treatment in obsessive-compulsive disorder: One-year follow-up. *Psychiatry Research, 49*(1), 63–75.

Dalton, E. J., Cate-Carter, T. D., Mundo, E., Parikh, S. V., & Kennedy, J. L. (2003). Suicide risk in bipolar patients: The role of co-morbid substance use disorders. *Bipolar Disorders, 5*(1), 58–61.

Dane, S., Caliskan, E., Karasen, M., & Oztasan, N. (2002). Effects of unilateral nostril breathing on blood pressure and heart rate in right-handed healthy subjects. *International Journal of Neuroscience, 112*(1), 97–102.

Davidson, J. R., Foa, E. B., Huppert, J. D., Keefe, F. J., Franklin, M. E., Compton, J. S., et al. (2004). Fluoxetine, comprehensive cognitive behavioral therapy, and placebo in generalized social phobia. *Archives of General Psychiatry, 61*(10), 1005–1013.

Davidson, J. R., Hughes, D. L., George, L. K., & Blazer, D. G. (1993). The epidemiology of social phobia: Findings from the duke epidemiological catchment area study. *Psychological Medicine, 23*(3), 709–718.

Davidson, J. R., Rothbaum, B. O., van der Kolk, B. A., Sikes, C. R., & Farfel, G. M. (2001). Multicenter, double-blind comparison of sertraline and placebo in the treatment of posttraumatic stress disorder. *Archives of General Psychiatry, 58*(5), 485–492.

Davidson, J. R., Tharwani, H. M., & Connor, K. M. (2002). Davidson trauma scale (DTS): Normative scores in the general population and effect sizes in placebo-controlled SSRI trials. *Depression and Anxiety, 15*(2), 75–78.

DelBello, M., Strakowski, S., Sax, K., McElroy, S., Keck, P., West, S., et al. (1999). Effects of familial rates of affective illness and substance abuse on rates of substance abuse in patients with first-episode mania. *Journal of Affective Disorders, 56,* 55–60.

Dement, W. (1993). Foreword to *Insomnia: Psychological assessment and management.* C. M. Morin (Ed.). New York: Guilford.

Dement, W., & Kleitman, N. (1957). Cyclic variations in EEG during sleep and their relation to eye movements, body motility, and dreaming. *Electroencephalography and Clinical Neurophysiology, supplement* 9(4), 673–690.

Drettner, B. (1970). Pathophysiological relationship between the upper and lower airways. *Annals of Otology, Rhinology, and Laryngology, 79*(3), 499–505.

Eccles, R. (2000). Nasal airflow in health and disease. *Acta Oto-Laryngologica, 120*(5), 580–595.

El-Zein, R., Abdel-Rahman, S., Hay, M., Lopez, M., Bondy, M., Morris, D., et al. (2005). Cytogenetic effects in children treated with methylphenidate. *Cancer Letters, 230*(2), 284–91.

Elbert, T., & Schauer, M. (2002). Burnt into memory. *Nature, 419*(6910), 883.

Faraone, S., Sergeant, J., Gillberg, C., & Biederman, J. (2003). The worldwide prevalence of ADHD: Is it an American condition? *World Psychiatry, 2,* 104–113.

Finkelhor, D. (1994). The international epidemiology of child sexual abuse. *Child Abuse and Neglect, 18*(5), 409–417.

Finkelhor, D., & Dziuba-Leatherman, J. (1994a). Victimization of children. *American Psychologist, 49*(3), 173–183.

Finkelhor, D., & Dziuba-Leatherman, J. (1994b). Children as victims of violence: A national survey. *Pediatrics, 94*(4 pt. 1), 413–420.

Finkelhor, D., Hamby, S. L., Ormrod, R., & Turner, H. (2005). The juvenile victimization questionnaire: Reliability, validity, and national norms. *Child Abuse and Neglect, 29*(4), 383–412.

Finkelhor, D., Ormrod, R., Turner, H., & Hamby, S. L. (2005). The victimization of children and youth: A comprehensive, national survey. *Child Maltreatment, 10*(1), 5–25.

Fischer, M., Barkley, R., Fletcher, K., & Patel, L. (2001). *Young adult outcomes of childhood ADHD: Costs to society.* Paper presented at the Annual Meeting of the American Academy of Child and Adolescent Psychiatry, exact date?, Washington, D.C.

Foa, E. B., Liebowitz, M. R., Kozak, M. J., Davies, S., Campeas, R., Franklin, M. E., et al. (2005). Randomized, placebo-controlled trial of exposure and ritual prevention, clomipramine, and their combination in the treatment of obsessive-compulsive disorder. *American Journal of Psychiatry, 162*(1), 151–161.

Fontaine, R., & Chouinard, G. (1989). Fluoxetine in the long-term treatment of obsessive compulsive disorder. *Psychiatric Annals, 19*, 88–91.

Ford, D. E., & Kamerow, D. B. (1989). Epidemiologic study of sleep disturbances and psychiatric disorders. An opportunity for prevention? *Journal of the American Medical Association, 262*(11), 1479–1484.

Freyd, J. J., Putnam, F. W., Lyon, T. D., Becker-Blease, K. A., Cheit, R. E., Siegel, N. B., et al. (2005). The science of child sexual abuse. *Science, 308*(5721), 501.

Friedell, A. (1948). Automatic attentive breathing in angina pectoris. *Minnesota Medicine, 31*, 875–881.

Fukuda, K., Straus, S. E., Hickie, I., Sharpe, M. C., Dobbins, J. G., & Komaroff, A. (1994). The chronic fatigue syndrome: A comprehensive approach to its definition and study. International chronic fatigue syndrome study group. *Annals of Internal Medicine, 121*(12), 953–959.

Furnival, C. M., Linden, R. J., & Snow, H. M. (1973). Chronotropic and inotropic effects on the dog heart of stimulating the efferent cardiac sympathetic nerves. *Journal of Physiology (London), 230*(1), 137–153.

Geddes, J. R., Freemantle, N., Mason, J., Eccles, M. P., & Boynton, J. (2000). SSRIs versus other antidepressants for depressive disorder. *Cochrane Database Systematic Reviews* (2), CD001851.

Gellhorn, E. (1967). *Principles of autonomic-somatic integration.* Minneapolis: University of Minnesota Press.

General, S. (1994). Health consequences of smoking cessation: A report of the surgeon general. Washington, D.C.: Government Printing Office, 24.

George, M. S., Sackeim, H. A., Marangell, L. B., Husain, M. M., Nahas, Z., Lisanby, S. H., et al. (2000). Vagus nerve stimulation: A potential therapy for resistant depression? *Psychiatric Clinics of North America, 23*(4), 757–783.

Ghodse, A. (1999). Dramatic increase in methylphenidate consumption. *Current Opinion in Psychiatry, 12*(3), 265–268.

Goldstein, L., Stoltzfus, N. W., & Gardocki, J. F. (1972). Changes in interhemispheric amplitude relationships in the EEG during sleep. *Physiology and Behavior, 8*(5), 811–815.

Goodman, W. K., Kozak, M. J., Liebowitz, M., & White, K. L. (1996). Treatment of obsessive-compulsive disorder with fluvoxamine: A multicentre, double-blind, placebo-controlled trial. *International Clinical Psychopharmacology, 11*(1), 21–29.

Goodman, W. K., McDougle, C. J., Barr, L. C., Aronson, S. C., & Price, L. H. (1993). Biological approaches to treatment-resistant obsessive compulsive disorder. *Journal of Clinical Psychiatry, 54 supplement,* 16–26.

Goodman, W. K., McDougle, C. J., & Price, L. H. (1992). Pharmacotherapy of obsessive compulsive disorder. *Journal of Clinical Psychiatry, 53 supplement,* 29–37.

Goodman, W. K., Price, L. H., Rasmussen, S. A., Mazure, C., Delgado, P., Heninger, G. R., et al. (1989). The Yale-Brown Obsessive Compulsive Scale. II. Validity. *Archives of General Psychiatry, 46*(11), 1012–1016.

Goodman, W. K., Price, L. H., Rasmussen, S. A., Mazure, C., Fleischmann, R. L., Hill, C. L., et al. (1989). The Yale-Brown Obsessive Compulsive Scale. I. Development, use, and reliability. *Archives of General Psychiatry, 46*(11), 1006–1011.

Goodwin, F., & Jamison, K. (1990). *Manic-depressive illness.* London: Oxford University Press.

Gorman, J. (2005). Benzodiaepines: Taking the good with the bad and the ugly. *CNS Spectrums: The International Journal of Neuropsychiatric Medicine, 10*(1), 14–15.

Grant, B., Harford, T., Dawson, D., Chou, P., Dufour, M., & Pickering, R. (1994). Prevalence of DSM-IV alcohol abuse and dependence: United States, 1992. *Alcohol Health and Research World, 18*(3), 243–248.

Grant, B. F., Dawson, D. A., Stinson, F. S., Chou, S. P., Dufour, M. C., & Pickering, R. P. (2004). The 12-month prevalence and trends in DSM-IV alcohol abuse and dependence: United States, 1991–1992 and 2001–2002. *Drug and Alcohol Dependence, 74*(3), 223–234.

Greenberg, P. E., Finkelstein, S. N., & Berndt, E. R. (1995). Calculating the workplace cost of chronic disease. *Business and Health, 13*(9), 27–28, 30.

Greene, R. W., Biederman, J., Faraone, S. V., Monuteaux, M. C., Mick, E., DuPre, E. P., et al. (2001). Social impairment in girls with ADHD: Patterns, gender comparisons, and correlates. *Journal of the American Academy of Child and Adolescent Psychiatry, 40*(6), 704–710.

Greist, J. H., Jefferson, J. W., Kobak, K. A., Katzelnick, D. J., & Serlin, R. C. (1995). Efficacy and tolerability of serotonin transport inhibitors in obsessive-compulsive disorder. A meta-analysis. *Archives of General Psychiatry, 52*(1), 53–60.

Group, M. T. A. (1999a). A 14-month randomized clinical trial of treatment strategies for attention-deficit/hyperactivity disorder. Multimodal treatment study of children with ADHD. *Archives of General Psychiatry, 56,* 1073–1086.

Group, V. N. S. S. (1999b). A randomized controlled trial of chronic vagus nerve stimulation for treatment of medically intractable seizures. *Neurology, 45,* 224–230.

Groves, D. A., & Brown, V. J. (2005). Vagal nerve stimulation: A review of its applications and potential mechanisms that mediate its clinical effects. *Neuroscience and Biobehavioral Reviews, 29*(3), 493–500.

Hamlin, R. L., & Smith, C. R. (1968). Effects of vagal stimulation on S-A and A-V nodes. *American Journal of Physiology, 215*(3), 560–568.

Hansen, R. A., Gartlehner, G., Lohr, K. N., Gaynes, B. N., & Carey, T. S. (2005). Efficacy and safety of second-generation antidepressants in the treatment of major depressive disorder. *Annals of Internal Medicine, 143*(6), 415–426.

Hanson, R. F., Resnick, H. S., Saunders, B. E., Kilpatrick, D. G., & Best, C. (1999). Factors related to the reporting of childhood rape. *Child Abuse and Neglect, 23*(6), 559–569.

Harford, T. (1992). The family history of alcoholism in the United States: Prevalence and demographic characteristics. *British Journal of Addictions, 89,* 931–935.

Harrison, L., Manocha, R., & Rubia, K. (2004). Sahaja yoga meditation as a family treatment programme for children with attention deficit-hyperactive disorder. *Clinical Child Psychology and Psychiatry, 9*(4), 479–497.

Hasegawa, M., & Kern, E. B. (1978). Variations resistance in man: A rhinomanometric study of cycle in 50 human subjects. *Rhinology, 16,* 20–29.

Hauri, P., & Fisher, J. (1986). Persistent psychophysiologic (learned) insomnia. *Sleep, 9*(1), 38–53.

Hayward, L., Zubrick, S., & Silburn, S. (1992). Blood alcohol levels in suicide cases. *Journal of Epidemiology and Community Health, 46,* 256–260.

Heetderks, D. R. (1927). Observations on the reaction of the nasal mucous membranes. *American Journal of the Medical Sciences, 174,* 231–244.

Henk, H. J., Katzelnick, D. J., Kobak, K. A., Greist, J. H., & Jefferson, J. W. (1996). Medical costs attributed to depression among patients with a history of high medical expenses in a health maintenance organization. *Archives of General Psychiatry, 53*(10), 899–904.

References

Hess, W. R. (1954). *Diencephalon, autonomic and extrapyridimal functions.* New York: Grune and Stratton.

Hirschfeld, R. M., Calabrese, J. R., Weissman, M. M., Reed, M., Davies, M. A., Frye, M. A., et al. (2003). Screening for bipolar disorder in the community. *Journal of Clinical Psychiatry, 64*(1), 53–59.

Hoge, C. W., Castro, C. A., Messer, S. C., McGurk, D., Cotting, D. I., & Koffman, R. L. (2004). Combat duty in Iraq and Afghanistan, mental health problems, and barriers to care. *New England Journal of Medicine, 351*(1), 13–22.

Hondeghem, L. M., Mouton, E., Stassen, T., & De Geest, H. (1975). Additive effects of acetylcholine released by vagal nerve stimulation on atrial rate. *Journal of Applied Physiology, 38*(1), 108–113.

Husted, D., & Shapira, N. (2004). A review of the treatment for refractory obsessive-compulsive disorder: From medicine to deep brain stimulation. *CNS Spectrum: The International Journal of Neuropsychiatric Medicine, 9*(11), 833–847.

ICSD. (1990). *International Classification of Sleep Disorders* (2nd ed.). city?: American Sleep Disorders Association.

Ischlondsky, N. (1955). The inhibitory process in the cerebrophysiological laboratory and in the clinic. *Journal of Nervous and Mental Disease, 121,* 5–18.

Jason, L. A., Richman, J. A., Rademaker, A. W., Jordan, K. M., Plioplys, A. V., Taylor, R. R., et al. (1999). A community-based study of chronic fatigue syndrome. *Archives of Internal Medicine, 159*(18), 2129–2137.

Jella, S. A., & Shannahoff-Khalsa, D. S. (1993). The effects of unilateral forced nostril breathing on cognitive performance. *International Journal of Neuroscience, 73*(1–2), 61–68.

Jenike, M. (1990). Illness related to obsessive-compulsive disorder. In M. A. Jenike, L. Baer, and W. E. Minichiello (Eds.), *Obsessive-compulsive disorders: Theory and mangement.* St. Louis, MO: Mosby.

Jenike, M., Baer, L., & Minichiello, W. (1986). *Obsessive-compulsive disorders: Theory and management.* Littleton, MA: Yearbook Medical.

Jensen, P. S., Garcia, J. A., Glied, S., Crowe, M., Foster, M., Schlander, M., et al. (2005). Cost-effectiveness of ADHD treatments: Findings from the multimodal treatment study of children with ADHD. *American Journal of Psychiatry, 162*(9), 1628–1636.

Jensen, P. S., & Kenny, D. T. (2004). The effects of yoga on the attention and behavior of boys with attention-deficit/hyperactivity disorder (ADHD). *Journal of Attentional Disorders, 7*(4), 205–216.

Judd, L. L., Akiskal, H. S., Schettler, P. J., Endicott, J., Maser, J., Solomon, D. A., et al. (2002). The long-term natural history of the weekly symptomatic status of bipolar I disorder. *Archives of General Psychiatry, 59*(6), 530–537.

Kabat-Zinn, J. (1990). *Full catastrophe living: Using the wisdom of your body and mind to face stress, pain, and illness.* New York: Delacorte Press.

Kales, A., Soldatos, C. R., & Kales, J. D. (1987). Sleep disorders: Insomnia, sleepwalking, night terrors, nightmares, and enuresis. *Annals of Internal Medicine, 106*(4), 582–592.

Kales, J. D., Kales, A., Bixler, E. O., Soldatos, C. R., Cadieux, R. J., Kashurba, G. J., et al. (1984). Biopsychobehavioral correlates of insomnia, V: Clinical characteristics and behavioral correlates. *American Journal of Psychiatry, 141*(11), 1371–1376.

Katzelnick, D. J., Kobak, K. A., DeLeire, T., Henk, H. J., Greist, J. H., Davidson, J. R., et al. (2001). Impact of generalized social anxiety disorder in managed care. *American Journal of Psychiatry, 158*(12), 1999–2007.

Kawase, T. (1952). Further studies on "pressure sweat reflex." *Japanese Journal of Physiology, 3,* 1–9.

Kayser, R. (1889). Uber den Weg der Athmungsluft durch die Nase. *Zeitschrift für Öhrenheilkunde., 20*(96–106).

Kayser, R. (1895). Die exacta Messung der Luftdurchgangigkeit der Nase. *Archives of Laryngology and Rhinology, 3,* 101–120.

Kennedy, B., Ziegler, M. G., & Shannahoff-Khalsa, D. S. (1986). Alternating lateralization of plasma catecholamines and nasal patency in humans. *Life Sciences, 38*(13), 1203–1214.

Kessler, R. C., Berglund, P., Demler, O., Jin, R., Koretz, D., Merikangas, K. R., et al. (2003). The epidemiology of major depressive disorder: Results from the national comorbidity survey replication (NCS-R). *Journal of the American Medical Association, 289*(23), 3095–3105.

Kessler, R. C., Sonnega, A., Bromet, E., Hughes, M., & Nelson, C. B. (1995). Posttraumatic stress disorder in the national comorbidity survey. *Archives of General Psychiatry, 52*(12), 1048–1060.

Kessler, R. C., Stein, M. B., & Berglund, P. (1998). Social phobia subtypes in the national comorbidity survey. *American Journal of Psychiatry, 155*(5), 613–619.

Keuning, J. (1968). On the nasal cycle. *Journal of International Rhinology, 6,* 99–136.

Khalsa, S. B. (2004). Treatment of chronic insomnia with yoga: A preliminary study with sleep-wake diaries. *Applied Psychophysiology and Biofeedback, 29*(4), 269–278.

References

Klein, R., & Armitage, R. (1979). Rhythms in human performance: 1 1/2-hour oscillations in cognitive style. *Science, 204*(4399), 1326–1328.

Klein, R., Pilon, D., Prosser, S., & Shannahoff-Khalsa, D. (1986). Nasal airflow asymmetries and human performance. *Biological Psychology, 23*(2), 127–137.

Kleitman, N. (1961). *The nature of dreaming.* London: Churchill.

Kleitman, N. (1967). *Phylogenetic, ontogenetic, and environmental determinants in the evolution of sleep-wakefulness cycles.* Baltimore: Williams & Wilkins Co.

Kleitman, N. (1982). Basic rest-activity cycle—22 years later. *Sleep, 5*(4), 311–317.

Knapp, M. (1997). Economic evaluations and interventions for children and adolescents with mental health problems. *Journal of Child Psychology and Psychiatry and Allied Disciplines, 38*(1), 3–25.

Kobak, K. A., Greist, J. H., Jefferson, J. W., Katzelnick, D. J., & Henk, H. J. (1998). Behavioral versus pharmacological treatments of obsessive compulsive disorder: A meta-analysis. *Psychopharmacology* (Berlin), *136*(3), 205–216.

Kocer, I., Dane, S., Demirel, S., Demirel, H., & Koylu, H. (2002). Unilateral nostril breathing in intraocular pressure of right-handed healthy subjects. *Perceptual and Motor Skills, 95*(2), 491–496.

Kohn, R., Saxena, S., Levav, I., & Saraceno, B. (2004). The treatment gap in mental health care. *Bulletin of the World Health Organization, 82*(11), 858–866.

Komaroff, A. L., & Buchwald, D. S. (1998). Chronic fatigue syndrome: An update. *Annual Review of Medicine, 49,* 1–13.

Komaroff, A. L., Fagioli, L. R., Geiger, A. M., Doolittle, T. H., Lee, J., Kornish, R. J., et al. (1996). An examination of the working case definition of chronic fatigue syndrome. *American Journal of Medicine, 100*(1), 56–64.

Kozak, M., Liebowitz, M., & Foa, E. (2000). *Cognitive behavior therapy and pharmacotherapy for obsessive-compulsive disorder: The NIMH-sponsored collaborative study.* London: Erlbaum.

Kraepelin, E. (1921). *Manic-depressive insanity and paranoia.* Edinburgh, Scotland: E. & S. Livingstone.

Kripke, D. F. (2000). Chronic hypnotic use: Deadly risks, doubtful benefit. *Sleep Medicine Reviews, 4*(1), 5–20.

Kristof, M., Servit, Z., & Manas, K. (1981). Activating effect of nasal airflow on epileptic electrographic abnormalities in the human EEG. Evidence for the reflect origin of the phenomenon. *Physiologia Bohemoslovaca, 30*(1), 73–77.

Kryger, M., Lavie, P., & Rosen, R. (1999). Recognition and diagnosis of insomnia. *Sleep, 22* (supplement 3), S421–S426.

Kupfer, D., Baltimore, R., Berry, D., & al., e. (2000). National Institutes of Health consensus development conference statement: Diagnosis and treatment of attention-deficit/hyperactivity disorder (ADHD). *Journal of the American Academy of Child and Adolescent Psychiatry, 39*(2), 182–188.

Kupfer, D. J., Frank, E., Grochocinski, V. J., Cluss, P. A., Houck, P. R., & Stapf, D. A. (2002). Demographic and clinical characteristics of individuals in a bipolar disorder case registry. *Journal of Clinical Psychiatry, 63*(2), 12–125.

La Rosa, M., Bucolo, M., Frasca, M., Fortuna, L., & Shannahoff-Khalsa, D. (2002). *MEG signals spatial power distribution and gamma band activity in yoga breathing exercises.* Paper presented at the Conference Proceedings of the IEEE Engineering in Medicine and Biology Society, October 23–26, 2002, Houston, TX.

Lasser, K., Boyd, J. W., Woolhandler, S., Himmelstein, D. U., McCormick, D., & Bor, D. H. (2000). Smoking and mental illness: A population-based prevalence study. *Journal of the American Medical Association, 284*(20), 2606–2610.

Leonard, H. L., Swedo, S. E., Lenane, M. C., Rettew, D. C., Cheslow, D. L., Hamburger, S. D., et al. (1991). A double-blind desipramine substitution during long-term clomipramine treatment in children and adolescents with obsessive-compulsive disorder. *Archives of General Psychiatry, 48*(10), 922–927.

Levy, M., & Martin, P. (1979). *Neural control of the heart.* In R. M. Berne, N. Sperelakis, & S. R. Geiger (Eds.), *Handbook of physiology, section 2: The cardiovascular system, vol. 1, the heart* (pp. 581–620). Bethesda, MD: American Physiological Society.

Levy, M. N., Ng, M. L., & Zieske, H. (1966). Functional distribution of the peripheral cardiac sympathetic pathways. *Circulation Research, 19*(3), 650–661.

Livnat, A., Zehr, J. E., & Broten, T. P. (1984). Ultradian oscillations in blood pressure and heart rate in free-running dogs. *American Journal of Physiology, 246*(5 pt. 2), R817–R824.

Lochner, C., du Toit, P. L., Zungu-Dirwayi, N., Marais, A., van Kradenburg, J., Seedat, S., et al. (2002). Childhood trauma in obsessive-compulsive disorder, trichotillomania, and controls. *Depression and Anxiety, 15*(2), 66–68.

Lopez-Ibor, J. (1968). *Intravenous perfusion of monochlorimipramine: Techniques and results.* Paper presented at the Proceedings of the 6th International Congress of the CINP, date?, Tarragone, Spain.

References

Luxenberg, T., Spinazzola, J., Hidalgo, J., Hunt, C., & van der Kolk, B. (2001). Complex trauma and disorders of extreme stress (DESNOS) diagnosis, Part two: Treatment. *Directions in Psychiatry, 21*, 395–413.

Maina, G., Albert, U., & Bogetto, F. (2001). Relapses after discontinuation of drug associated with increased resistance to treatment in obsessive-compulsive disorder. *International Clinical Psychopharmacology, 16*(1), 33–38.

Mann, R., Borowsky, I., Stolz, A., Latts, E., Cart, C., & Brindis, C. (1998). *Youth violence: Lessons from the experts.* Washington, D.C.: Maternal and Child Health Bureau; Health Resources and Services Administration; Public Health Service; U.S. Department of Health and Human Services.

Marks, I. (1981). *Cure and care of neuroses: Theory and practice of behavioral psychotherapy.* New York: Wiley.

Meador, K. J., Loring, D. W., Ray, P. G., Helman, S. W., Vazquez, B. R., & Neveu, P. J. (2004). Role of cerebral lateralization in control of immune processes in humans. *Annals of Neurology, 55*(6), 840–844.

Meyer, V. (1966). Modification of expectations in cases with obsessional rituals. *Behaviour Research and Therapy, 4*(4): 273–80.

Miller, J. J., Fletcher, K., & Kabat-Zinn, J. (1995). Three-year follow-up and clinical implications of a mindfulness meditation-based stress reduction intervention in the treatment of anxiety disorders. *General Hospital Psychiatry, 17*(3), 192–200.

Mohan, S., & Wei, L. (2002). Modulation of pulse rate by unilateral nostril breathing. *Journal of Indian Psychology, 20*(1), 32–37.

Mohan, S. M., Reddy, S. C., & Wei, L. Y. (2001). Modulation of intraocular pressure by unilateral and forced unilateral nostril breathing in young healthy human subjects. *International Ophthalmology, 24*(6), 305–311.

Monuteaux, M. (2005). *A five-year follow-up of female youth with and without ADHD.* Paper presented at the 52nd Annual Meeting of the American Academy of Child and Adolescent Psychiatry, October 18–23, Toronto, Ontario.

Morin, C. (1993). *Insomnia: Psychological assessment and management.* New York: Guilford.

Mulrow, C., Ramirez, G., Cornell, J., & Allsup, K. (2001). Defining and managing chronic fatigue syndrome. In AHRQ Pulication No. 02-E001, *Agency for Healthcare Research and Quality.*

Murdock, D., Phil, R., & Ross, D. (1990). Alcohol and crimes of violence: Present issues. *International Journal of the Addictions, 25*, 1065–1081.

Murray, C. J., & Lopez, A. D. (1996a). Evidence-based health policy: Lessons from the global burden of disease study. *Science, 274*(5288), 740–743.

Murray, C. J. L., & Lopez, A. D. (1996b). *The global burden of disease: A comprehensive assessment of mortality and disability*. Cambridge MA: Harvard University Press.

Naveen, K. V., Nagarathna, R., Nagendra, H. R., & Telles, S. (1997). Yoga breathing through a particular nostril increases spatial memory scores without lateralized effects. *Psychological Reports, 81*(2), 555–561.

NCSDR. (1993). *Wake up America: A national sleep alert, executive summary and executive report submitted to the United States Congress and to the Secretary Department of Health and Human Services, vol. 1*. Washington, D.C.: National Commission on Sleep Disorders Research.

Neveu, P. J. (1988). Cerebral neocortex modulation of immune functions. *Life Sciences, 42*(20), 1917–1923.

NFCMH. (2003). *Achieving the promise: Transforming mental health care in America* (Final Report, DHHS Pub. No. SMA-03-3832). Rockville, MD: New Freedom Commission on Mental Health, U.S. Department of Health and Human Services.

NHTSA. (1991). *General estimates system 1990: A review of information on police-reported traffic crashes in the United States, Doc HS 807 781*. Washington, D.C.: National Highway Traffic Safety Administration.

Nutt, D. J. (2005). Overview of diagnosis and drug treatments of anxiety disorders. *CNS Spectrums: The International Journal of Neuropsychiatric Medicine, 10*(1), 49–56.

O'Connor, K., Todorov, C., Robillard, S., Borgeat, F., & Brault, M. (1999). Cognitive-behaviour therapy and medication in the treatment of obsessive-compulsive disorder: A controlled study. *Revue Canadienne de Psychiatrie, 44*(1), 64–71.

Ohayon, M., Caulet, M., & Lemoine, P. (1996). Sujets âgés, habitudes de sommeil et consommation de psychotropes dans la population francaise. *L'Encéphale, 22*, 337–350.

Ohayon, M. M., & Shapiro, C. M. (2000). Sleep disturbances and psychiatric disorders associated with posttraumatic stress disorder in the general population. *Comprehensive Psychiatry, 41*(6), 469–478.

Orr, W. C., & Hoffman, H. J. (1974). A 90-minute cardiac biorhythm: Methodology and data analysis using modified periodograms and complex demodulation. *IEEE Transactions on Biomedical Engineering, 21*(2), 130–143.

Pato, M. T., Zohar-Kadouch, R., Zohar, J., & Murphy, D. L. (1988). Return of symptoms after discontinuation of clomipramine in patients with obsessive-compulsive disorder. *American Journal of Psychiatry, 145*(12), 1521–1525.

Pauls, D. (1990). *Gilles de la Tourette syndrome and obsessive compulsive disorder: Familial relationships*. In M. A. Jenike, L. Baer, & W. E. Minichiello (Eds.), *Obsessive- compulsive disorders: Theory and management* (pp. 149–153). St. Louis: Mosby.

Pelham, W. (1982). Childhood hyperactivity: Diagnosis, etiology, nature, and treatment. In R. Gatchel, A. Baum, J. Singer (Eds.), *Handbook of psychology and health: Clinical psychology and behavioral medicine: Overlapping disciplines* (Vol. 1, pp. 261–327). New Jersey: Lawrence Erlbaum Associates.

Pernanen, K. (1991). *Alcohol in human violence*. New York: Guilford.

Pilkington, K., Kirkwood, G., Rampes, H., & Richardson, J. (2005). Yoga for depression: The research evidence. *Journal of Affective Disorders, 89* (1–3): 13–24

Pollack, C., Perileck, D., Linsner, J. (1990). Sleep problems in the community elderly as predictors of death in nursing home placement. *Journal of Community Health, 15*, 123–135.

Popper, C. (1988). *Disorders usually first evident in infancy, childhood, or adolescence*. Washington, D.C.: American Psychiatric Press.

Power, A. K. (2005). Achieving the promise through workforce transformation: A view from the center for mental health services. *Administration and Policy in Mental Health, 32*(5–6), 489–495.

Putnam, F. W. (2003). Ten-year research update review: Child sexual abuse. *Journal of the American Academy of Child and Adolescent Psychiatry, 42*(3), 269–278.

Pynoos, R., & Fairbank, J. (2004). *Child and trauma in America: A progress report of the national child traumatic stress network*. Los Angeles, CA and Durham, NC: National Child Traumatic Stress Network.

Rao, S., & Potdar, A. (1970). Nasal airflow with body in various positions. *Journal of Applied Physiology, 28*(2), 162–165.

Rapoport, J. L. (1989). *The boy who couldn't stop washing*. New York: E. P. Dutton.

Rapoport, J. L. (1990). The waking nightmare: An overview of obsessive compulsive disorder. *Journal of Clinical Psychiatry (51 supplement)*, 25–28.

Rasmussen, S., & Eisen, J. (1990a). *Epidemiology and clinical features of obsessive compulsive disorder*. In M. A. Jenike, L. Baer, and W. E. Minichiello (Eds.), *Obsessive-compulsive disorders: Theory and management* (pp. 10–27). St. Louis: Mosby.

Rasmussen, S., Greenberg, B., Noren, G., Marshano, R., & Eisen, J. (2003). *Neurosurgical approaches to treatment-intractable OCD: Symposium #65, new research and novel therapeutic strategies for OCD*. Paper presented at the 156th American Psychiatric Association Annual Conference, May 17–22, San Francisco, CA.

Rasmussen, S. A., & Eisen, J. L. (1990b). Epidemiology of obsessive compulsive disorder. *Journal of Clinical Psychiatry, (51 supplement)*, 10–13, discussion 14.

Rasmussen, S. A., Eisen, J. L., & Pato, M. T. (1993). Current issues in the pharmacologic management of obsessive compulsive disorder. *Journal of Clinical Psychiatry, (54 supplement)*, 4–9.

Rattenborg, N. C., Amlaner, C. J., & Lima, S. L. (2000). Behavioral, neurophysiological, and evolutionary perspectives on unihemispheric sleep. *Neuroscience and Biobehavioral Reviews, 24*(8), 817–842.

Regier, D. A., Farmer, M. E., Rae, D. S., Locke, B. Z., Keith, S. J., Judd, L. L., et al. (1990). Comorbidity of mental disorders with alcohol and other drug abuse. Results from the epidemiologic catchment area (ECA) study. *Journal of the American Medical Association, 264*(19), 2511–2518.

Regier, D. A., Goldberg, I. D., & Taube, C. A. (1978). The de facto U.S. mental health services system: A public health perspective. *Archives of General Psychiatry, 35*(6), 685–693.

Rennison, C. (2000). *Criminal victimization 1999: Changes 1998–99 with trends 1993–99.* (No. NCJ 182734). Washington, D.C.: U.S. Department of Justice.

Rice, D. (1993). The economic cost of alcohol abuse and alcohol dependence: 1990. *Alcohol Health and Research World, 17*(1).

Rice, D. P., & Miller, L. S. (1998). Health economics and cost implications of anxiety and other mental disorders in the United States. *British Journal of Psychiatry, supplement, 34*, 4–9.

Richters, J. E., Arnold, L. E., Jensen, P. S., Abikoff, H., Conners, C. K., Greenhill, L. L., et al. (1995). NIMH collaborative multisite multimodal treatment study of children with ADHD: I. Background and rationale. *Journal of the American Academy of Child and Adolescent Psychiatry, 34*(8), 987–1000.

RINCB. (1998.). *Report of International Narcotics Control Board for 1997.* New York: United Nations Publication.

Robinson, W. D., Geske, J. A., Prest, L. A., & Barnacle, R. (2005). Depression treatment in primary care. *Journal of the American Board of Family Practice, 18*(2), 79–86.

Rush, A. J., George, M. S., Sackeim, H. A., Marangell, L. B., Husain, M. M., Giller, C., et al. (2000). Vagus nerve stimulation (VNS) for treatment-resistant depressions: A multicenter study. *Biological Psychiatry, 47*(4), 276–286.

Sachs, G., & Thase, M. (2000). *Bipolar disorder: A systematic approach to treatment.* London: Martin Dunitz.

References

SAMHSA. (2004). 2003 *National survey on drug use and health: Results.* (No. Publication SMA 04-3964). Rockville, M.D.: Office of Applied Studies.

Samzelius-Lejdstrom, I. (1939). Researches with the bilateral troncopneumograph on the movements of the respiratory mechanisms during breathing. *Acta Otolaryngology, supplement, 35,* 3–104.

Sanders, B., Lattimore, C., Smith, K., & Dierker, L. (1994). Forced single-nostril breathing and cognition. *Perceptual and Motor Skills, 79*(3 pt. 2), 1499–1506.

Saper, C. B., Loewy, A. D., Swanson, L. W., & Cowan, W. M. (1976). Direct hypothalamo-autonomic connections. *Brain Research, 117*(2), 305–312.

Sapuppo, F., Umana, E., Frasca, M., La Rosa, M., Shannahoff-Khalsa, D., Fortuna, L., Bucolo, M. (2006). Complex spatio-temporal features in MEG data. *Mathematical Biosciences and Engineering, 3*(4), 697–716.

Satcher, D. (1999). *Mental health: A report from the Surgeon General* (No. GPO Order No: 2005113001100). Washington, D.C.: SAMHSA's National Mental Health Information Center.

Schiff, B. B., & Rump, S. A. (1995). Asymmetrical hemispheric activation and emotion: The effects of unilateral forced nostril breathing. *Brain and Cognition, 29*(3), 217–231.

Schulberg, H. C., Katon, W. J., Simon, G. E., & Rush, A. J. (1999). Best clinical practice: Guidelines for managing major depression in primary medical care. *Journal of Clinical Psychiatry, 60 (supplement 7),* 19–26, discussion 27–18.

Sercer, A. (1930). Research on the homolateral reflex of the nasal cavity on the lung. *Acta Otolaryngology, 14,* 82–90.

Servit, Z., Kristof, M., & Strejckova, A. (1981). Activating effect of nasal and oral hyperventilation on epileptic electrographic phenomena: Reflex mechanisms of nasal origin. *Epilepsia, 22*(3), 321–329.

Shaffer, D., Fisher, P., Dulcan, M. K., Davies, M., Piacentini, J., Schwab-Stone, M. E., et al. (1996). The NIMH diagnostic interview schedule for children version 2.3 (DISC-2.3): Description, acceptability, prevalence rates, and performance in the MECA study. Methods for the epidemiology of child and adolescent mental disorders study. *Journal of the American Academy of Child and Adolescent Psychiatry, 35*(7), 865–877.

Shannahoff-Khalsa, D. (1991a). Lateralized rhythms of the central and autonomic nervous systems. *International Journal of Psychophysiology, 11*(3), 225–251.

Shannahoff-Khalsa, D. (1991b). *Stress technology medicine: A new paradigm for stress and considerations for self-regulation.* In M. Brown, C. Rivier, & G. Koob (Eds.), *Stress: Neurobiology and neuroendocrinology* (pp. 647–686). New York: Marcel Dekker.

Shannahoff-Khalsa, D. (1993). The ultradian rhythm of alternating cerebral hemispheric activity. *International Journal of Neuroscience, 70*(3–4), 285–298.

Shannahoff-Khalsa, D. (1996). *Sounds for transcendence: Yogic techniques for opening the tenth gate.* In R. R. Pratt & R. Spintge (Eds.), Music Medicine II (pp. 351–360). Gilsum: NH: Barcelona Publishers.

Shannahoff-Khalsa, D. (1997). *Yogic techniques are effective in the treatment of obsessive compulsive disorders.* In E. Hollander & D. Stein (Eds.), *Obsessive-compulsive disorders: Diagnosis, etiology, and treatment* (pp. 283–329). New York: Marcel Dekker.

Shannahoff-Khalsa, D. (2001). Unilateral forced nostril breathing: Basic science, clinical trials, and selected advanced techniques. *Subtle Energies and Energy Medicine Journal, 12*(2), 79–106.

Shannahoff-Khalsa, D. (2003). Kundalini yoga meditation techniques in the treatment of obsessive compulsive and OC spectrum disorders. *Brief Treatment and Crisis Intervention, 3*(3), 369–382.

Shannahoff-Khalsa, D. (2004). An introduction to Kundalini yoga meditation techniques that are specific for the treatment of psychiatric disorders. *Journal of Alternative and Complementary Medicine, 10*(1), 91–101.

Shannahoff-Khalsa, D. (2005). Patient perspectives: Kundalini yoga meditation techniques for psycho-oncology and as potential therapies for cancer. *Integrative Cancer Therapies, 4*(1), 87–100.

Shannahoff-Khalsa, D., & Beckett, L. R. (1996). Clinical case report: Efficacy of yogic techniques in the treatment of obsessive compulsive disorders. *International Journal of Neuroscience, 85*(1–2), 1–17.

Shannahoff-Khalsa, D., & Bhajan, Y. (1988). Sound current therapy and self-healing: The ancient science of Nad and mantra yoga. *International Journal of Music, Dance, and Art Therapy, 1*(4), 183–192.

Shannahoff-Khalsa, D., & Bhajan, Y. (1991). The healing power of sound: Techniques from yogic medicine. In R. Droh & R. Spintge (Eds.), *MusicMedicine* (pp. 179–193). Gilsum, NH: Barcelona Publishers.

Shannahoff-Khalsa, D., Boyle, M. R., & Buebel, M. E. (1991). The effects of unilateral forced nostril breathing on cognition. *International Journal of Neuroscience, 57*(3–4), 239–249.

Shannahoff-Khalsa, D., Gillin, J. C., Yates, F. E., Schlosser, A., & Zawadzki, E. M. (2001). Ultradian rhythms of alternating cerebral hemispheric EEG dominance are coupled to rapid eye movement and non-rapid eye movement stage 4 sleep in humans. *Sleep Medicine, 2*(4), 333–346.

References

Shannahoff-Khalsa, D., & Kennedy, B. (1993). The effects of unilateral forced nostril breathing on the heart. *International Journal of Neuroscience, 73*(1–2), 47–60.

Shannahoff-Khalsa, D., Kennedy, B., Yates, F. E., & Ziegler, M. G. (1996). Ultradian rhythms of autonomic, cardiovascular, and neuroendocrine systems are related in humans. *American Journal of Physiology, 270*(4 pt. 2), R873–R887.

Shannahoff-Khalsa, D., Kennedy, B., Yates, F. E., & Ziegler, M. G. (1997). Low-frequency ultradian insulin rhythms are coupled to cardiovascular, autonomic, and neuroendocrine rhythms. *American Journal of Physiology, 272*(3 pt. 2), R962–R968.

Shannahoff-Khalsa, D., Ray, L., Levine, S., Gallen, C., Schwartz, B., & Sidorowich, J. (1999). Randomized controlled trial of yogic meditation techniques for patients with obsessive compulsive disorders. *CNS Spectrums: The International Journal of Neuropsychiatric Medicine, 4*(12), 34–46.

Shannahoff-Khalsa, D., & Yates, F. E. (2000). Ultradian sleep rhythms of lateral EEG, autonomic, and cardiovascular activity are coupled in humans. *International Journal of Neuroscience, 101*(1–4), 21–43.

Shimada, S. G., & Marsh, D. J. (1979). Oscillations in mean arterial blood pressure in conscious dogs. *Circulation Research, 44*(5), 692–700.

Shire, U. I. (2004). Behavioral briefs: ADHD has repercussions throughout adulthood. *Drug Benefit Trends, 16,* 426.

Simos, G. (2002). *Medication effects on obsessions and compulsions.* Oxford, UK: Elsevier.

Sonne, S., Brady, K., & Morton, W. (1994). Substance abuse and bipolar affective disorder. *Journal of Nervous and Mental Disease, 182,* 349–352.

Spencer, T. (2005). *A ten-year follow-up of males with and without ADHD.* Paper presented at the 52nd Annual Meeting of the American Academy of Child and Adolescent Psychiatry, October 18–23, 2005, Toronto, Ontario.

Spivak, H., Christoffel, K., Gray, H., Hayes, M., Jenkins, R., Montes, L., et al. (1999). Task force on violence, American Academy of Pediatrics. The role of the pediatrician in youth violence prevention in clinical practice and at the community level, policy statement. *Pediatrics, 103,* 173–181.

Stancak, A., Honig, J., Wackermann, J., Lepicovska, V., & Dostalek, C. (1991). Effects of unilateral nostril breathing on respiration, heart rhythm, and brain electrical activity. *Neurosciences, 17,* 409–417.

Steketee, G. (1993). *Treatment of obsessive-compulsive disorder.* New York: Guilford.

Stinson, F., Dufour, M., Staffens, R., & Debakey, S. (1993). Alcohol-related mortality in the United States, 1979–1989. *Alcohol Health and Research World, 17,* 251–260.

Stoksted, P. (1960). Obstructions in the nose and their influence on the pulmonary functions. *Acta Otorhinolaryngology, supplement, 158,* 110.

Stoksted, P. (1953). Measurements of resistance in the nose during respiration at rest. *Acta Otolaryngology, supplement, 109,* 143–58.

Sutker, P. B., Allain, A. N., Jr., & Winstead, D. K. (1993). Psychopathology and psychiatric diagnoses of World War II Pacific theater prisoner of war survivors and combat veterans. *American Journal of Psychiatry, 150*(2), 240–245.

Telles, S., Nagarathna, R., & Nagendra, H. R. (1994). Breathing through a particular nostril can alter metabolism and autonomic activities. *Indian Journal of Physiology and Pharmacology, 38*(2), 133–137.

Telles, S., Nagarathna, R., & Nagendra, H. R. (1996). Physiological measures of right nostril breathing. *Journal of Alternative and Complementary Medicine, 2*(4), 479–484.

Tillman, R., & Geller, B. (2003). Definitions of rapid, ultrarapid, and ultradian cycling and of episode duration in pediatric and adult bipolar disorders: A proposal to distinguish episodes from cycles. *Journal of Child and Adolescent Psychopharmacology, 13*(3), 267–271.

Tsai, S., Chen, C., Kuo, C., Lee, J., Lee, H., & Strakowski, S. (2001). 15-year outcome of treated bipolar disorder. *Journal of Affective Disorders, 63*(1–3), 215–220.

Vaitl, D., Birbaumer, N., Gruzelier, J., Jamieson, G. A., Kotchoubey, B., Kubler, A., et al. (2005). Psychobiology of altered states of consciousness. *Psychological Bulletin, 131*(1), 98–127.

Van Balkom, A., Van Oppen, P., Vermeulen, A., Van Dyck, R., Nauta, M., & Vorst, H. (1994). A metaanalysis on the treatment of obsessive compulsive disorder: A comparison of anti-depressants, behaviour, and cognitive therapy. *Clinical Psychology Review, 14,* 359–381.

Van der Kolk, B. A. (2001). The psychobiology and psychopharmacology of PTSD. *Human Psychopharmacology, 16*(S1), S49–S64.

van der Kolk, B. A., Dreyfuss, D., Michaels, M., Shera, D., Berkowitz, R., Fisler, R., et al. (1994). Fluoxetine in posttraumatic stress disorder. *Journal of Clinical Psychiatry, 55*(12), 517–522.

Velikonja, D., Weiss, D. S., & Corning, W. C. (1993). The relationship of cortical activation to alternating autonomic activity. *Electroencephalography and Clinical Neurophysiology, 87*(1), 38–45.

Vgontzas, A. N., & Kales, A. (1999). Sleep and its disorders. *Annual Review of Medicine, 50,* 387–400.

Voeller, K. K. (2004). Attention-deficit hyperactivity disorder (ADHD). *Journal of Child Neurology, 19*(10), 798–814.

Von Korff, M., Katon, W., Unutzer, J., Wells, K., & Wagner, E. H. (2001). Improving depression care: Barriers, solutions, and research needs. *Journal of Family Practice, 50*(6), E1.

Wagner, D., Nisenbaum, R., Heim, C., Jones, J. F., Unger, E. R., Reeves, W. C. (2005). Psychometric properties of the CDC symptom inventory for the assessment of chronic fatigue syndrome. *Population Health Metrics, 3,* 1–8. Also retrievable from http://www.cdc.gov/ncidod/diseases/cfs/index.htm, and http://www.cdc.gov/ncidod/diseases/cfs/treat.htm

Walsh, J., & Ustun, T. B. (1999). Prevalence and health consequences of insomnia. *Sleep, 22 (supplement 3),* S427–S436.

Werntz, D. A., Bickford, R. G., Bloom, F. E., & Shannahoff-Khalsa, D. S. (1980). *Cerebral hemispheric activity and autonomic nervous function.* Paper presented at the 10th Annual Meeting Society for Neuroscience, November 9–14, 1980, Cincinnati, Ohio.

Werntz, D. A., Bickford, R. G., Bloom, F. E., & Shannahoff-Khalsa, D. S. (1981). *Selective cortical activation by altering autonomic function.* Paper presented at the Western EEG Society Meeting, Abstract, February 21, 1981, Reno, Nevada.

Werntz, D. A., Bickford, R. G., Bloom, F. E., & Shannahoff-Khalsa, D. S. (1983). Alternating cerebral hemispheric activity and the lateralization of autonomic nervous function. *Human Neurobiology, 2*(1), 39–43.

Werntz, D. A., Bickford, R. G., & Shannahoff-Khalsa, D. (1987). Selective hemispheric stimulation by unilateral forced nostril breathing. *Human Neurobiology, 6*(3), 165–171.

White, K., & Cole, J. (1990). *Pharmacotherapy.* New York: John Wiley & Sons.

WHO. (2001). *The World Health report: 2001: Mental health: New understanding, new hope.* Geneva, Switzerland: World Health Organization.

Wiezorek, W., Welte, J., & Abel, E. (1990). Alcohol, drugs, and murder: A study of convicted offenders. *Journal of Criminal Justice, 18,* 217–227.

Williams, J. W., Jr., Mulrow, C. D., Chiquette, E., Noel, P. H., Aguilar, C., & Cornell, J. (2000). A systematic review of newer pharmacotherapies for depression in adults: Evidence report summary. *Annals of Internal Medicine, 132*(9), 743–756.

Willoughby, M. T., Curran, P. J., Costello, E. J., & Angold, A. (2000). Implications of early versus late onset of attention-deficit/hyperactivity disorder symptoms. *Journal of the American Academy of Child and Adolescent Psychiatry, 39*(12), 1512–1519.

Winokur, G., Coryell, W., Akiskal, H., Maser, J., Keller, M., Endicott, J., et al. (1995). Alcoholism in manic-depressive (bipolar) illness: Familial illness, course of illness, and the primary-secondary distinction. *American Journal of Psychiatry, 152*, 365–372.

Wotzilka, G., & Schramek, J. (1930). Tierexperimentelle untersuchungen uber den weg des inspirationsstromes jeder nasenseite in die lunge. *Monatsschrift für Ohrenheilkunde und Laryngo-Rhinologie, 64*, 580–585.

Zimmerman, M., Chelminski, I., & Posternak, M. (2004). A review of studies of the Montgomery-Asberg depression rating scale in controls: Implications for the definition of remission in treatment studies of depression. *International Clinical Psychopharmacology, 19*(1), 1–7.

Zisook, S., Rush, A. J., Albala, A., Alpert, J., Balasubramani, G. K., Fava, M., et al. (2004). Factors that differentiate early vs. later onset of major depression disorder. *Psychiatry Research, 129*(2), 127–140

Index